CONDITIONING
For Combat Sports

CONDITIONING
For Combat Sports

By
Steve Scott
and
John Saylor

 Turtle Press Santa Fe, NM

To contact the author or to order additional copies of this book:
Turtle Press
500 N. Washington St #1545
Rockville MD 20849
www.TurtlePress.com

ISBN 978-1-934903-19-3
LCCN 2010018260

Printed in the United States of America

Warning-Disclaimer

This book is designed to provide information on the strength, fitness and conditioning for martial arts and other sports. It is not the purpose of this book to reprint all the information that is otherwise available to the author, publisher, printer or distributors, but instead to compliment, amplify and supplement other texts. You are urged to read all available material, learn as much as you wish about the subjects covered in this book and tailor the information to your individual needs. Anyone practicing the skills, exercises, drills or techniques presented in this book should be physically healthy enough to do so and have permission from a licensed physician before participating.

Every effort has been made to make this book as complete and accurate as possible. However, there may be mistakes, both typographical and in content. Therefore, this text should be used only as a general guide and not as the ultimate source of information on the subjects presented here in this book on any topic, skill or subject. The purpose of this book is to provide information and entertain. The authors, publisher, printer and distributors shall neither have liability nor responsibility to any person or entity with respect to loss or damages caused, or alleged to have been caused, directly or indirectly, by the information contained in this book. If you do not wish to be bound by the above, you may return this book to the publisher for a full refund.

This book is about getting results and achieving success. Your technical expertise is based on your body being physically able

Cataloging in Publication data
Scott, Steve, 1952-
Conditioning for combat sports / by Steve Scott and John Saylor.
    p. cm.
ISBN 978-1-934903-19-3
1. Hand-to-hand fighting--Training. 2. Mixed martial arts--Training. I. Saylor, John. II. Title.
GV1111.S345 2010
613.7'148--dc22
                    2010018260

Contents

SECTION ONE: WHY FUNCTIONAL TRAINING WORKS   17

To be physically, mentally and emotionally able to compete at the level you wish to excel, you must first, and foremost, be physically able to pull it off. If, for no other reason than pride, show up in shape. Your ability to compete, and win, at your best level is directly related to your fitness level.

SECTION TWO: EXERCISES & DRILLS: HOW THEY HELP YOU WIN ON THE MAT   69

This section's main purpose is to present a variety of exercises, drills, movements, games or other physical activities that you can use in your training. In addition to that, we will show why and how these specific exercises work and how they translate to winning performances on the mat.

ACKNOWLEDGEMENTS

The authors wish to thank Louie Simmons, Bob Corwin, Becky Scott, Bryan Potter, Chris Garlick, Sean Daugherty, Dr. Dan Rinchuse, Mike Hallman and Drew Hills CSCS, for technical advice as well as the Sylvester Powell Community Center, Westside Barbell Club, Bally's Fitness and Kansas City North Community Center for the use of their facilities. Special thanks go to Patricia Saylor and Becky Scott for their help in editing this book, as well as Brad Eppler and Melissa Stage for their additional technical assistance. Also, many thanks to all the athletes at Welcome Mat, the Barn of Truth, Shingitai Jujitsu Association, Big Al's Gym, Jackson Weightlifting Club and Westside Barbell Club who patiently posed for the photographs in this book.

Terry Smemo, Sharon Vandenberg, Dr. Al Myers, Thom VanVleck, Dr. Dan Rinchuse, Louie Simmons, Jake Pursley, Mike Hallman, Jorge Garcia, Mike Schmidt, Sean Daugherty, Fritz Goss, John Saylor and Steve Scott provided photographs for this book.

FOREWORD BY LOUIE SIMMONS

This book can lead one to a path of excellence for all forms of fighting. The authors have spent years in perfecting their training not only in the Judo, Jujitsu and Sombo arts but how to build a base starting with G.P.P. (General Physical Preparedness) to S.P.P. (Special Physical Preparedness).

Steve Scott is a two time national Sombo champion, as well as having coached three world champions in Sombo. When a coach can make three world champions he is indeed a great teacher. With his experience and expertise in Sombo he has also coached a number of U.S. international Judo teams. His vast experience in training and actual combat that is conveyed in this text can help the aspiring novice or the most advanced combat enthusiast. His philosophy and advice for organizing a proven program is priceless. You will learn how to increase your cardiovascular endurance, muscular endurance and learn the basics to the most advanced techniques to become a champion.

Along with John Saylor, a man I have known for over 15 years, this book is a must read. John was a three time U.S. national champion in Judo and he was also an international caliber Judo fighter. Along the way he was the coach of the U.S. National Judo Training Squad at the Olympic training center for seven years. Not only is he a master at fighting, John is also an expert at conditioning and preparing for combat. He is a fully certified at the Westside Barbell for strength training from explosive, speed strength, strength endurance as well as absolute strength.

Through this text Steve and John will show the athlete how to bridge the gap from learning general exercises and training methods to winning on the mat, in the cage or in the street if you must. A pyramid is only as tall as its base. This concept is a reality as the authors show functional training methods based on winning. Without a plan, you plan to fail. This is where this book separates itself from the rest. It takes you through the four classic training periods in preparing for any combat sport.

The first period is Accumulation where a wide base of activity takes place, getting the fighter into shape. Next is Intensification. Here John and Steve show how to eliminate some G.P.P. and direct the fighter to more fighting skills. This causes the transformation period when you have transformed into a fighter. And finally, the fourth period is the Delayed Transformation Period. This is when and how much rest before the match. This text will indeed help you fulfill your dream.

Louie Simmons
Owner of Westside Barbell (one of the world's strongest gyms)
Former National Champion
One of five men to total Elite in five weight classes

More Books by STEVE SCOTT

Tap Out Textbook - Ultimate Guide to Submissions for Grappling

Tap Out Textbook: The Ultimate Guide to Submissions for Grappling is packed with hundreds of armlocks, chokes and leglocks that you can use to make any opponent tap out. This book offers hardcore, serious, practical instruction on submitting an opponent in a wide variety of grappling and fighting situations.

Armlock Encyclopedia

This book specializes in the armlocks used in all forms of submission grappling, jujitsu, judo, MMA, sambo, martial arts and any other combat sports of fighting. The specifics of why armlocks work are examined in depth.

Grappler's Book of Strangles & Chokes

This is a comprehensive study of both "gi" and "no gi" strangles and chokes. The differences between strangles and chokes are explained as well as the physiological reasons why these techniques work, and why they are dangerous.

Vital Leglocks

Ankle, knee and other lower body submissions are presented in this book. Taken from sambo, jujitsu, old-time legitimate professional wrestling and catch wrestling, the theory and technique of lower body submissions are presented in this book.

Groundfighting Pins & Breakdowns

This book is a comprehensive and thorough presentation of many positions and situations and how to set an opponent up, break him down and get him on his back to pin him. A huge number of hold-downs and pins used in judo, jujitsu, sambo, submission grappling and MMA are shown in this book. This book serves a dual purpose in that it not only shows how to break an opponent down to hold him, but it is also one of the most comprehensive studies of position grappling on the market.

Throws And Takedowns

You have to get your opponent to the mat or ground before you can apply a submission technique on him and this book shows many ways to do it. How and why a throwing technique works as well as the difference between a throw and a takedown are examined. Both common and unique throwing techniques and takedowns are shown in this book.

Drills For Grapplers

If you want to master a move, you have to drill on it. This book shows many drills, games and exercises that you can use on the mat. Drills for all ages and skill levels are presented. This book was written for both coaches and athletes.

Championship Sambo. Submission Holds and Groundfighting

If you're interested in the Russian sport of sambo, this book offers a history of sambo, its technical basis and a variety of groundfighting techniques used in all levels of competition. One of the few books on sambo published in the United States, it has a variety of armlocks, hold-downs and leglocks commonly seen in sambo.

Championship Sambo: The DVD

This DVD, about 2 ½ hours in length, shows a variety of groundfighting skills as well as numerous throws and takedowns native to Russian sambo.

To order the books and DVD listed above, visit Turtle Press at www.TurtlePress.com.

INTRODUCTION
BY STEVE SCOTT

to perform, and perform under pressure.

Athletic performance, especially performance in combat sports or self-defense can be summed up in three primary principles. The first is *shin*, the mental and emotional factors that are the driving force behind all of us. It's the will, strength of character or fighting heart that is necessary for anyone to push his body to extremes to produce a successful or desired result. Additionally, an athlete will perform better if he understands why he is doing something, and how it can benefit him. This mental/emotional factor is necessary for the next principle, and that is *gi*, which translates to mean the applied technical skill necessary to get the job done. It's the practical application of a technique whether it's in a sporting context or in a self-defense situation. It's technical expertise realistically performed. But that second principle can't be complete, or even accomplished, without the third principle; *tai*, or the body, meaning physical ability to perform it. This third principle is what much of this book is about. You must be able to function under pressure and have the endurance, strength, speed and coordination necessary to apply your skills against a fit, skilled and resisting opponent during a stressful, competitive or real-world situation. It's this functional fitness that is the basis of this book.

All three of these principles build on each other and work together in unison. This concept of shin, gi and tai, formed together, is called Shingitai, and has been around for a long time but is the core premise for the approach to training that both John Saylor and I adhere to. While this book focuses on the tai aspect, I hope you remember that all three principles work together.

I want to personally thank my wife Becky Scott, as well as Drew Hills, Bryan Potter, Chris Garlick and Jake Pursley for their technical input, in addition to Louie Simmons for his expertise. My sincere thanks go to Bob Corwin, who has been an advocate of sports performance training for judo athletes for years. His innovative training methods influenced me greatly. The athletes and coaches at Welcome Mat, as always, were both supportive and patient during the many photo sessions. Thank you to every one of them. Sharon Vandenberg, Terry Smemo, Jake Pursley and Jorge Garcia are responsible for the great action photos used in this book and I thank them very much. Sincere thanks are also in order to Cynthia Kim at Turtle Press. The professionalism and support that Turtle Press has shown during this entire project is very much appreciated. When Cynthia first discussed the idea of me writing a book on fitness and conditioning for the martial arts, my first thought was to include John Saylor in the project.

This leads me to offer a few words about my co-author John Saylor. For years, John Saylor and I have collaborated on our coaching efforts and this book is part of that long-standing relationship. John is one of my closest friends. He is also one of the most innovative coaches in any sport or martial art that I know of and it's my belief that John is one of the most knowledgeable people anywhere on the subject of conditioning and fitness training for combat sport and self-defense athletes. As an athlete, it's a simple fact that John was one of the best heavyweights in the history of judo in the United States. He's too modest to say it himself, but it's true. John was known not only for his technical skill, but also for his extreme fitness level and dedication to training. Had it not been for a career-ending injury in 1982, I am certain John would have represented the United States in the Olympic Games in Los Angeles in 1984. As a coach, he personally developed many U.S. national and international champions and medal-winners in the sport of judo during his tenure as the Head Coach for the Judo Squad at the U.S. Olympic Training Center in Colorado Springs, Colorado. After leaving his post at the Olympic Training Center, John devoted his attention to the Shingitai Jujitsu Association and has been a respected and innovative force in the development of sport combat and self-defense athletes at his headquarters in Perrysville, Ohio.

This book is divided into two sections. The first section pretty much presents the nuts and bolts of functional, effective fitness training for combat sports. The second section shows how the nuts and bolts fit together to complete the project. To get the most out of the second section, make sure that you thoroughly read the first section. As with all of the books I've written, this isn't the complete word on this subject, so take what we present on these pages and make it work for you. This book is the result of many mistakes as well as many successes over the course of our lives as athletes and coaches.

We've done our best to learn from both and offer to you some hard-earned advice and valid information on how to be successful. Both John and I firmly believe in functional training and how that translates into success and have spent our lives training hard and then pondering what we have done as well as learned what others have done. Some of the methods we advocate may not be considered normal, but then, as Louie Simmons has said, "It takes abnormal training to get abnormal results."

INTRODUCTION
BY JOHN SAYLOR

My goal in writing this book is to help you achieve your full physical potential for martial arts. Whether you're involved in judo, jujitsu, sombo, submission wrestling, MMA, self-defense, or some other martial art, this book will detail exercises and training programs that will transform your body into a finely-tuned fighting machine. Some of the methods are traditional ones that were used by the fighters of old; others are based on the cutting-edge research of sports sciences from the former Soviet Union and other Eastern Bloc countries. Still others come from recent innovations from one of the world's best strength and conditioning coaches, Louie Simmons.

All of these methods have one thing in common—they work. Well, let me restate that: If you do the work, these exercises and training methods will work for you.

A huge gap seems to exist between fighters and coaches on the one hand, and modern athletic training methods and research on the other. This is a shame since it may just be that this research contains the keys to overcoming the very obstacles that are standing in the way of your progress. Steve Scott and I hope to bridge that gap. We hope you will use this book as a training guide and reference for years to come, and that it helps you become a winner in your chosen martial arts discipline.

Best of luck as you embark on the path to physical mastery.

Acknowledgements

I'm very happy to be writing this book with my good friend Steve Scott, who has a wealth of knowledge from decades of training in judo, sombo, and jujitsu. Steve has trained all over the world, and has also coached the U.S. National (Under 21) Judo Team at the Junior World Championships and coached the U.S. Team at the 1983 Pan American Games in sombo, as well as having personally coached 3 World Sombo Champions and was a U.S. national sombo champion himself. For the last couple decades Steve has also taught and coached jujitsu at his nationally renowned Welcome Mat Judo and Jujitsu Club in Kansas City, MO. Steve has produced more national and international champions in judo, Sombo, and jujitsu than he or I can even count.

Steve and I became friends in the early 1980s when we were chosen by the governing body of judo to attend the U.S. Olympic Committee Coach's College. Throughout that session and the USOC Coach's College the following year, I was highly impressed with Steve's knowledge and coaching ability. Ever since, we've shared ideas on training and coaching, and have remained lifelong friends. I am honored to co-author this work with Steve.

I am also very grateful for the opportunity to publish this work through Turtle Press, and for the unwavering professionalism and spirit of helpfulness shown us by our editor, Cynthia Kim.

No One – Size – Fits - All Training

A lot of martial artists and fighters copy the program of some champion, usually something printed up in one of the martial art magazines. Although you can get some good exercises and ideas this way, it is usually wrong to copy the champion's program verbatim. First of all, the champion probably has a higher level of background training, different strengths and weaknesses, a different body type, and so on. His program works fine for him, obviously, but may not be at all appropriate for you. Instead, I recommend that you start with a personal **needs analysis**. Your needs analysis should answer such questions as the following:

1) What are your short and long-term goals? (Is your main interest self-defense or are you more geared toward competition? When are your most important competitions?)

2) What is your body type? (Do you need to gain muscular body weight? Or do you need to lose weight to improve your endurance or to compete in a lower weight category?)

3) How old are you? (As a 14 year old you shouldn't attempt to copy the program of a 30-year-old champion. Conversely, if you're 40 years of age or older, for example, you must adjust the amount of work you do, especially the amount of high intensity work.)

4) How many years have you been training? (Are you a beginner, intermediate, or advanced trainee? The percentages of general, directed, and specific training will depend on the level you have attained in your particular discipline.)

5) What are your strengths and weaknesses? (If, for example, you're too slow to catch the 7-year itch, don't lie to yourself. Admit it, and then work hard to develop explosive speed. If you find yourself running out of gas in practice or in a match, devote more time and effort to endurance training.) Whatever your weakness—strength, speed, endurance, flexibility, skill—once you've identified it, **work to bring your weakness up to the level of your strengths**.

6) Do you have any injuries or medical conditions that require special attention? (Obviously you need to be in overall good health to undertake serious training, so make sure you resolve any medical issues that may interfere with your training. Also, any injuries you may have sustained will require special attention. The most common injury sites in grappling, for example, are knees and shoulders. So even if you're now injury-free, pay special attention to strengthening these areas.)

By answering these types of questions you will gain a better understanding of your training needs and can then design your program accordingly.

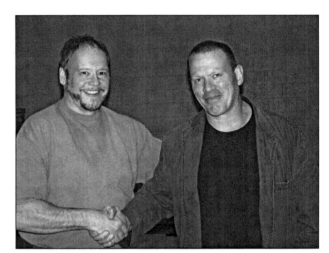

AUTHORS STEVE SCOTT AND JOHN SAYLOR

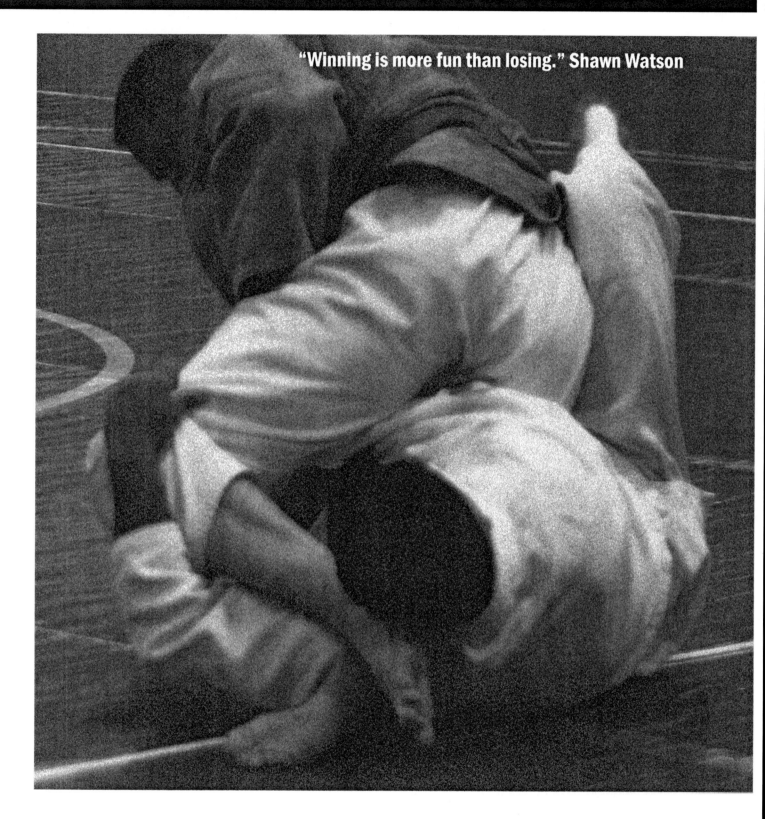

"Winning is more fun than losing." Shawn Watson

SECTION ONE
WHY FUNCTIONAL TRAINING WORKS

SECTION ONE: PART 1. SHOW UP IN SHAPE

• • • "Just run. Get up, put on your shoes and go run. Do it every day." Mike Swain

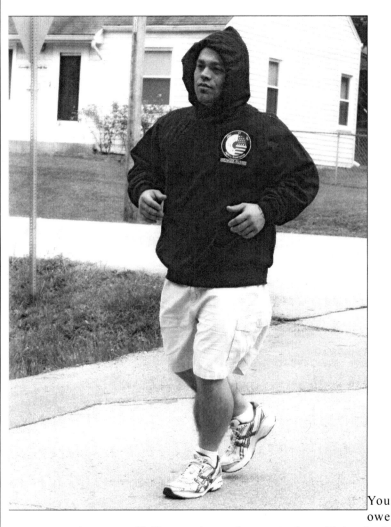

On the other hand, when you're in shape, and you know it, you actually feel yourself gaining in strength and confidence as the fight progresses. Your skills will work better, a lot better, when you are physically able to make them work against a skilled, resisting, fit and motivated opponent.

IT'S A FIGHT, NOT A GAME

This book is about training for grapplers and fighters. It doesn't matter what combat sport or martial art you specialize in, showing up in shape is mandatory. Your work ethic, willingness and ability to withstand harsh physical training and ability to absorb punishment all directly affect your success in grappling or fighting.

Remember, it's a fight, not a game. You're training to win a fight, not simply win a game. Some games are rougher than others, but in the end, they're just games. Fighting somebody, whether it's in a sporting context or on the street, is far more personal than simply playing a game. Winning is more personal, and so is losing.

YOUR BODY IS THE IMPLEMENT THAT ENABLES YOU TO ACHIEVE YOUR GOALS

You're not training to have the physique of a bodybuilder; you're training to be a fighter. A fighter's physique may not win a trophy in a bodybuilding contest, but our purpose in developing our bodies is to win fights or matches on the mat or in a cage, and even in a real self-defense situation. If, in the course of your training, you develop the type of physique that could win a bodybuilding contest, so be it. The bottom line is to understand that your body is the implement that enables you to achieve your goals as a grappler, fighter or self-defense athlete.

You owe it to yourself, if no on else, to show up in shape. To be physically, mentally and emotionally able to compete at the level you wish to excel, you must first, and foremost, be physically able to pull it off. If, for no other reason than pride, show up in shape. Your ability to compete, and win, at your best level is directly related to your fitness level.

Years ago, the great football coach Vince Lombardi said, "Fatigue makes cowards of us all." There is nothing that any coach ever said that was truer. If you are not in shape, you won't have the will to do what it takes to beat another human being in a test of combat whether it's sport combat or the real thing. You won't be able to perform your technical skills, make your strategy work or even have time to think straight if you're not physically prepared.

TRAINING FOR GRAPPLING AND COMBAT SPORTS

Combat and grappling sports, in all their variations, are demanding on the human body. Whether you do jujitsu, judo, submission grappling, boxing, wrestling, MMA or any martial art or fighting sport, your fitness level directly determines how well you perform the skills of your sport. If you don't show up in shape, you'll quickly discover that your opponent will take advantage of it. You simply cannot perform the skills of your sport at a functional level against a resisting, skilled opponent unless you are physically capable of performing them. Your body is your most important weapon in your arsenal. This book examines and presents information on how to get the most out of your body, especially when under stressful situations in fighting.

Training for any type of fighting isn't a static thing. Your training methods will undergo continual, constant change. In some cases, it will be big change, and in some cases, small change, that will refine and fine-tune your performance. It's all about results and achieving success. For this reason, we sincerely believe that success is an on-going process. The advice in this book is the result of years of training, coaching and learning. The information we present is meant to be practical, so make any necessary changes to make this information work best for you in your own specific situation. And, as said earlier, training isn't static. What may not work for you right now, may work for you at a later time. As you progress, evolve and develop in the many ways every athlete (or coach) does, the information in this book will serve you well. We hope you use this book as a reliable reference resource for many years to come.

While this book focuses on the physical factors of training effectively for fighting, your mental and emotional approach dictates what your body will do. It takes discipline to achieve success and it takes discipline to force yourself to do what it takes to physically prepare to achieve success. It's not really "normal" to push your body to the extremes necessary to reach your athletic potential. The human body naturally prefers "homeostasis" or the act of remaining as it is. In other words, you have to force your body to physically perform the tasks necessary to be a better fighter. That's what training is all about.

Bat Masterson, a lawman in the Wild West, once said; "It's not the one who is the fastest or most accurate. It's the one most willing.. He was talking about winning gunfights, but it's the kind of advice that can be used here as well. If you have the will, you can develop the discipline, and if you have the discipline, you will push yourself to do what it takes to achieve success, and ultimately, excellence in your chosen field of endeavor. Our chosen field of endeavor is fighting in some way or another.

Along with your will and discipline, remember that combat sports aren't like playing a baseball game. It's fighting another human being. As said before, it's not a game; it's a fight. Because of that, there's more stress involved. How you handle that stress depends largely on how confident you are of your physical ability and your skill level as a fighter or grappler.

If you've trained hard and trained smart, you'll be more confident. The more confidence, the less stress. This is why coach Lombardi said what he did about fatigue making cowards of us all. You'll be far less likely to be a coward if you are in excellent physical condition, and know that you are. Besides that, you trained your butt off. Take it out on the guy facing you on the mat!

GENERAL FITNESS EXERCISES AND TRAINING: THE CORE CONCEPTS

What we'll be initially discussing in this section is general fitness exercises and training. Before you go on to more specific, directed training, it's necessary to have a solid base to build on. This general fitness is that base. Don't skip over this part of the book and go on to the more advanced information before you have a good, overall and general fitness level. In the same way you learn new techniques or skills, you need a good foundation. What we're talking about here is that foundation.

General Aerobic (Cardio) Fitness

Aerobic fitness, also called cardiovascular endurance, is the foundation of a fighter's training program. Let's look at it this way: your car can have the best engine in the world, but if you don't have the gas to make it run, it won't go very far and it certainly won't go very fast.

To develop general, overall effective cardio endurance, participate in activities such as biking, running, swimming or other moderate exercises that will make your hear work at approximately 130 to 150 beats per minute.

A good way to figure your maximum heart rate is to subtract your age from 220. Choose a steady, moderate exercise that will make you work between 60 to 85% of your maximum heart rate.

Also, when you are grappling or working out on the mat, make it a rule to train with partners who buy into the idea that you all need to train at a steady, moderate pace. There's plenty of time and opportunity to go full-bore, but structured drill-training and structured live training (randori) will benefit you more than seeing who's the toughest guy on the mat all the time. We recommend that when training on the mat, you should train for 20 to 60 minutes straight at a steady pace. A good rule of thumb, no matter what type of cardio training you are doing, is to work out at a pace so that you can have a conversation during the workout. Bryan Potter calls this "smiling randori. If you and your training partner can smile during your live (randori) session, both you and your partner are working at a moderate, steady pace. This allows you to move freely, try new things, and use your randori time wisely. It's not a gym fight, it's randori. Use it for what it's meant to be, and it's meant to be training.

General Muscular Endurance

Another important part of your general fitness training is muscular endurance. Actually, you will most likely develop some muscular endurance by training in your sport or martial art. Doing your sport will certainly develop the muscles necessary to perform that sport, at least on a moderate, functional level. However, if you want to develop your full potential in muscular endurance, do high repetition bodyweight and other repetition exercises outside of your regular martial arts workouts.

Your body adapts to this training by developing miles of capillaries. These tiny blood vessels carry the oxygen-enriched blood to your muscles and flush the carbon dioxide, lactic and pyruvic acids (along with other wastes) from your muscles. This is what muscular endurance is all about: making sure that your muscles have enough oxygen to work effectively. The better you build your capillary system, the better your muscular endurance will be.

GENERAL ENDURANCE

To succeed in any fighting art you need a large base of cardiovascular and muscular endurance. In a moment we'll take a look at how to develop general endurance, but first let's examine what endurance is comprised of. Very simply, to have a high level of endurance you need the following:

1) A large powerful motor—your heart.

2) A lighter frame. In other words, keep your body weight and percentage of body fat low. Of course, those competing in heavier weight classes may need to add, not lose, muscular body weight. But make sure the increased weight is lean body mass. From an endurance standpoint there is no benefit to gaining fat. Remember, your heart needs to work much harder to pump blood and oxygen through all that extra mass, so keep your percentage of body fat low.

3) An efficient oxygen transport system. By this we are referring to your vascular system—arteries, veins, and miles and miles of capillaries to bring fresh blood and oxygen to your working muscles and to remove fatigue products like lactic and pyruvic acid.

DEVELOPING GENERAL CARDIOVASCULAR ENDURANCE

To develop general cardiovascular endurance simply pick an activity like running, biking, or swimming, and sustain it for 20 to 30 minutes. Do this 4 to 6 times per week. Occasionally do a longer workout on the weekend, say a 40 to 60 minute cross-country run, or some equivalent with biking or swimming. To develop an aerobic base, try to maintain a heart rate of about 150 beats per minute throughout your workout.

Note: If you choose running for your cardiovascular training avoid unnecessary pounding on your joints by running on softer surfaces whenever possible.

As you can see, developing general cardiovascular endurance is not rocket science. You just need to discipline yourself to get out on the trail, or the bike, or the pool, and do it.

Several years ago we hosted Mike Swain for a training camp at the Shingitai Training Center in Perrysville, Ohio. Mike was a World Judo Champion in the 156 lb. weight category in 1987, and an Olympic medallist. At one point during the camp the subject turned to training off the mat. One guy asked Mike what he did to stay in shape outside of judo practice itself. Mike mentioned doing some circuit training, but went on to say, "I run almost every day." Another person asked, "So, do you run distance, or sprints, or interval training, or what?" Mike replied, "Just run. Get up, put your shoes on, and go run. Do it every day. Then you can worry about sprints, intervals, and all that."

Mike was telling the campers not to overanalyze things but just to get out and run every day. Then once they've got that part down and have a base built up, to tweak the program by adding some anaerobic sprints and intervals.

In later chapters we will discuss directed and specific endurance training, but for now, work on building your aerobic base.

GENERAL PHYSICAL PREPARATION

General Physical Preparation (GPP) is the foundation of your career as a martial artist and fighter. It is the base from which you will build your body so that you can withstand the more intense and specific training of the future.

Think of your training as a pyramid. If the base of your pyramid is narrow, the peak cannot be very high. But if the base is strong and wide, you can build a tall pyramid with a high peak. The same holds true with your training. A wide base of GPP will ensure that you make more consistent progress, and with fewer injuries, as you advance to the directed and specific training to come. A high level of GPP will also ensure more stable results throughout your competitive career, and a much higher peak performance when you need it most.

> **TECHNICAL TIP.** It's important to understand why the methods of training presented in this book work, but don't simply leave it at that. The only way they work is to do them. Just get up and run, lift or train on the mat. Your actions speak louder than our words.

NO WEAK LINKS IN THE CHAIN

GPP is designed to ensure that there are no weak links in your body. Your goal during GPP training is to develop all-around balanced muscular development, an efficient cardiovascular system, and good general flexibility, agility, balance, and speed. To accomplish this you will employ a wide variety of exercises and methods, many of which are not directly related to your event.

If you are a more advanced martial artist or fighter you will still include GPP training in your schedule, although not as much. This will help you to maintain your base and to enhance recuperation from the more intense and specific training you've been doing.

Note: The base of the pyramid, GPP, is the foundation of your training. The training gradually becomes more specific as you go up the pyramid.

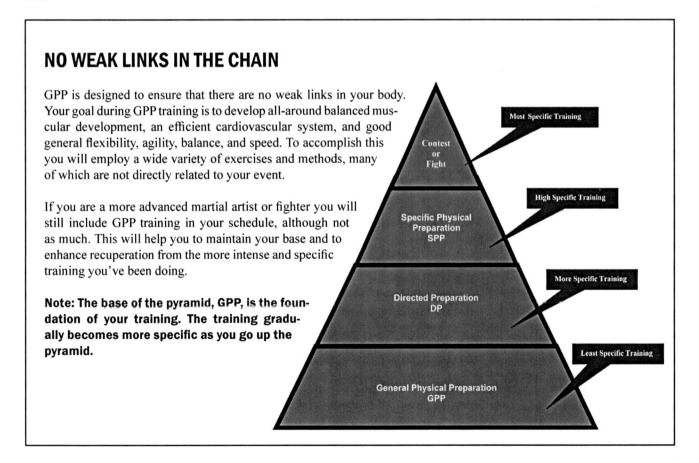

Although the following visual aids are not meant to be used in an overly strict manner, the percentages of GPP to SPP training would roughly look like this:

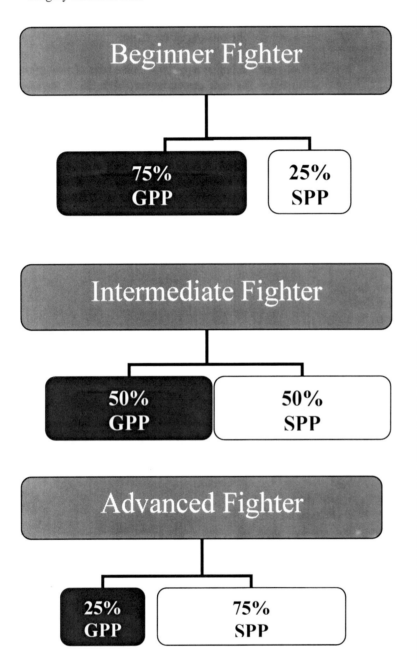

Beginner Fighter

| 75% GPP | 25% SPP |

Intermediate Fighter

| 50% GPP | 50% SPP |

Advanced Fighter

| 25% GPP | 75% SPP |

TECHNICAL TIP: A STUDY IN CULTURES-GENERAL PHYSICAL PREPARATION (GPP) IN THE FORMER SOVIET UNION VS. THE U.S. APPROACH

In the United States children start sports at a very young age, often 8 to 10 years old. Check out any neighborhood park and you will find dozens of kids playing soccer, football, baseball, or basketball, depending on the season. Rarely, though, is there any program to get them in shape for that sport prior to the season. Almost all their training is sport-specific.

This approach produces fast results initially. But because these young athletes have no general foundation their progress stagnates within a few years. And unless they go back and do some serious work on GPP their progress will remain stunted. Since specific exercises and training methods are not designed to provide balanced all-around development, the young U.S. athletes are also much more vulnerable to injuries.

In contrast, promising young people in the former Soviet Union, at about age 12, were enrolled in sports schools. But unlike their U.S. counterparts, the Soviet youth were not allowed to play their sport yet. Rather, they were put through a well-organized, systematic program of GPP consisting of general strength, endurance, flexibility, agility, balance, and hand/eye coordination.

Note: You'll notice that we didn't include a graph for Directed Preparation. This is because Directed Preparation or Exercises are basically a transition between GPP and SPP training. Directed Exercises duplicate a similar movement pattern, energy system, or muscle group, but they are not exactly the same as your technique or event. But these directed exercises do allow you to concentrate on certain weaknesses in your technique, or event as a whole, and therefore will more fully prepare you to practice your event.

WHAT THE EXPERTS SAY REGARDING
GENERAL PHYSICAL PREPARATION (GPP)

Dr. Steve Fleck: sports researcher, author and head exercise physiologist at the Olympic Training Center in Colorado Springs.

While John Saylor was the judo coach of the U.S. National Training Squad at the Olympic Training Center Dr. Fleck told him, "You just can't play your way into shape." Dr. Fleck wisely advised athletes to build a base through GPP before undertaking actual practice in their sport.

Louie Simmons: strength and conditioning coach and author.

In a published article, Louie Simmons listed the following GPP exercises that young Soviet Sports School athletes worked on. Among others, these were: pushups, pull-ups, rope climbing, medicine ball work, kettle bell work, running and short sprints. Louie noted that through this program "they produced the model athlete for their sports system."

Ryzard Zenewa: former Polish National Judo Coach.

From John Saylor's talks with Ryzard Zenewa, It was learned that young athletes in the Eastern Bloc countries, in addition to the type of training Louie described, played other sports and games such as soccer, basketball, and various track and field events, to improve GPP.

Compare this to the typical U.S. approach in which young athletes are started in a certain sport without any prior general physical preparation (GPP). Although certain athletes who are genetically encoded for that sport may reach a level of success, the overwhelming majority won't get very far, or even worse, will suffer debilitating injuries. And what about those gifted few who do actually achieve a measure of success; are they going to reach their full potential? Not likely.

To sum it up, by building and maintaining a solid base through GPP you will:

*   Achieve more reliable results.
*   Sustain fewer injuries.
*   Make continual progress toward your ultimate goal.

PROGRESSION OF EXERCISE

You will progress through three phases of training as you progress as an athlete. The first is the General Phase, sometimes referred to as the "Accumulation Phase.. The second is the Directed Phase, also called the "Intensification Phase. The third is the Specific Phase, or "Transformation Phase." For those of you who compete you will also have a Peaking Phase, or "Delayed Transformation Phase. The first three phases will be discussed below. The Peaking or Delayed Transformation Phase will be discussed later in this book.

Note: The terms, "accumulation, intensification, transformation, and delayed transformation, are discussed in Thomas Kurz' excellent book, Science Of Sports Training. These terms are also used by Louie Simmons, and now by us, because they briefly describe the main goal of each phase.

GENERAL PHYSICAL PREPARATION (GPP) or "Accumulation Phase"

This first phase of training is all about accumulating a solid base. This phase is vital to the success of the other two phases that build on this solid foundation. There are five primary areas of development that take place in this General Phase. They are:

1. Develop cardiovascular endurance.
2. Develop muscular endurance.
3. Develop muscular strength (including ligament and tendon strength).
4. Develop functional flexibility.
5. Develop all-around athletic ability & coordination.

DIRECTED PHYSICAL PREPARATION (DPP) or "Intensification Phase"

Directed exercises and training methods are those that are in some way specific to your technique or event, but are not specific in every way. Interval Training with running, for example, can be set up to use the same energy systems as those used in a competitive grappling or martial art contest. So in terms of energy systems it can be said to be a Directed Training Method. But interval training with running is not specific in other respects such as movement patterns, muscle groups, muscular endurance, and so on. It can, however, serve as a transition from the long slow distance running used to build up a base of general cardiovascular endurance, and the more intense anaerobic work required in high level grappling, MMA, and martial arts practice and competition. In other words, during DPP you will be intensifying your training in preparation for the specific training to come.

In strength training, for example, a general exercise for the abs might be a standard Sit Up or Leg Raise. A directed exercise would be the Danek Twist, or Vertical Bar Twists done on The Grappler. The latter exercises mimic the movement patterns of the twisting motions of all forward throws and of other throws involving a twist to the rear. These directed exercises will help you develop a strong finish to your throw. Directed exercises allow you to strengthen some weakness in your technique or physical preparation. But a directed exercise is not the technique or event in its entirety. It doesn't exactly duplicate the entire movement, type of fatigue, speed, and the like, of your technique. In other words, a directed exercise is not completely specific. Rather, directed training is a transition from general exercises and training methods to the specific exercises and training methods you will be using at actual practice on the mat or in the ring.

SPECIFIC PHYSICAL PREPARATION (SPP) or "Transformation Phase"

This phase of training is extremely specific and aimed at your unique needs as an athlete within the parameters of your particular sport or martial art. It is sometimes called the "transformation phase" because during this phase you will transform the general and directed training of the previous two phases into your actual fighting ability.

The objectives of this phase are as follows:

1. Strengthen the muscle groups used in your sport and specifically used in the techniques you use best. A good example is your grip strength. If you are in a grappling sport using jackets such as judo, jujitsu or sambo, grip fighting and gripping your opponent's jacket is a vital skill. You need a strong grip. Make it a habit to incorporate some different grip strength exercises in your training routine on a regular basis. Also, examine specific situations you will be in during an actual match or fight and determine which muscle groups are most often used. An example is when fighting on the bottom in the guard; you should develop your core strength. Work on your abdominals, lower back, hips, glutes, upper leg muscles and any other major (or minor) muscle group you will use.

2 Incorporate training that duplicates the fatigue and physical stress in your sport. If you are an MMA fighter and go five 5-minute rounds in a championship fight, duplicate your training so that you are used to the physical fatigue and stress of an actual fight. Use situational drills where you put yourself in a specific situation and have to work out of it. This helps your physical adaptation and response to the situation as well as your technical adaptation and response.

3. Select exercises that improve specific speed, strength, flexibility and coordination for your event. A good example is your flexibility. Do you need the flexibility of an elite gymnast to be a good grappler? No, but you need to be supple enough to perform the skills of your sport at an elite level against resisting, skilled, fit opponents. Another example is foot speed. If you are a judo athlete and specialize in throws, you need to increase the quickness of your foot movement. Hitting in with a fast, powerful Uchi Mata throw requires tremendous foot speed. Use a "quick-foot" ladder to increase lower body coordination, especially your feet and legs.

4. Strengthen the movement patterns of your whole technique or the component parts of it. In other words, if you specialize in the double leg takedown, you will see a major improvement in your takedown if you drill on it using resistance bands, a throwing dummy or resistance drills with training partners. Perform your takedown drills with resistance training.

OPTIMAL SURPLUS: THE KEYS TO RELIABLE PERFORMANCE

Throughout this book we will be using the term, "Optimal Surplus." We first came across this idea in the book, GYMNASTICS: HOW TO CREATE CHAMPIONS, by Arkaev and Suchilin (2004, Meyer and Meyer Sport Ltd.). This concept seemed the perfect way to describe what we're striving for in combative sports and arts. Simply put, "optimal surplus" means that you have more of certain psychological, technical, and physical qualities than you actually need for your event.

Optimal surplus for a martial artist or fighter does not require you to have the **strength** of a world-class powerlifter, or the general **endurance** of a Marathoner, only more strength and endurance than you actually need to attack with speed and power throughout your fight. As for **flexibility**, you don't need to be a contortionist; you just need more flexibility than you need to complete your techniques with complete freedom of movement. You also need an optimal surplus of **technique, mental toughness, and tactical preparation**, as well as **overall good health**. Although some of these factors are beyond the scope of this book, the optimal surplus of conditioning that you will build by following the methods described will definitely affect your skill, mental toughness, and health in a positive way.

Abundance of Strength and Optimal Surplus

Louie Simmons once wrote an article for the magazine, POWERLIFTING USA, in which he spoke of developing an **abundance of strength**. In this article he mentioned the Soviet Olympic Lifter and World and Olympic Champion, David Rigert. Rigert, when his feet were out of position in the bottom of the Snatch and with the weight held overhead, would squat walk into the correct position before driving up to a standing position to complete the lift, often setting a world record in the process. This was only possible, Louie wrote, because Rigert had developed an abundance of strength through special exercises, one of which was to squat walk across the floor with a barbell held overhead. **This abundance of strength compensated for small technical flaws or lapses and enabled him to win Olympic and World Gold Medals.**

Although Louie Simmons used the word "abundance" when speaking of Rigert, we are essentially saying the same thing when we speak of "optimal surplus." Again, you need to develop more of the required physical qualities than what you actually need to execute your skills or compete in your event. To paraphrase Arkaev and Suchilin, "Only through an optimal surplus of physical, technical, and psychological preparation can we achieve reliability of performance."

OPTIMAL SURPLUS IN COMBAT SPORTS

How many times have you seen a top international-level judo, sambo or MMA fighter finish a forward throw even when his hip wasn't in a perfect textbook position. If you follow MMA, judo, sambo or jujitsu, you've seen this happen often. Many times author John Saylor witnessed U.S. Olympian and World Military Games Champion, Leo White, finish his forward Soto Makikomi (Outer Winding Throw) even when he didn't have his hip completely across in an ideal throwing position; and sometimes this was against a World or Olympic Champion. This was the case in the 1984 Los Angeles Olympics when Leo threw 1980 Olympic Champion Robert Van de Walle of Belgium for a major score and then maintained his lead to win the match.

How did Leo White do this? Even though his hip position wasn't perfect—after all, his world-class opponents were defending strongly—the rotation of his torso was so strong that he completed the throw anyway! In other words, the overwhelming strength of his finish compensated for the small technical flaw of his hips not being in deep enough.

> **TECHNICAL TIP.** Many times, the overwhelming strength of your finish will compensate for minor technical flaws in your throw, takedown, submission hold, pin, punch or kick.

By doing the exercises and training programs in this book you will develop this kind of optimal surplus in your strength, endurance, and technique.

Many times we've witnessed wrestlers and submission grapplers get blocked and stretched out when their opponents sprawled against their leg shot, often do a Double or Single Leg Takedown. Once they got stuck in this unfavorable position the opponent invariably took the attacker's back, or worse.

Many time World and Olympic Champion John Smith, on the other hand, would shoot his trademark Low Single, get on an opponent's leg, and even when it looked as though his opponent had stopped his shot, Smith would relentlessly find a way to finish. John Smith knew that the fight had just begun when the opponent temporarily blocked his initial shot.

The ability to finish a technique from an unfavorable position is one of the marks of a champion. Much of John Smith's, or any great champion's, ability to finish a technique and get the score comes from having voluntarily put themselves in these unfavorable positions and fighting out of them hundreds of times in practice. **They put themselves in these tough positions many more times than they would actually occur in**

a match or in regular wrestling practice. Not only does this situation drilling make them streetwise against the various holds and positions of a match, it also develops an **optimal surplus** of mental toughness, tactics, technique, and physical strength and endurance in that position.

You will find that the champions in any fighting art or sport have an optimal surplus of the various physical and mental qualities necessary for success in their event. Now, let's move forward and look at how you can develop this kind of optimal surplus and go on to reach your full potential in whatever fighting art or sport you practice.

TRAINING FOR GENERAL MUSCULAR ENDURANCE

Any method in which you work against resistance for prolonged periods of time, anywhere from 3 to 30 minutes, will develop muscular endurance. The length of your exercise rounds will depend on what type of exercise or routine you are doing. But as a general rule, when developing muscular endurance work against moderate resistance, anything from body weight only to 50% of your 1 rep max, and take very few rest breaks.

There are many types of exercises and programs to develop muscular endurance. The following pages contain a few of them that you can use to develop effective muscular endurance.

THE SHINGITAI SIX-PACK

The Shingitai Six-Pack is discussed again later in this section, but it's the type of training circuit that typifies what we mean when talking about General Muscular Endurance. The Shingitai Six-Pack consists of: 1) Neck Bridges, 2) Hindu Squat, 3) Glute Ham Raises, 4) Sit Ups, 5) Push Ups, 6) Pull Ups.

> **TECHNICAL TIP: The Shingitai 6 Pack consists of 6 exercises that you can do with a minimum of equipment, and which will build considerable strength and muscular endurance throughout your entire body. You don't need a gym membership to do it. You just need 15 to 40 minutes and the willingness to work hard.**

NECK BRIDGE

The neck is one of the most neglected areas in the average fighter's routine. A weak neck is an invitation for your opponent to do a snap down to a go-behind, or a Guillotine Choke,

or Thai Clinch to a knee to your head, or any number of bad things. On the other hand, a strong neck can give you a few extra seconds to fight out of chokes, and can help you maintain your posture to resist the type of techniques just mentioned. It can also help you absorb a punch better, and will lessen your odds of getting neck injuries.

One of the best exercises for neck development is the **neck bridge**. The neck bridge will also develop your hips, legs, back, and abs.

To perform the neck bridge, get a stopwatch, lie down on the mat, and gradually bridge back on your head until your nose touches the mat. This flexibility won't happen overnight, so just bridge as far back as is comfortable, and gradually try to go a little further back each time you bridge. Until you develop sufficient neck strength, use your hands to take a little of the resistance off your neck. As you get stronger you will no longer need your hands. Depending on your goals and fitness level, hold the bridge between 1 and 5 minutes.

For added variety and more complete development you should occasionally do the **front bridge**. To perform the front bridge simply face downward, put the top of your head on the mat, and with your hands behind your legs or back come up onto your head. You can simply hold that position, or as you get stronger you can slowly rock forward and back, and from side to side. Be sure to place your hands on the mat to remove some of the resistance until you're strong enough to do the exercise with your neck alone.

THE HINDU SQUAT

The Hindu Squat is one of the best exercises to develop muscular strength and endurance in the lower body. In fact, its benefits are not limited to the lower body. Hindu Squats, when done in high repetitions, will develop a fair amount of cardiovascular endurance as well. When done in high repetitions, say from 100 to 500 reps, you will also develop miles and miles of extra capillaries throughout the muscles of your lower body. These extra capillaries serve as an oxygen transport system that brings in blood and oxygen to the working muscles, and removes fatigue products like lactic acid. Since your legs are furthest from your heart, these extra capillaries are important in your quest to develop superior endurance.

Another benefit of high repetition Hindu Squats, and other super high rep exercises, is increased tendon and ligament strength. Tendons and ligaments have a very poor blood supply. Therefore, super high reps are required to bring blood and oxygen to these tissues. Thomas Kurz, in his excellent book, SCIENCE OF SPORTS TRAINING, recommends between 100 and 200 reps on various exercises to strengthen tendons and ligaments.

To perform Hindu Squats let your hands hang loosely by your sides and stand with your feet about shoulder width apart.

With your hips under you and your back straight, lower yourself into a squat. With a scooping motion of your hands, rise up to the starting position. Get into a steady rhythm and focus on your breathing as you do the allotted number of reps. Experiment with various breathing patterns throughout the weeks ahead, but start with inhaling on the way down and exhaling on the way up.

Sets and Reps: Work up to between 100 and 500 reps in one continuous set.

At first you may not be able to do this many continuous reps. Don't worry about it. Just start where you're at and keep adding reps over the coming weeks.

3-WEEK WAVES

Exercises in the **Shingitai 6 Pack** should be done in 3-week waves. This is especially true after you've built up to a more advanced level. Let's say you can do 500 consecutive Hindu Squats in good form. If you keep doing 500 reps every workout you will not get stronger or gain more endurance. In fact, accommodation will set in and you will start to feel worse, and eventually your performance will decline. To avoid this use a 3-week wave like the following:

Week 1: 300 Hindu Squats (60% of Volume).

Week 2: 400 Hindu Squats (80% of Volume).

Week 3: 500 Hindu Squats (100% of Volume).

On Week 4 go back to 60% and do another 3 week wave. 3-week waves will help you avoid accommodation and staleness.

Another strategy in combating accommodation is **The Conjugate Method of Training**. We will have more to say on The Conjugate Method elsewhere in this book, but for now just be sure to rotate other lower body exercises into your routine. In other words, when you're getting sick of Hindu Squats rotate another comparable exercise into your schedule for a while. This should be an exercise that essentially works the same muscle groups, but slightly differently. A few good choices would be Sumo Squats, Duck Walks, Hindu Squats with a staggered stance, Hindu Box Squats or Hindu Squat with added band resistance, high rep 1-leg Squats, and many more.

BUILD THE HOUSE FROM THE BASEMENT UP

Back around 1977 author John Saylor was lifting weights in the old weight room under Ohio State's football stadium. At the time, an Austrian shot-putter whom I knew only as Ernst was doing squats with some impressive weight, around 800 lbs. Over the weeks I noticed that Ernst really concentrated on Squats. When I asked him why, he simply told me, "You build a house from the basement up." He went on to explain that the shot put, like many movements in sport, is not done with muscles working in isolation. Rather, it is a **chain reaction movement**. "The shot put," he explained, "is started with the lower body, goes up through the torso, and is then released through the upper body."

If you think about it, the same is true of most throws and takedowns. Take any hip throw, for example. After you position yourself for the throw, it starts from your lower body, goes through your torso, and is assisted with your upper body. Pick-Up Throws are similar. Any pick-up throw is started by positioning your hips under your opponent's hips. Then you start the lift with your hips and legs, continue it through your torso, and complete the throw with your upper body. So, make sure you build the house from the basement up.

GLUTE-HAM RAISES

Hindu Squats are great, but they don't provide enough concentrated work on the hamstring muscle group. One of the main reasons athletes suffer knee injuries and hamstring pulls is because they have a muscular imbalance between the quads and hamstrings. Usually their quads are much stronger than their hamstrings. The hamstrings should be at least 60% of your quad strength.

Glute-Ham Raises will go a long way toward strengthening your hamstrings, glutes, and to a lesser extent your calves. They will also give you greater jumping ability and will increase explosiveness.

Sets and Reps: Perform Glute-Ham Raises at least 2 times per week.

On the first workout of the week (Max Effort Day) use added weight or band tension and perform 2 to 3 sets o. 10 to 30 reps.

On Dynamic Day, about 72 hours later, do high rep Glute-Ham Raises after your main workout. Work up to 1 set of 60 to 100 reps.

Again, use a 3-week wave, as follows:

Week 1: 60 reps (60% of Volume).

Week 2: 80 reps (80% of Volume).

Week 3: 100 reps (100% of Volume).

On week 4, wave back down to 60% and begin another 3-week wave.

If you aren't yet able to perform that many reps, just figure out your percentages based on your top number of reps.

SIT UPS

The sit-up is an old standard exercise that we're sure you're familiar with. Just secure your feet and keep your hands by the side of your head or crossed in front of your chest, and sit up and back. You can sit straight up touching both elbows to your knees, or you can alternately touch one elbow to the opposite knee on one rep, then the other on the next rep, and so on.

Sets and Reps: Work up to as many as 200 reps per set.

To inject variety from week to week be sure to rotate other sit-up variations and ab exercises into your workout.

As with your other exercises, be sure to use a 3-week wave on your total volume.

PUSH-UPS

The standard push-up is one of the oldest exercises around, but it's still a good one. Make sure you keep your core rigid and straight throughout the movement. Simply lower yourself until your chest almost touches the floor and then press yourself back to the starting position.

Sets and Reps: You can use any set and rep scheme you like, but try to work up to around 200 total reps per workout.

More advanced athletes may choose to do more total reps, but should remember to use the 3-week wave as described on Hindu Squats. In other words, use 60% of volume on week 1, 80% of volume on week 2, and 100% of volume on week 3. Then drop back to 60% and start another wave on week 4.

Also, be sure to employ the conjugate method and rotate different push-up variations from week to week. There are a lot of different ones to choose from, many of which you can find in this book. All of them work you slightly differently, and by rotating them into your schedule you will get better all-round development, and will avoid going stale.

PULL-UPS

The pull-up is an excellent exercise for the arms, lats, shoulders, and all the pulling muscles of the upper body. Pulling is vitally important in all grappling arts, both in standing work and on the ground.

There are many different pull-up variations, but to start out grab the bar with a reverse grip (palms facing away from you) and perform reps to near-failure. To perform a pull-up, simply hang from the bar and then pull yourself up until your chin is above the bar.

Sets and Reps: The reps will vary from person to person. Heavier athletes, for example, will often not be able to perform as many pull-ups as lighter athletes, but they will gain great strength because they are handling greater resistance. Whether you are heavy or light, your goal should be to handle your body weight for at least 8 to 10 reps. If you are lighter, set your goal much higher.

Depending on your fitness level and goals, perform 2 to 4 sets per workout.

As with the other exercises in the **Shingitai 6 Pack**, be sure to rotate other pull-up variations into your schedule on a regular basis. These variations are demonstrated elsewhere in this book, but a few you can start with are: underhand grip (both hands facing you), parallel grip, from overhead rings, with rock climbing grips, rope climbing, or gi or towel pull-ups. The gi pull-ups are a great grip developer for those of you competing in grappling events with the gi.

Add further variety by varying the width of your grip, doing isometric holds in several positions, adding weight or band resistance, or varying the angle.

TECHNICAL TIP. Athletes in uniform such as our armed forces, special operations, law enforcement officers and others who by the very nature of their dangerous jobs or situations rely on their strength, conditioning, speed, coordination and flexibility. Equally important, the ability to withstand physical punishment, abuse and deprivation is a by-product of your physical fitness, strength and conditioning. Winning in combat sports is a passion we all share, but when it comes down to it, winning in a real fight, in a life or death confrontation or being able to withstand the shock and abuse of physical injury in an accident is vital to us all.

PERIODIZATION, TRAINING CYCLES AND TRAINING WAVES

Basically, what is called "periodization" is a progression of your overall training program, divided into specific time frames, each accomplishing different goals in the overall scheme of things. Covered extensively by Dr. Tudor Bompa and others, periodization has been used by athletes and coaches in a variety of sports. Also known as a "cycling of training" this concept of dividing your training program in a progressive manner starts with general conditioning, then leads into more directed training, and ultimately into the specific phase of training; all leading up to your competitive event. This is also called by some "training waves" with the concept being that, much like a wave, your training rises and lowers in intensity and volume depending on where you are at in the yearly cycle.

When embarking on a training cycle, it is important that you have a solid base of fitness and skill. Periodization training isn't for novices; so don't start a training cycle unless you are physically ready to do it.

TECHNICAL TIP. How To Turn In Your Best Performance At Contest Time: The Art and Science Of Peaking

First of all, to peak properly requires that you've done a lot of training earlier in the training year or period. Think of it like money in the bank. If you haven't made your deposits, you can't make a big withdrawl when you need it. The same is true in training. A high peak is built upon the foundation of a high volume of training. Or look at it like this: if you're building a pyramid, the height of the peak is determined by the size of the base. So, before you even think about peaking make sure you've done plenty of general and specialized physical preparation.

As for the peaking itself, remember the following guidelines:

- To achieve a high peak you need plenty of general and specific physical preparation (GPP & SPP) behind you.
- About 4 to 6 weeks out from your major contest, **gradually reduce the total amount of training while increasing the intensity.**
- Include a 2 to 3 week unloading phase in which you'll **reduce both the volume and intensity** of your training. Middleweights and below seem to do best on a 2-week unloading phase, while heavy weights often require 3 weeks of unloading to be at their best for a contest. This unloading phase ensures that you will achieve what Russian sports scientists call **"supercompensation."** In other words, if you unload properly your physical abilities will climb far above your previous levels, thereby bringing you to a high peak.

Keep in mind that the 3-week wave itself can be used to bring you to a minor peak for the smaller events. Just time your wave so that a light week precedes your fight or contest. You can even modify it to a 2-week wave if time doesn't permit a full 3-week wave—no big deal. Don't try to hit a full peak more than 2 or 3 times per year. Save the major peaks for your most important fights or contests. For the smaller contests just use the 3-week wave.

There's absolutely no point in leaving your best performances in the gym. By adhering to the above guidelines you will be able to mobilize all your mental and physical forces toward one end—victory at the big events!

TWO APPROACHES TO PERIODIZATION

We're going to present two different approaches to periodization, both are successful and the authors have used both of them through the years with their athletes. The first approach is what we call the "wave" approach where you have an established baseline of fitness and training and have multiple training cycles or "waves" during a season. This is the type of training that wrestlers must use during a wrestling season where they have to make weight regularly for dual meets and for major tournaments. It's also useful for a judo or sambo athlete that may have a fairly short notice of a tournament and needs to be as sharp as possible for it. This approach is also good for boxers and MMA fighters who don't have an established "season" and may have to fight on short notice.

The second one is the standard approach to periodization. It's effective for athletes who are training for one specific event or fight and can focus directly on the one event. Both approaches to periodization are useful, depending on your combat sport and how much time or notice you have to train for it. This is why we're presenting both approaches for your information.

SHORT TRAINING WAVES

A practical approach to periodization is using short-term training cycles of 3 weeks in duration. This is useful for athletes who may not have a set schedule or season and have to stay in shape pretty much year-round.

This approach to peaking for a fight or tournament is based on the fact that you must stay in good shape most of the year. You need to stay at about 80% in shape most of the year to make this work. This provides a solid base of fitness and skill. Remember, you're working out on a regular basis with about 2 days a week where you go live or randori with intensity and 3 or 4 other days per week on your technical training and fitness training. You're also working on your skills on a regular basis and your cardio and strength levels are good. Basically, you're working out 4 to 6 days per week, taking 1 or 2 days off to rest. Think of it this way: your goal is to stay in about 80% shape most of the year. You'll take some time off from practice once in a while to keep from going stale and over-training, and to recover from injuries, but you will usually be in good shape throughout the year; good enough shape so that you can step up your training routine when it's necessary to work into 100% shape for a fight or tournament. When you get the call for a fight or tournament, you may have only 3 or 4 weeks notice. In this case, you will use a Short Training Wave to peak for the event.

The first 2 weeks of this 3-week training wave consist of situational drilling where you place yourself in specific situations that actually come up in a fight or match and work on them. An example might be if you are an MMA fighter and know that your opponent likes to put his opponents with their backs to the cage, you will work on skills to keep him from putting you in that position. You might also work on having your training partners put you with your back to the cage and you work on fighting out of that situation.

These 2 weeks will also see you step up more cardio work on the mat or in the gym. An example is that you may go five 2-minute grappling rounds with a new training partner each round. This is truly fighting yourself into shape in the strictest sense. This is also the time for you to focus on your tactics and sharpen your defensive skills.

The last week is devoted to light drill training with the emphasis on doing the skills you do. Practices during this last week should be short and sweet. You want to mobilize all your physical and mental energy for the fight. If necessary, this last week might be devoted to travel and settling in so you feel as comfortable as possible where you are fighting.

Basically, you came into this short training cycle at about 80% and these 3 weeks serve to get you as close to 100% as you possibly can. Realistically, many of you reading this book will most likely use this type of periodization.

THE STANDARD TRAINING CYCLE OR PERIODIZATION

The "standard" approach to periodization or setting up a training cycle is presented here using a 16-week training cycle. If you're training for one specific fight or event, this is an effective way to prepare for it.

Plan Your "Season"

It's important to sit down with your coach or teammates and plan out the events you want to fight in for the upcoming year. Create and plan your own "season" in the same way a college wrestling team would do and then do what it takes to be successful at it. Plan for about 12 months out so you can select the tournaments or events you want to fight in, and allow yourself the time to train for them. Here's an example of a "season" using the 2009 season for our judo/jujitsu/sambo team at Welcome Mat.

> **Year:** 2009
> Late March: Welcome Mat Games or Arnold Classic
> Late July: AAU Grand Nationals
> Mid-August: AAU Nationals
> Late October: State Championships
> Late November: AAU Freestyle Nationals

We selected five primary events to train for. If something else came up and team members were ready to compete in it, the guys competed in it, but these five events were the ones we set our training cycle for. This planning provided the athletes (as well as coaches) a focused and planned schedule to follow. After a short layoff from mid-December to the first week of January, the guys got back to it with their overall training on the mat and in the weight room, as well as on the cardio

> **TRAINING TIP.** You need about 2 to 3 days rest between intense bouts of training. In other words, if you go live, spar or randori on an intense basis, you will get the most out of your training if you do it no more than twice or three times a week. The general public, who doesn't know what intense training feels like or does to the body, thinks that a fighter or grappler can fight hard every day. You may be able to go about an hour of daily randori, sparring or going live during a short-term training camp, but you sure don't want to have a training cycle where you fight hard every day just before a major tournament or fight. Athletes who bang on each other full blast every workout either end up hurt all the time or are the guys easy to beat in a tournament. The old saying "Don't leave your fight in the gym" is certainly true. Train hard...real hard, but it's also important to train smart as well.

training. This foundation is necessary to get the most out of a training cycle when starting into it. When the time came to start the first training cycle, everyone was ready and willing to get with the program and bear down on having a successful season.

After establishing our "season" we can now set up a training cycle with specific goals in mind.

Training Camp

This 16-week training cycle is similar to the concept of a training camp used for years by professional boxers, and now with MMA fighters. We all know about fighters secluding themselves and their team of trainers, sparring partners and others in a remote area for three or four months of hard, specialized training for a big fight. What they have done for years, and continue to do, is periodization. It may not have been called "periodization" years ago when Joe Louis or other famous fighters did it, but that's what it was and continues to be.

THE 3 PHASES OR CYCLES OF PERIODIZATION

There are 3 primary phases or cycles in a standard training cycle. They are:

General Phase (High Volume Phase)
> also known as Accumulation Phase

This phase develops basic strength and endurance, and other general athletic abilities, as well as the selection and development of skills that you, as the athlete, want to work on. During the GPP Phase you will be accumulating a solid, all-round general base. This phase of training can start as far as a year away from the event you are training for, but more often starts about 4 months out. Think about your training cycle this way; start your training cycle about 16 weeks (4 months) prior to your event. Count down starting at week 16 and culminating in week 1 (and then the day of your event). This initial, general phase of training should last from week 16 up to, and including, week 11; in other words, the first 6 weeks of your training. Your general fitness training should increase in intensity as each week goes by. You should also work hard on your technical phase of training during this period of time. Perform a large number (high volume) of drills and exercises that emphasize overall fitness, but especially cardio fitness as well as technique development.

Directed Phase (DP)
> also known as the "Intensification Phase"

As you progress in your strength, endurance and speed, you also establish the techniques or skills that will work best for you at the event you are training for in this second cycle of training. This directed phase of training will last for 6 weeks,

from week 11 through and including week 5. This second phase is the time that you concentrate on the physical skills and overall strategy you will use for your event. You're now concentrating on the gym exercises, drills on the mat and cardio work which are in some way related to your sport and what you need to do to win at it. This is the time you really work on drill training so that your skills are instinctive and performed with an increasing level of skill. This is also the time that you mold your techniques so that they fit you like a glove. This phase of training is intense as you are going live or doing randori with real intensity. These 6 weeks of directed training are important in the sense that this is the time when you fit all the pieces together.

Specific Phase (SP)
> also known as the "Transformation Phase"

If you were to think of training as a pyramid, this is the tip of the pyramid. This specific phase of your training cycle lasts 4 weeks. Week 4 and into week 3, you should finalize everything you're been working toward. Taper back on the intensity during randori or going live and work on randori or fighting drills where you key in on your tactics, grip-fighting and defense. Work a lot on situational drills where you are behind in the score, ahead in the score or your coach puts you in specific situations that you have to adapt or react to. This is when you work on your tactics and make sure you have as many answers to as many questions as possible.

The last 10 to 14 days of this phase is when you taper down (back off on your training intensity) so that you avoid injuries, keep your intensity level high, and are pretty much at the weight you plan on fighting at. This is the time to work out any last-minute details in your tactics or fight plan as well. Your workouts should be short and to the point. Don't go live or randori during these last 10 to 14 days, and by all means, don't do anything that will get you injured. Make sure your training partners are all on board as well. There's nothing worse than having a training partner pull some macho cheap shot the last week before your major fight or tournament and injure you.

These last 2 weeks or so in your training cycle are often the toughest mentally and emotionally. You've been training your butt off and now you have to taper back and maintain your peak. The last 2 to 3 days of this tapering phase should be used for resting your body and maybe just work on some tactics or easy technique work. If you're cutting weight, keep working on making sure you're on weight.

This is a good time to work on your final mental preparation. A good idea is to "fight" your matches in your mind with you always winning and doing the techniques or skills that you've been working on. These mental fights always end up with you standing on the podium or having your hand raised as the winner. Plan any travel that you might have to do during this last tapering period of your training cycle. If you have to travel overseas, your last few days might be in a foreign country, so make sure to plan for cutting weight, your diet, jet lag or other factors.

Piggy Backing In a Training Cycle

In some cases, you may have trained for a specific event and need to keep your edge for another tournament or fight that is scheduled several weeks after the first event. In this case, you will want to keep your "peak" for the second event as well, and this isn't impossible to do. This is what is called "piggy backing" from one event to another. There may be two events that are important to you and it's important to think about that when planning out your season. Say, for instance, the second event is 3 weeks after the first. In this case, it's good to think of your training as a "wave" where you rise and recede in the intensity of your training. After competing in the initial event where you've gone through 16 weeks of periodization, you can take a week off before the second event to rest and recover (but don't forget that you may have to make weight again, so don't over-eat). You're not going to lose your "peak" physically, so don't go crazy on the running or lifting.

Then, the final 2 weeks before the second event, keep your training intensity up by working on specific drills for your sport and performing light randori (going live) with teammates who are willing to take some falls or tap out for you. This open (randori) training should be "smiling randori" so that it's about 60% intensity (or so you can actually smile when doing it). Keep your cardio fitness level maintained with light roadwork. The hardest part about fighting in events so close to each other is to keep the intensity level up for the second one. The final 2 or 3 days before this second event should be like the final 2 or 3 days before your first event. Don't get hurt, make sure your weight is controlled and be rested and ready to fight.

AN OVERVIEW OF PART 2 AND PART 3

We're now putting into practice what was explained earlier in this section. The next part of Section 1 presents some basic, functional stretches that you can use as an effective warm-up for your grappling or fighting workout or for a lifting or cardio workout. This book's main goal isn't to present stretching or flexibility training in its entirety. If you're looking for a book that offers excellent advice on stretching for a variety of martial arts, the authors recommend ULTIMATE FLEXIBILITY by Sang H. Kim and published by Turtle Press. However, functional stretching is part of every athlete's overall training program, and because of this, this book presents some stretches that are generic, yet effective.

Then, in Part 3 of this first section, we present a variety of workouts that have proven effective for athletes in combat sports. These workouts will be different and they are effective and will include workouts you can do in the gym, on the mat or outside. When putting together a workout routine, look at what your goals are, and then attempt to do what is necessary to fulfill those goals. These routines are presented to serve as guides for you when you design your own training program or work with a coach or trainer in developing a training program.

SECTION ONE: PART 2: FUNCTIONAL STRETCHING, WARM-UPS AND COOL-DOWNS

• • • "Warm up, stretch out and then get at it." Shawn Watson

WARM-UPS AND COOL-DOWNS

Effective Warm-Ups

Before tackling a hard training session, your body must be prepared to handle the stress you will place on it. Warming up your muscles, as well as preparing your body to handle the rigors of a hard workout, is a vital first step in every training session. Remember, your body will take hard falls on the mat, have joints and muscles stretched, take bumps, bruises and hard shots, and generally take a beating every time you train. If your body isn't physically prepared, and just as important, if your mind isn't mentally prepared, you won't have an effective workout and you may even sustain injuries. Every warm-up should include:

1. Light exercises, drills or games to physically warm the muscles of your body up before stretching. Many of these exercise, drills and games are featured in Section 2. Take a few minutes for this phase of your workout. Your muscles are now physically warmed up and ready to stretch.

2. Functional stretching for your entire body. Work within your range of motion, and as you gain in flexibility, your range of motion will gradually increase to meet the demands of your sport. Stretch out as thoroughly as possible, making sure to work your entire body. It should only take a few minutes, but don't limit yourself by time; make sure you stretch thoroughly.

3. Fitness drills or exercises that transition into your drill training for skill and technique development. This is the transition from the warm-up phase of your workout to the drill-training phase of your workout. Many of these exercises, drills and games are explained in Section 2 of this book. These are the drills that help prepare your body for the harder workload it will endure later in the workout. We recommend doing breakfalls, tumbling and games and drills that feature some body contact with other members of your training group. Spend a few minutes in this phase of your workout and transition directly to your drill training.

Effective Cool-Downs

After a hard workout, take a few minutes to cool down or finish. This is a good time to allow your body to physically cool down and return to a more normal state. When it's cold outside, a cool-down is even more important. Let the body settle down, cool down and calm down before leaving the gym, especially in cold weather. You should not be physically sweating when you leave the gym or dojo after a workout whether it's cold outside or not. Your cool-down should allow you to lower your heart rate and body temperature. Your cool-down should include:

1. Light exercises, drills or games to flush out waste products in the muscles. This is a good time to let your heart rate gradually slow down and allow your body temperature to lower.

2. Light stretches that help decrease muscle soreness increase flexibility and slow down your heart-rate. Lower your body temperature and allow your body time to literally "cool off". Light and mild stretching after a workout will flush out waste products from your muscles and help increase your range of motion.

FUNCTIONAL STRETCHING

Functional stretching is best defined as being flexible enough to easily move within the range of motion in a joint or group of joints. In other words, you need to be flexible enough to get the job done as a grappler or fighter. Flexibility is one part of your overall fitness level including cardio endurance, muscle endurance, strength, speed, balance, agility, coordination, skill, and other physical, mental and emotional attributes. The flexibility needs we have as grapplers and fighters are very different than those of gymnasts, runners or athletes in other events. Stretch your muscles so that they can perform their desired function. To be able to perform grappling or fighting skills at your highest possible level, you must be physically able to perform them. If you're not flexible, you won't be able to mount a good offense or offer a good defense, plain and simple.

THE 3 BIG BENEFITS OF STRETCHING

1. **Your Range of Motion Increases:** By increasing the length of your muscle, a reduction in overall muscle tension takes place and this increases your range of motion.

2. **Additional Power and Explosive Strength:** By increasing your muscle length, you are increasing the distance over which the muscles are able to contract. This translates into more efficient ability to produce power.

3. **Muscle Soreness and Fatigue Lessened:** Being sore is part and parcel of the after effects of a hard workout. This soreness is the result of micro tears within the muscle fibers and the pooling of blood and various waste products. If you stretch as part of your cool-down, you'll go a long way in cutting down the soreness by lengthening the individual muscle fibers, increasing circulation of blood and helping flush out waste products. Along with being sore, fatigue sets in after strenuous training. Muscles that are flexible work more efficiently and aren't forced to put forth as much force against opposing muscle groups.

> **TECHNICAL TIP: Flexibility is simply how we refer to the range of movement in a joint or group of joints. Flexibility is one part of your overall fitness level including cardio endurance, muscle endurance, strength, speed, balance, agility, coordination and skill, among other aspects. The flexibility needs we have as grapplers and fighters are very different than those of gymnasts, runners or athletes in other events.**

STATIC, BALLISTIC AND PNF STRETCHES

There are a number of different types of stretching, but for most grapplers and fighters, stretching falls into 3 basic categories:

1. Static stretching is a safe and effective way to stretch, both before and after a hard workout. Basically, in a static stretch, you don't "bounce" when you stretch. Hold your stretch to the point of mild tension or tightness, but not where it's painful. By doing this, you're staying within your safe range of motion. Hold the stretch for 10 to no more than 60 seconds. Most grapplers hold the stretch for about 30 seconds. Stretch in a slow, controlled way and gradually increase your range of motion. In most cases, static stretching is what you will do in your workouts.

2. Ballistic stretching isn't recommended, but is the oldest form of stretching used in athletics. Bouncing, swinging or fast, rapid movements of the body or appendages are potentially dangerous. Ballistic stretching and bouncing when you stretch will not allow your muscles time to adapt to the stretched position.

3. PNF stretching is an advanced form of stretching that allows the muscle being stretched to both stretch and contract. Done with a partner, PNF (Proprioceptive Neuromuscular Facilitation) stretches involve the muscle being stretched, and then relaxed. Repeated use of this will gradually increase the range of motion. Your partner will hold you in a stretched position for a specified time period, and then release the tension in the stretch allowing your muscle to relax. Eventually, your range of motion increases.

BASIC STRETCHES FOR GRAPPLERS

The following exercises are pretty general, and are good, effective stretches that can be used before or after a workout. As mentioned before, the primary purpose of this book isn't in the area of flexibility, but functional flexibility is necessary for all grapplers and fighters. For a more complete presentation of stretching and flexibility, refer to ULTIMATE FLEXIBILITY by Sang H. Kim and available from Turtle Press. The stretching routine shown here is one used by many grapplers trained by the authors. Take about 10 minutes to stretch before a workout as part of a good, effective warm-up, and then when you're done working out, take a few minutes to stretch as part of your cool-down.

ARM STRETCH

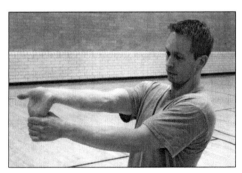

This stretch is important if you train on a lot of armlocks. Extend one arm and grab the fingers of that arm with your other hand. Pull back on your fingers. This stretches most of the muscles in the arm.

ARM GRAB SHOULDER STRETCH

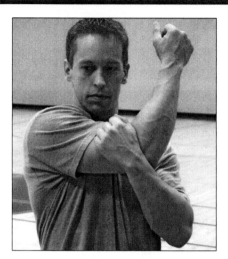

Place one arm across your body and use your other hand and arm to hook or grab it, pulling it to your opposite shoulder. This is a good stretch for your trapezius, rhomboids, latissimus dorsi and rear deltoid. It's also good for the rotator cuff and general shoulder area.

FOOT STRETCH

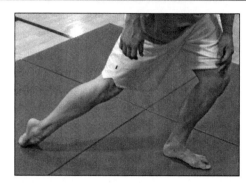

Place the top of your foot on the mat as shown and push your ankle forward. This is a good stretch for the muscle sin your shins and the top of your foot. This is especially important to fighters in sports where kicking is used as well as grapplers where foot sweeps and reaps are used.

KNEELING TRUNK ROTATION

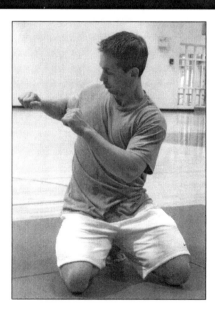

Kneel on the mat and gently rotate from one side to the other as shown. Turn as far as possible each way, before rotating to the other side. This works the abdominals and obliques, as well as the many muscles that also run along the spine in the back.

KNEELING QUAD STRETCH

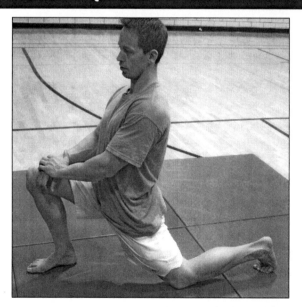

Kneel on one leg with the other propped up as shown. Lean your hips far forward. This is a good stretch for the quadriceps, hip flexors and some of the other muscles in the abdominal and lower back areas.

INNER THIGH STRETCH

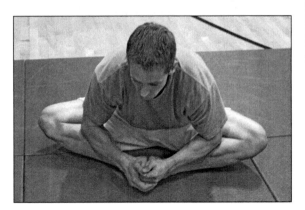

Sit on the mat with your knees wide and feet pulled in as close as possible to your crotch. Grab your feet with your hands and use your elbows and forearms to push down on your legs. Try to get the knees as flat to the mat as possible. This stretches your inner thighs well.

TORSO ARCH

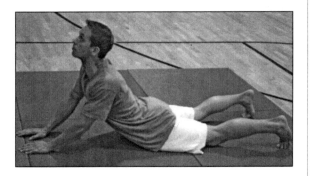

Lie on your front on the mat and extend your hands out to your front as shown. Keep your hips on the mat as you arch up and raise your head to look at the ceiling. This is a really good stretch for the intercostals, obliques, abdominals and the muscles in the hip and lower back.

STANDING HAMSTRING STRETCH

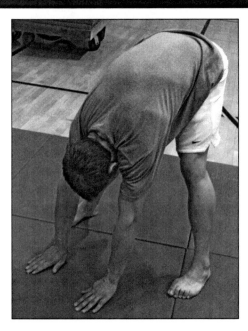

Stand with your feet about shoulder width and your knees as straight as possible. Bend forward and let your body weight dictate how far you bend over. As you gain flexibility, you will be able to touch the mat with your palms. This is a good stretch for the hamstrings, gastrocnemius (calf and lower leg), glutes in your rear end and illicostalis lumbrorum in your lower back and the muscles along your spine.

LEGS SPREAD WIDE STRETCH

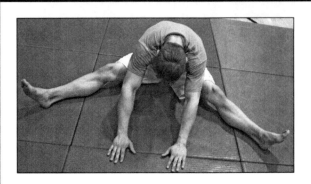

Sit on the mat with your legs spread out as wide as possible, making sure to keep your knees straight. Lean forward as shown and use your hands to pull your body forward. This stretches the adductors, gracilis and other inner thigh muscles.

HURDLER'S STRETCH

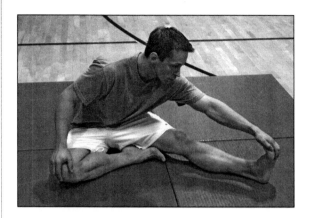

Sit on the mat with one leg extended out to your side as far as possible with your toes pointing up. Place your other foot up to your knee as close to your crotch as you can. Use one hand to grab the extended foot and pull back on the toes as you flew your toes forward. With your other hand, push down on your bent knee. Lean your body forward. This stretch works your biceps femoris (hamstrings) and the many muscles in the inner thigh as well. It also stretches the flexors in your lower leg and Achilles tendon. It's a good stretch for your obliques and muscles in your rib, core and hip areas.

KNEE HOOK ROTATION STRETCH

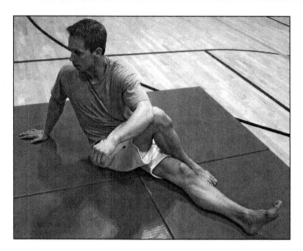

Sit with one leg straight and the other leg crossed over your extended leg at the knee. Turn your shoulders and place your arm over your bent knee push a bit to rotate your body. This stretch mostly works the glutes, outer hips and the muscles along the spine.

QUAD STRETCH LAYING ON YOUR SIDE

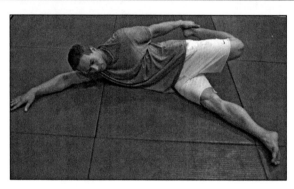

Lie on your side and pull your top leg behind you as close to your buttocks as you can. Try to push your hips forward as you do the stretch. This works the rectus femoris, vastus medialis, lateralis and intermedius muscles in the upper leg. This is a good upper leg stretch that you should include.

KNEELING REACH AND FLATTEN STRETCH

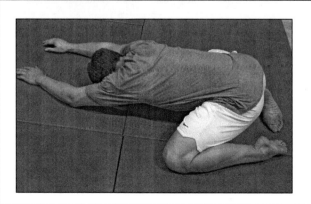

Kneel on the mat with your knees as wide as possible with your feet in close. Get your pelvis as low to the mat as possible. Try to touch your chest to the mat as you reach forward as far as you can. This works your latissimus dorsi in the upper back and adductors (inside of your thighs), your entire glute area and your entire shoulder area.

BACK ARCH

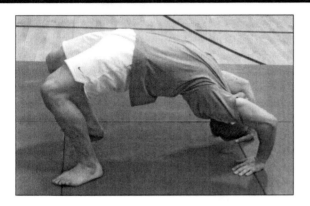

From a lying position on your back, use your hands to reach above your head and place them on the mat as shown. Make sure your feet are firmly placed on the mat as shown as well. Arch up as shown. This works your entire lower back, shoulder area, triceps and core region. It also stretches your glutes, hip flexors and upper leg muscles.

NECK BRIDGES (WRESTLER'S BRIDGE)

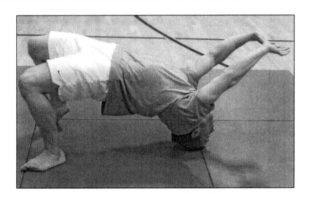

Don't do this exercise unless you are capable of it and have sufficient strength in the traps and back. Ease down onto the top of your head from the Back Arch exercise. Roll gently on the top of your head and make sure to keep your feet on the firmly on the mat. A good way to add more effort to this exercise is to reach forward with your hands as shown.

SHOULDER BRIDGES

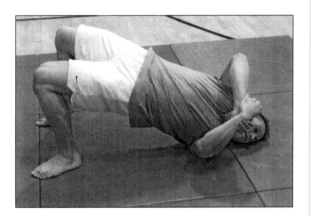

Lie on your back, arch up as shown, and grab your hands together. Rotate from one shoulder to the other without letting your butt touch the mat.   As with the Back Arch, this exercise works your entire body.

LEG TO SIDE SQUATTING STRETCH

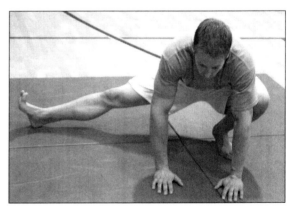

Squat on the mat and extend one leg directly to the side as shown. Lean forward and squat low while extending your other leg out to the side as far as possible. The adductors are the primary muscle group stretched.

SECTION ONE: PART 3: WORKOUT ROUTINES AND TRAINING ADVICE

• • • "To be weak is miserable." John Milton

If you want to become stronger, get to the gym or dojo and train. We're glad you're reading this book, but the goal of this book is to get you in a dojo or gym and work out! This part of Section 1 includes an explanation of the different types of training and some advice on how to get the most out of your time when working out, as well as some practical information that may be of interest to you. Also included are a variety of workout routines that have long proven valuable for a lot of athletes. There is no "magic" routine that will make you stronger, fitter or tougher than the other guy. The workout routines listed here are ones the authors have used, or seen used by others, that worked for them. In the course of your career, you will use many different routines; some better than others. All of us, through trial and error, find the workout routines that work for us.

TRAINING WITH WEIGHTS

Both authors grew up in an era when many coaches would tell athletes that weight training would "make you slow" or would "tighten your muscles." While every good coach in the business today advocates strength training for athletes, including the authors, there is some validity to what the old-timers said. But then, weight training has progressed and has come a long way since then. We've learned how to train both harder, and just as important, train smarter since then. However, the objections the old coaches had to being "slow" or "tight" are still true. Many athletes don't train efficiently in the weight room, and we hope to present some information in this book that will help you train both hard and train smart; and as a result, train efficiently.

Be honest. How many people have asked you, "How much can you bench?" A lot of people spend way too time bench pressing. Don't miss our point, there's nothing wrong with that particular lift. What is wrong, however, is the over-emphasis people give it. Doing too many bench presses is largely a waste of time for most fighters and grapplers.

Also, the weight training of most athletes produces danger-ous muscle imbalances that can, and will, come back to hurt them.

> **TECHNICAL TIP: When training with weights, you must work opposing muscle groups to avoid an im-balance of development. An imbalance of develop-ment leads to injuries.**

An athlete who performs Squats on a regular basis but doesn't balance it out with hamstring work is just asking for knee in-juries and hamstring pulls!

Also, because a lot of athletes have been told that explosive weight training is dangerous, they aren't training fast in their lifts. How they come to believe that they can get fast by train-ing slow is a mystery. If you want to become fast, you must train fast.

Louie Simmons is a respected strength and Powerlifting coach who has produced numerous National and World Powerlifting Champions and is known for his work in speed-strength development for athletes in a variety of sports. Louie has influenced much of what the authors present in this book. For those of you who are serious about weights and weight training, we suggest you pick up a copy of Louie's DVD, THE REACTIVE METHOD, where he shows how to train with weights with added bands and chains for maximum de-velopment of speed-strength. You can find this DVD at www. westside-barbell.com. The approach we take in this book is similar to Louie Simmons' approach to training for strength and speed.

THE "BIG 3" OF TRAINING: INTENSITY, DURATION AND FREQUENCY

An effective training routine or workout has 3 elements to it. They are:

1. **Intensity:** How hard the training session is on you. In-tensity can be measured in terms of percentage of a 1-rep max, or by percentage of maximum heart rate.

2. **Duration:** How long the workout lasts. How long does it take to complete the workout?

3. **Frequency:** How often during the week that the workout takes place. It's how many times you actually work out during the week.

Every phase of training, whether it's on the mat, in the gym, or anywhere, has its roots in the Big 3 listed above. All 3 ele-ments work together and are dependant on each other. They all build on each other as well. If you're "hit and miss" in your workouts, you have a big hole in the Frequency of your training habits. On the other hand, if you show up on a regu-lar basis, but only go through the motions, then you're lack-ing in Intensity. Someone might be very intense in his efforts, but fail to complete the workout, and in this case, the Duration of the workout is cut short and ineffective. Look at every phase of your training: on the mat, in the gym and elsewhere. Are the Big 3 elements met? If not, make it a point to correct the situation and include them all. In doing so, you'll have a more well-rounded approach to your overall development.

> **TECHNICAL TIP: Train to attain a "fighter's physique."** If you're a grappler, MMA fighter, wrestler, judo, jujitsu or self-defense athlete, you're not a bodybuilder, weightlifter, long-distance runner or cyclist; you're all of that, and more. You're training for fighting. Big pecs or big biceps don't win fights. Will you see an increase in muscle mass or a definite improvement in your physique as a result of hard and consistent training? Of course! However, an improvement in how you look is secondary to your main goal of training to succeed in your combat sport. Use your strength and fitness training as an instrument to help you become a better fighter.

THE VALUE OF HARD WORK: SACRIFICE FOR SUCCESS

Some coaches rightly call it your "training ethic". That's another way of saying "work ethic". Your success lies in direct relation to how hard you work. Additionally, it's how "smart" you work that plays a vital role. By training smarter, you also train harder. You train in a systematic, structured way that makes you work harder and yield greater rewards for your efforts. Lazy athletes may get by on natural talent for a while, but eventually, the athlete who works harder will surpass the one who isn't willing to make the sacrifice for success.

Hard, physical work does more for you than simply make you strong. It toughens you up physically, mentally and emotionally. If you're training for combat sports, you realize that an important part of your training must include things that make you physically tougher and harder in order to sustain the severity of abuse you will sustain in a match, fight, or even in a tough training session.

When you walk into the gym or step outside for some outdoor training, the idea is to work hard. Don't make a big show of it; simply work your butt off. Yelling, grunting, cussing, dropping weights and acting macho during a gym workout, or any workout anywhere (including on the mat) only makes you look bad. Serious athletes don't put on a show. They don't have to; they just train hard. If you have to grunt when pushing up out of a heavy squat, that's one thing, but don't put on a show. Anybody who's been around knows what's going on.

On the other hand, sweating and being workmanlike and serious is what will make your stronger, fitter and tougher. One time, Thom VanVleck, a friend of author Steve Scott, was asked to not come back to a gym by the manager because Thom perspired too much and "scared the clients". Thom was out of town on a business trip and dropped by the gym that was near his hotel. Thom, a top Highland Games athlete and Strongman competitor who has worked out in gyms all across the United States, was aware that this gym wasn't a "hard core" gym but rather a commercial venture catering to an upscale clientele. Knowing that, he was respectful, friendly, kept to himself and followed all the rules of the gym. The one thing Thom did was to work hard, and as a result, he did indeed sweat. Although Thom made it a point to clean anything he perspired on with the sanitizer provided, he still seemed to "scare the clients". After being informed of his lapse of civility, Thom politely thanked the gym manager for letting him work out there and found somewhere else to train while on his trip.

The point here is that not everyone has the same goals as you, or will work out as intensely as you, and if this is the case, find a gym where you feel comfortable and can make progress.

Any activity can and should be considered a form of training. Don't limit your view of training to what can be done in a gym or on a mat. Rock climbing, hiking, cutting wood, and hard physical labor all make you stronger, fitter and tougher. Anyone who has baled hay knows the meaning of hard work. Author John Saylor has, for years, cut his own wood and towed it from the forest to his barn for use in his wood-burning furnace. If you don't have access to this type of activity, create your own hard work. That's where flipping big tires, lifting and carrying stones, barrels and heavy objects can come in handy as part of your overall training. Even in the gym, create hard work by using your imagination when using the barbells, dumb-bells and machines available to you.

SAFETY WHEN TRAINING

The best workout is one in which nobody goes home injured. Whether you're in the gym or in the dojo, respect your training partners and do everything possible to accommodate each other. We're all in this together, so if we respect each other, we all benefit. Respecting other people in the dojo or gym goes a long way toward everyone being safe as well. Here are some other safety rules you should always follow when lifting in the gym:

1. Use a spotter, especially when lifting heavy. Always use a spotter when bench pressing or squatting.

2. Use good lifting technique. Bad lifting technique or form will cause injuries. Learn how to perform all the lifts and

exercises correctly.

3. When lifting with barbells or dumb-bells, use the collars or locks. Weights can slide off bars and cause serious injuries.

4. Don't drop weights. Weights land on things, such as your foot or somebody else's foot. Don't slam the weights down when using a machine. Slamming weights on the stack can damage them.

5. Wear shoes when lifting in a gym. Shoes protect your feet.

6. Breathe when you lift. Don't hold your breath.

7. Don't bounce or jerk the barbell or dumb-bell, especially in the bottom position of a Squat. Poor lifting form such as jerking, swinging or bouncing the weight gets poor results and can cause injuries.

8. Make sure you are clear of other people when lifting. If the gym is crowded, be careful not to invade anyone else's training space.

THE RULES OF THE ROOM: GYM AND DOJO RULES

Every gym, club or dojo has its own rules and if you want to work out there, follow them. It's wise to keep in mind that grappling, MMA, judo, jujitsu and any martial art are "group" activities. While not a team sport, what we do depends (to a large degree) on having other people to do it with. Anywhere people gather to work out, train or learn, there are "rules of the room," "gym rules," or "dojo rules." Each place has its own atmosphere, culture and norms that reflect the attitude, work ethic and philosophy of the head coach, club owner or the people who train there. If their work ethic or philosophy does not match yours, find somewhere else to work out, but if they do, you have a home away from home and will spend a lot of your life in that place. Check with the head coach or gym owner to learn the rules of the room when first joining to avoid any embarrassing situations.

KEEP A TRAINING LOG OR WORKOUT JOURNAL

Keep a workout journal or training log to record your exercises, sets, reps, the amount of weight you used and anything else you want to put in there. A workout journal helps you organize your training. Both authors have each kept a workout journal for many years and use the information they jotted down as an effective tool in setting goals, seeing what worked (and didn't work) for them previously or using the information they wrote down to help them motivate themselves. Some athletes keep a log of all their workouts, including what they do on the mat or in the dojo as well. Your training journal will also let you know when you're not making progress and will provide excellent feedback and source of useful information for you. Keeping a training log or workout journal really provides you with the organization necessary to coordinate your training efforts.

TIPS ON BREATHING WHEN TRAINING WITH WEIGHTS

As you progress, you'll find that you breathe at your own rhythm when lifting, but there are some basic guidelines to follow when training with weights as far as breathing is concerned.

Don't hold your breath when lifting. Holding your breath stops the flow of oxygen to your brain, which will cause you to pass out. Holding your breath is especially dangerous if you have high blood pressure or other medical concerns. It's also a good idea to breathe through both your nose and mouth. Get as much oxygen as possible when lifting.

Here's an exception to the rule. For highly trained, fit, younger athletes who are trying for a personal record on a major lift, it is desirable to hold the breath. This holding of the breath creates intra-abdominal pressure and helps protect the spine during the strain of a max effort lift. But again, holding the breath should only be used by those who are fit and healthy, and then only sparingly during max effort work. Otherwise the rule remains as stated above: keep your breathing steady and uninterrupted.

OVERTRAINING

You want to train hard, but you also want to train smart. Sometimes, and it happens to all of us, you will train too hard…and that means you haven't been training smart. We're not mentioning this to insult anyone, because overtraining is common. One of the basic concepts of training is that you want to overload your body so that it responds by an increase in strength, muscular endurance and an efficient aerobic or cardio capacity. You are progressively increasing your workload, and because of this, you run a very real risk of what is referred to as "overtraining". Most of us who are involved in combat sports are probably "Type A" personalities and as a result of this, we are susceptible to demanding too much from our bodies from time to time.

Overtraining is the result of physical, mental and emotional factors that lead to staleness. We're not only talking about the stress you place on yourself in the gym or the dojo, but also the stress in your daily life. It all adds up, so consider everything when you undertake a training program. It's hard to get the most out of your training if things at home or at work are in turmoil. Additionally, heat exhaustion is a physical factor that leads to overtraining, so consider the weather when training outside, or the temperature of the dojo or workout room. Dropping on the floor from heat exhaustion isn't macho or a sign of hard training; it's a sign of highly ineffective training which can have serious consequences.

Along with training hard, make sure you balance it out with good rest and recovery time as well as with good nutrition. Variety of training and workouts, cross training, recovery and good nutrition are vital in avoiding overtraining. Remember, the harder you train, the more intense the after-effects of that training. This is why it's crucial for you to actively make the effort to rest and recover, as well as have good nutritional habits.

When working out in no longer enjoyable, or if you have difficulty in concentrating, experience mood swings, and have a general sense of fatigue, you are overtrained.

TECHNICAL TIP: Signs of Overtraining include, but are not limited to the following:

• **Irritability, mood swings, anger and "not being yourself."**

• **An increase in getting a head cold or getting sick, increased aches and pains.**

• **Your sleep pattern changes and you wake up tired.**

• **Lack of motivation to work out. You lose interest in your sport or martial art.**

• **Your performance lessens, not only on the mat, but also in every aspect of life.**

• **You get sore and tired from what used to be light to moderate workouts.**

• **Reflexes, strength, skill, speed and cardio endurance are lessened.**

• **You stay tired for days after a workout.**

• **You look for reasons not to train or work out.**

TIPS ON AVOIDING OVERTRAINING

A good way to avoid overtraining is to sit down with your coach or teammates and develop training goals. Use training cycles or periodization when training for a major event,

fight or tournament. Stay in decent shape when not training for a major event. Use a workout journal or training log to record your on-mat training, what you do in the weightroom or for your cardio training. Keeping a record of what you do. Adding comments as to how you feel, in a workout journal, is a useful tool in maintaining an effective overall training program. When cutting weight, do it intelligently. Don't go on a starvation diet and then expect not be burned out from training!

Follow these common-sense tips on training to avoid overtraining or even a slump in your training.

1. Balance periods of work and rest. This means rest, recovery and nutrition between training sessions, as well as alternating rest and recovery periods during your actual training session or workout. Doing this helps you adapt to the training load you are placing on yourself. In other words, Interval Training is efficient and helps in not only working you hard, but also in helping you rest effectively during the workout.

2. Don't make huge jumps in the level of intensity in your training. Gradually increase how hard you push yourself.

3. You need rest, recovery and nutrition to not only make gains but to help avoid overtraining. Adequate rest and quality nutrition help you recover and make progress in your training.

4. Consider your age. Older athletes require more recuperation time than younger athletes.

5. Female athletes usually recover at a slower pace than males because of differences in the endocrine system.

6. Consider the altitude, climate and weather of where you are training.

7. In most cases, athletes and grapplers who are more experienced require less time to recover. This is due mostly to the fact that experienced athletes generally have faster and more efficient physiological adaptation to intense training. In other words, if you're new to this type of training, take your time and make gradual increases in your training. This ties in directly to number 2.

8. Your diet is important. Especially when cutting weight, make sure that you eat nutritious food and use quality supplements to assist food metabolization more efficiently in your body.

9. Vary the way you work out. Change the order of exercises you do, and the amount of resistance you use. Alter

the speed of execution in your exercises. Actually vary the exercises in your workout routine. Constantly rotate the assistance exercises you use in your workout routine. Rotate your exercises on a regular basis so that they don't become boring or stale. In fact, no two workouts should be exactly alike.

If you think you're overtraining, cut back in the intensity of what you are doing, and in very rare cases, you may need to take a lay-off to get some much-needed rest. If you're really burned out, take some time for what the former Soviets used to call active rest. Active rest is any light to moderate activity that promotes circulation, maintains some degree of general fitness, and most importantly, is fun. This might be in the form of some other sport or game, hiking in the forest, going for a bike ride, or swimming. Water training, especially in a natural setting, is especially good for restoration. In extreme cases, especially if a fever is present, you may need to take a lay off. It's better to take a few days off when you're pushing it too hard than to get so bad that you have to take an extensive lay-off and not only lose the gains you made, but possibly even lose your interest in training. Some athletes confuse overtraining with working hard. If you're a motivated individual and have a good work ethic, this won't be a problem.

Overtraining leads to injuries and injuries can end an athletic career. Take overtraining seriously and if you are overtraining, take some time off, rest, rehabilitate, recover, and then return to the dojo or gym.

TECHNICAL TIP: When you overtrain, do the following:
- **REST**
- **REHABILITATE**
- **RECOVER**
- **RETURN**

INJURIES

Donn Draeger, who authored many books on the martial arts, once said, "Judo is the great crippler." He, like every other serious judo athlete, knew that there is a 100% injury rate in what we do. Bumps, bruises, joint injuries, getting choked out, broken bones, concussions; it all seems to happen due to the nature of this rough world we live in.

One of the best ways to avoid injuries, or at least lessen their severity, is to be in the best shape possible. Not only might you have the physical ability to withstand abuse or injury, your body might physically compensate and an uninjured body part might help a injured body part from sustaining further or more severe injury.

The best advice to give you is to say that when you are injured, accept the fact that you're injured and deal with it intelligently and analytically. All the griping and cussing in the world won't make you uninjured, so deal with it and get on with what it takes to get you back on the mat again. Be analytical about it and take the time off necessary to heal, rehabilitate and recover. Take the injury seriously. Training or competing with a serious injury will do you more harm than good. Also understand that just about everyone who fights or participates in a combat sport or martial arts always has some kind of "ding" that we have to deal with. Make sure that you receive proper, professional medical and therapeutic care. It's always a good idea to find out who the good sports orthopedic doctors are in your area.

Know the difference between pain and the soreness from training, as well as the difference between being genuinely injured and just a bit dinged up. When you are recovering from an injury, follow your physical therapy plan to the letter and consider that as part of your training. Don't get re-injured by "testing" yourself or the injured body part when still injured. Let your body heal. One of the most common reasons athletes get re-injured is that they don't rehabilitate the initial injury well enough. However, if you can train around the injury without hurting yourself, plan on doing that. When you come back after an injury, take your time and gradually get back into the swing of things. Watch your weight when you are recovering from an injury. Don't gain too much weight, and conversely, don't take this time to cut weight. Your body needs rest and nutrition to recover fully. Learn from your mistakes, or at least learn from how or why you were injured and plan on not letting that happen again!

SOME THOUGHTS ON DIET, NUTRITION AND HYDRATION

A healthy body is a prerequisite for every athlete and your diet is a key factor in making sure your body is healthy. Good nutrition will provide you with increased energy and allow you to recover from heavy training. What you ingest is the fuel that provides energy to your body. We're not dieticians, but here are some common sense dietary tips that we believe will keep you healthy and enable you to recover more efficiently and quickly from heavy training.

Eat plenty of fresh (and raw) vegetables, fruits and juices. While this is obvious, not all that many people do it. Vitamin or nutritional supplements or pills don't take the place of real food. When shopping, keep in mind that the food you put in your cart is the fuel you will put in your body. Salty, fried chips, carbonated beverages and fatty foods provide sludge and not the high-octane you need to fuel your engine. If you can afford it, get a good quality juicer and use it.

Eliminate hydrogenated oil from your diet. You need fat in your diet, but use such fats as olive or flaxseed oil rather than what's more commercially available. Eat less animal fat. Our culture had conditioned us to salivate at the sight and smell of a big, juicy hamburger and fries, but consider what you're eating and make it a point to drive by the burger joint and save your arteries from clogging.

Foods containing white sugar, white flour and to a lesser extent, salt, are full of empty calories. They offer very little nutrition and detract from your health. Simple adjustments in your diet such as cutting out soda pop, candy and white bread will go a long way in reducing your intake of empty calories. Examine your diet carefully to see what you're eating that's not contributing to your health.

Drink plenty of water. About 50% of your body is made of water and it's essential for sustaining life. As an athlete, you place a great amount of stress on your body and need an adequate supply of water. A good rule of thumb is to drink a glass of water (about 8 ounces) every hour. Using commercially available drinks to replace electrolytes is okay, but nothing beats water. When you go out running or go to the gym, make it a habit to take a bottle of water with you and to drink it as needed. Your body needs to be constantly rehydrated during strenuous training. It's not a sign of weakness to have a bottle of water near the mat and to take a drink now and then as needed. Don't gulp it, but drink water during a tough training session to sustain yourself and have a more efficient workout. Don't substitute carbonated beverages for good, clean water.

Use supplements wisely. There are many different supplements on the market, so research and know what you put in your body. Vitamins are essential for everyone. Vitamins are organic food products and are not made by the body. There are about 20 vitamins that are present in different amounts in foods, with each vitamin essential for overall good health. Minerals are contained in all of our bodily tissues and fluids and are vital for good health. All bodily functions require minerals, as do nerve cells, blood, bones, and muscles.

The authors are certainly not experts on nutrition or supplements, so we're offering only generic advice on the subject. But as a serious athlete, take the time to research the subject of nutrition and supplements or seek the advice of a professional in the field.

PRE-FIGHT MEAL AND TOURNAMENT NUTRITION

Eat a meal high in complex carbohydrates before your fight or tournament. Carbohydrates are digested easily and provide for a normal level of blood glucose and glycogen before your match. This is especially important if you've been cutting weight and need to get your blood sugar levels back to normal. Stay away from high protein foods such as steak before a tournament or fight. It takes too much energy to digest that steak and you need all the energy you can get for your fight; eating a high protein meal before your match will make you sluggish. Digesting all that protein also dehydrates your body during exercise as well and it takes a lot of water to digest that much beef in your system. Not only that, and while this sounds a bit personal, you really need to have as clean of a colon as possible when you walk onto the mat for your match. A big lump of steak simply doesn't pass through your digestive system in time. A carbohydrate meal the evening before your fight not only supplies you with the necessary nutrition, it is more easily eliminated.

When at the tournament, take a supply of carbohydrate snacks and plenty of water. Don't use the "energy" supplements or drinks commercially available. One reason is that if you are competing in an event where they perform a drug test, the energy drink or supplement you just took may be the reason you might possibly flunk the drug test.

We're not saying all drinks or supplements will cause you to test positive on a drug test, but it has happened to people we know. More likely (and important), however, is the fact that many of these energy drinks and supplements last for a while and then cause a "crash" in your system. That "sugar high" or "caffeine high" is always followed by a serious reverse rebound and results in a dull performance.

DRUGS AND ANABOLIC STEROIDS

Both authors have seen too many strong, vital athletes ruin their health by using drugs. We're not talking about the morality of the subject or if it's "cheating" if an athlete uses performance enhancing drugs. Steroid abuse is a matter of health and life or death. We've both known and seen too many people get sick, have heart attacks or die because they abused performance enhancing and recreational drugs or substances. Both the physiological and psychological effects of drug abuse ruins lives; not only the life of the athlete taking them, but the lives of family, friends and training partners. Don't use them.

DIFFERENT TYPES OF TRAINING

When you work out, you want to train both hard and train smart. Get the most out of your training times, whether it's on the mat, in the gym or elsewhere. Presented here is an explanation of the various types of training you can do, and how you can incorporate them into your overall program of preparing for martial arts. The authors don't want to turn you into exercise physiologists, and honestly, with a few exceptions, a discussion with a talkative exercise physiologist is about as exciting as a root canal. With this in mind, we'll try to offer information on the essentials of how to train effectively.

Briefly, remember that using maximum power for short bursts of movement most efficiently develops **Strength. Muscular Endurance** is most efficiently developed by power performed over a longer period of time than in strength training. **Cardio Endurance** is best developed over extended periods of training. **Flexibility** is the range of motion in your joints. **Balance, Agility, Speed** and **Coordination** are the factors that determine how fast you act and react and are essential for all fighters and grapplers.

TRAINING BASICS FOR GRAPPLERS AND FIGHTER

Training with weights, body weight exercises, bands, and other implements with heavy resistance are the best all-around ways of developing strength, but there are also other factors necessary for overall conditioning in combat sports. Some basic guidelines are:

- Develop Strength by using heavy resistance and low repetitions.

- Develop Muscular Endurance by using low to moderate resistance and high repetitions.

- Develop Cardio Endurance by running, various machines, and other methods done at a steady pace for longer periods of time, or through shorter, more intense intervals.

- Develop Flexibility by stretching and other methods.

- Develop Balance, Agility, Speed and Coordination by using body weight exercises, jumping, tumbling and other gymnastics exercises, and other methods.

AEROBIC ENDURANCE

The word aerobic means "with oxygen" and should be the foundation of your training. Commonly called "cardio training" this means that when you train aerobically, your heart rate is somewhere between 60% to 85% of your maximum, and for our purposes is kept somewhere in the target zone for 15 to 60 minutes. The energy you expend comes from the oxidation of carbohydrate and fat.

Marathon running is the ultimate example of an aerobic sport or activity. Remember, though, training for a marathon is very different than training for fighting and the type of training a marathon runner performs isn't the type of endurance training a fighter or grappler needs. As a martial artist or fighter, you need an aerobic base so that you can recover quickly between intense bouts or matches that can last for the entire day if competing in a tournament. Because of our unique, and very demanding needs as fighters, we have to understand that there is a point of diminishing return at which more aerobic training detracts from the development of explosive power and strength. Fighting, especially in matches or rounds of 5 minutes or less in duration, is largely anaerobic in nature. These matches are often made up of a number of short bursts of attacking and defending, with periods of lesser activity in between.

ANAEROBIC ENDURANCE

The word anaerobic means "without oxygen". When training anaerobically, you build up an oxygen debt, and in the same way someone may run up too much credit card debt, it needs to be paid off. A product called lactic acid accumulates in your muscles when you work them hard and if you don't ease up, your muscles will cramp and shut down. When training at high intensity anaerobically, your body is unable to get enough oxygen to your muscles and gets some of the energy for muscular working from carbohydrates that are stored as glycogen in the muscles.

When you include anaerobic training, you do 2 things:

1. You train your body to recover to a lower heart rate more quickly between periods of intense exercise, such as in between intense flurries of attacks in a match or fight.

2. By training anaerobically, you train your muscles to tolerate lactic acid (and other wastes) for longer periods of intense effort before shutting down. It also trains your muscles to drain off lactic acid and conditions your heart to bring in fresh oxygen-rich blood more efficiently.

Anaerobic training enables you to make stronger and more frequent attacks throughout the fight or match. One of the best ways to train for anaerobic endurance is Interval Training.

INTERVAL TRAINING

You can't sustain a near maximum heart rate for very long. Doing so is dangerous and lactic acid (and other factors) will eventually shut down your muscles. Instead, in order to keep the quality (intensity) of your work at a high level, you should perform repeated, high intensity bouts or some activity that elevates your heart rate, followed by a rest **interval**. Let's call this your "work:rest ratio." For example, if you run a 110 yard sprint in 15 seconds and then rest 45 seconds before running another sprint, you will have a 1:3 work: rest ratio. The concept of the rest interval is to allow your heart to return to about 120 beats per minute before doing another bout of exercise. This allows you to put out repeated high intensity efforts. As your anaerobic fitness improves, you will probably be able to reduce your work: rest ratio to 1:2, and eventually to 1:1.

Exercises that you can use when performing Interval Training are running, cycling or swimming, but an even more efficient way to train could be to use some element of your martial art or fighting style. Here's an example for a judo or sambo fighter using a throwing drill at high intensity. Perform this drill as hard a possible for a specific number of repetitions or time, followed by a timed rest interval. Here's an example:

Using a forward throwing technique, perform as many Uchikomis (Fit Ins) as possible in the allotted time. You can substitute working on Lunge Steps, working the heavy bag or any movement used in your sport or martial art.

- 20 seconds: Do forward throw Uchikomis.
- 20 seconds: Your partner does his Uchikomis.
- 20 seconds: Rest before repeating the sequence.

Repeat this drill for 3 to 10 sets depending on your needs and level of fitness. After this, go on to step 2 as follows:

- 10 seconds: Do forward throw Uchikomis
- 10 seconds: Your partner does forward throw Uchikomis.
- 10 seconds: Rest before repeating the sequence.

Repeat this drill for 3 to 10 sets depending on your needs and level of fitness.

This drill gives you a 1:2 work:rest ratio. In other words, you'll rest twice as much as you work, and as you get in better shape, you can eliminate the rest period and just get your rest as your partner does his Uchikomi attacks giving you a 1:1 work:rest ratio. When you get to this point, you'll be grinding opponents into the mat.

TRAIN LIKE A DECATHLETE

When fighters ask author John Saylor's help in designing training programs, he always starts by telling them to train like a decathlete. Think about the Decathlon for a moment. It is comprised of the following events:

1. The 100 Meter Run
2. The Long Jump
3. The Shot Put
4. The High Jump
5. The 400 Meter Run
6. The Hurdles
7. The Discuss
8. The Pole Vault
9. The Javelin
10. The 1500 Meter Run

Not only does the training for many of these individual events not benefit the other events, it often actually detracts from the results in other Decathlon events. Take The Shot Put and The 1500 Meter Run, for example. These two events are diametrically opposed to each other! The trick then, for the decathlete, is to balance his training. In other words, the aspiring decathlete must devote just the right percentage of the training pie to each event. This is not only a science, but an art. When the decathlete sees his results in the 400 Meter or 1500 Meter Run going down because of too much max effort strength work, for example, he must devote more training time to these events, even if it means reducing the volume of his strength work somewhat. Conversely, if his Shot Put and Discuss distances are below his best, the decathlete must add more strength and explosive speed work to his schedule. For the successful decathlete these kinds of adjustments need to be made all the time. The same holds true for all grappling, MMA, and self-defense athletes.

To Be A Champion You Need Balanced Development

Many observers believe Mixed Martial Arts (MMA) is one of the most demanding sports there is. To reach the top of the food chain in MMA you can no longer have a weak range of fighting. In the early days of MMA this wasn't necessarily true, and we often saw a great grappler defeat a striker. Then the strikers started balancing their game by studying jujitsu and other grappling arts, and by learning to defend the takedown. This cross training made them much more dangerous. Today MMA has evolved to a whole new level, and to be competitive you must be very well balanced both in your physical and technical training. Again, as far as your physical conditioning is concerned, train like a decathlete. That will give you the all-round development you need to make it to the top.

INTERVAL TRAINING FOR GROUNDFIGHTING

When author John Saylor was the Head Coach for the U. S. National Judo Training Squad at the Olympic Training Center in Colorado Springs, Colorado, he would regularly have the squad do Interval Training groundfighting. If the length of your contest or match is 5 minutes, add an extra minute so that you build extra stamina and confidence. Perform a specific number of 6-minute rounds. The judo squad would perform 10 to 12 six-minute rounds with a 1 to 2 minute rest interval between each round. These can also be done as regular Randori, and this drill was often performed in the late afternoon practice.

The morning workouts usually emphasized drills for groundfighting and standing skills such as throwing and grip fighting. Depending on the time of the year and how close it was to a major tournament, the team often did the same type of timed rounds with groundfighting.

The general rule was that during the off-season, the team performed lots of low-intensity continuous work with only one or two short, higher intensity rounds thrown in so that the athletes didn't forget how to turn up the heat. However, as a major event or tournament approached, the team gradually increased the intensity and did randori, drill training and groundfighting with timed rounds and rest periods. This, along with training at the high altitude in Colorado, got the team into excellent shape. As you can see, this type of training is a definite form of Interval Training.

INTERVAL TRAINING FOR BOXERS AND KICKBOXERS

Boxers and kickboxers train in interval-style rounds much of the time and this routine follows that format. During the 3-minute rounds, the fighters work on the various bags, use the focus mitts, shadow box, jump rope, perform calisthenics or actually do some sparring.

A typical workout looks something like this:
- 3 minutes: Jump rope
- 1 minute: Rest
- 3 minutes: Heavy bag work
- 1 minute: Rest
- 3 minutes: Calisthenics (Push Ups, Crunches, Medicine Ball work, and other exercises)
- 1 minute: Rest
- 3 minutes: Heavy bag work again
- 1 minute. Rest
- 3 minutes: Focus Mitts
- 1 minute: Rest
- 3 minutes: Top and Bottom Bag or Speed Bag
- 1 minute: Rest
- 3 minutes: Shadow Boxing

MMA fighters can add rounds of Thai Pad work, as well as various grappling-based drills such as pummeling or Uchikomi.

THE MONDAY-FRIDAY ROUTINE: WEIGHT TRAINING FOR MAXIMUM STRENGTH AND SPEED

The focus here is on concentrated weight work on exercises that work the lower body, back, and torso, and on chain reaction exercises that work the entire body in a coordinated way. The goals of our weight workouts are to develop maximum strength and to develop explosive speed.

This program devotes Monday to maximum strength and Friday to the development of explosive speed. The rest of the week, our extra workouts revolve around conditioning workouts (such as freehand or body weight exercises for high reps), circuits, extra drill training and other aspects of training that enhance our fitness.

MAX EFFORT DAY (USUALLY MONDAY)

On Monday, select a major Squat movement for 2 weeks (for instance, the Front Squat) or partial squats off the power rack pins, or use some form of Good Morning exercise. Then, for the next 2 weeks, do a pulling movement such as Clean Pulls from the floor and from various hang positions, or Deadlifts. You can alternate back and forth between 2 weeks of a squatting exercise, and then 2 weeks of a pulling exercise, and so on. Whatever the major exercise for that week, try to work up to a personal record of some sort, either for a single rep or double reps. Follow this with several assistance exercises that are chosen to work specific weak points you may have in your lift or in your fighting technique. Although you won't be doing max singles or doubles on your assistance exercises, you should use heavier resistance. We'll give you some specific examples later in the book.

Rotate your assistance exercises every 1 to 2 weeks. This is called the Conjugate Method and is how you can train heavy all year long without going stale. The Conjugate Method is the way you can make continual gains year after year and insures a more balanced, all-around development. This translates into better performance with fewer injuries.

How To Choose Assistance Exercises

Once you've finished your core lift on max effort or dynamic effort day, perform 3 to 5 assistance exercises. You should choose your assistance exercises to accomplish three goals. 1) To achieve balanced, all-around development. 2) To work your weaknesses and bring any lagging muscle groups up to the level of your strength. 3) To strengthen weaknesses and flaws in your techniques. In Section 2 you will learn many different assistance exercises to choose from.

Pointers For Max Effort Day

1. Avoid psyching up for your lifts. It only fatigues your central nervous system. You need to save that added energy for the contest.

2. In his excellent book, THE WESTSIDE BOOK OF METHODS, Louie Simmons recommends that you limit the number of lifts over 90% to 2-3. "Do one with 90%, one with 95-98%, and then try for a record," he advises. This may not be an all-time personal record (PR), but the most you are capable of that day.

3. If you have a fight coming up you don't need to do max effort work every week. You need to conserve your energy going into a contest. Don't worry about losing your strength. Remember, you should be doing some very specific max effort work in your actual practice sessions that will make you very strong where it counts, on the mat. Also, you should be maintaining strength with your circuits. After all, the idea is to display maximum strength throughout your fight, not leave everything you've got in the weight room on max effort day.

4. Employ the conjugate method of training and rotate max effort exercises each week. This doesn't mean you have to do a totally different exercise, but vary something about it. Say, for example, you're doing Dead Lifts as your max effort exercise. You can vary it by pulling from different height pins each week, adding bands, chains, or both, and by varying your stance. You could also stand on foam as you pull, which gives the muscles more work. Or do Straight Leg or Sumo Style Dead Lifts. All of these variations work you differently and will help you avoid accommodation. After 2 weeks of Dead Lifts, switch to a squat of some sort. Then after a few more weeks rotate some type of extension movement into your max effort workout, say a Good Morning or Back Raise (a.k.a. Hyperextensions). Whatever the lift, vary something about it from week to week. No two workouts should be the exactly the same.

5. Keep your max effort work short and sweet. Work up to your max single for that day and move on to your assistance exercises. Try to finish your entire max effort workout in less than 45 minutes. Remember, you're also using your muscles at practice.

Sample Max Effort Day Workouts

Max Effort Sample Workout #1

1. **Zercher Squat:** Work up to a max single.
2. **Glute-Ham Raises while holding a weight to your chest:** 1 to 2 sets of 15 to 20 reps.
3. **Push Ups with Alternate KB Rows:** 3sets of 12 to 20 Push ups with 6 to 10 KB Rows on each arm.
4. **Leg Raises (on Leg Raise Apparatus):** 1 or 2 sets of 30 to 50 reps

Max Effort Sample Workout #2

This is an example of the Max Effort Method followed by the repetition method using circuit training.

* Note: This is a method author John Saylor used with the U.S. National Judo Training Squad at the Olympic Training Center with great results.

<u>Monday</u>

Good Mornings – Work up to a max triple.

1. **Hindu Jump Squats** – 30 seconds
2. **Incline Sit Ups** – 30 seconds
3. **Hindu Push Ups** - 30 seconds
4. **Seated Leg Curls w/Bands** – 30 seconds
5. **Side to Side Leg Raises** – 30 seconds
6. **Pull Ups** – 30 seconds
7. **Back Raises (Hypers)** – 30 seconds
8. **Alternate DB or KB Overhead Press** – 30 seconds
9. **Regular Push Ups** – 30 seconds
10. **Bent Rows w/ DB's or KB's** – 30 seconds

* Note: More advanced athletes can do 45 sec. or 1 minute on each exercise.

Sample Max Effort Day Workouts

Max Effort Sample Workout #3

* Note: After you've built up your work capacity somewhat it's time to start using chains, bands or both.

1. **Dead Lift** from various pin heights in the power rack. Set your bar at a certain pin height, say #2 in the rack. **Attach 1 or 2 sets of heavy chains** on the end of the bar and **work up to a max single**. Note: To avoid accommodation you can vary the height of the pin for a few weeks, add bands, and vary your stance.

2. Follow your max effort work with 2 to 3 sets of **ab work.**

3. Finish with **Heavy Towing**. Tow the sled walking forward with long deliberate strides. Also, tow backwards. Do 2-arm rows, alternate hand rows, or any of the other towing sled exercises described in this book. Since the sled weight is heavier on max effort day you won't tow as far, and will need to take more frequent rest breaks.

Max Effort Sample Workout #4

1. **Box Squats w/ Added Band Tension:** Attach bands to the bar and to the bottom of the power rack and **work up to your best single**. Note: Vary the height of the box week to week, from below parallel all the way to quarter squat height.

2. **Glute-Ham Raises With Added Band Tension:** 1 or 2 sets of 15 to 20 reps.

3. **Back Raises (Hypers) w/Twist:** Place a weight behind your head, or place bands behind your neck, and do 2 to 3 sets of 15 to 20 reps.

4. **Forward Throw Twist w/Band:** Attach a medium to strong band on a post and perform the twisting motion of your forward throws. **Do 3 to 5 sets of 20 reps on each side.** This will strongly work your abs, obliques, and all the rotational muscles of your upper body, and will greatly improve the finish of your forward throw.

5. **Rope Climbing:** Finish with as much rope climbing as you can in a 6-minute round. Rest when you need to. **But keep it short.** Get right on another set as soon as you can. Continue to climb the rope interspersed with very short, say 15 second, rests until the 6 minutes are up.

Other Exercises To Use On Max Effort Day

1. **Good Morning Squat:** With a barbell on your shoulders, bend over at the waist, and while remaining bent over, do a squat. When you come up out of the squat complete the Good Morning by returning to an upright position. **Note:** This is a tough combination exercise and should only be attempted after you have built a good all-round strength base.

2. **Seated Good Mornings:** Sit on a bench and perform your Good Mornings. This exercise is a great alternative when you have sore or injured knees.

3. **Belt Squat:** The Belt Squat is a great alternative when your back is sore or injured since it actually serves as traction. It also places more emphasis on the thigh muscles than the Box Squat and some of the other forms of squatting.

4. **Heavy Sled Work:** Occasionally just make heavy lower body and upper body towing your **Max Effort Lift** for the day.

5. **One-Arm Kettle Bell Clean and Press:** You could do this from the floor, or from a hanging position just above the knee. Be sure to use both arms. In other words, **work up to a max single on each side.**

6. **Push Ups With A Band:** Drape a band across your back and hold an end in each hand. Choose a band tension that only allows a couple of reps. Assume the push up position and work up to a couple of sets. Assume the push up position and perform several sets.

7. **Variations:** Vary something about the push up itself. Vary the height or angle of your feet, for example. Do the push ups on rings, or on the mat or on foam. You can also vary the spacing of your hands, do jumping push ups, or elevate your upper body slightly. Use your imagination.

8. **Pull Ups With Added Weight:** Attach weight around your waist and work up to a heavy double. If you are strong enough, you could do 1-Arm Pull Ups instead of weighted pull-ups.

Note: These are just a few of many max effort exercises you can work into your program. You'll find many others throughout this book.

Jump Training

Although we often do jump training before or after our max effort workout and dynamic workouts, we occasionally eliminate the box squats and focus solely on some very concentrated jump training like that described in this book. Section 2 features a variety of plyometric and jump training exercises.

DYNAMIC EFFORT DAY (SPEED DAY)

Your second concentrated weightroom workout of the week in this training program is your speed day; usually done on Friday. The goal on Friday is to use lighter weight; 50% to 60% of your maximum poundage for a single rep in that particular lift. Choose some form of Box Squat for your major exercise on Friday. Use that in a 3-week "wave" starting with 50% on week number 1 for 12 sets of 2 repetitions. On week number 2, use 55% for 10 sets of 2 reps. On week number 3, use 60% for 8 sets of 2 reps.

Rest about 30 to 45 seconds between each set. Remember, in a fight or match, you'll be required to make strong, explosive attacks for the duration of the contest without the luxury of complete recovery between attacks. This is a form of Interval Training. The lighter weights, using 50% to 60% for only 2 reps per set, allow us to move the bar **explosively**. Always apply maximum speed and force on each rep, even though you are using a lighter weight. Dr. Fred Hatfield calls this "compensatory acceleration" and it is one of the keys to developing explosive speed. In every combat sport, whether it's a grappling-based activity, a striking activity or a combination (such as MMA), you gain nothing by training slow. Always train to be fast.

In the dynamic effort method you will use sub-maximal weights, somewhere in the 50 to 75% range, as explosively as possible. Although the bar is relatively light you must still generate maximum force by moving the bar as fast and explosively as possible. Again, this is called **compensatory acceleration**.

> **TECHNICAL TIP: If possible, schedule your dynamic effort, or "speed day," on Friday. This will give you 72 hours of recovery between your maximum effort and dynamic effort days.**

One exercise you can keep in your schedule throughout the year, and which you can use on speed day, is the **Box Squat**. The box squat is one of the best ways to develop explosive speed and power in the lower body. It is particularly useful for developing explosive and starting strength in throws, takedowns, and kicks. Also, box squats, when done properly, are easier on the knees than conventional squats.

When incorporating box squats into your schedule on speed day use a 3 week wave. On week 1, use 50% of your 1-rep max for a **regular back squat**. On week 2, use 55%, then 60% on week 3. So, the Box Squat workout looks like this:

Week 1: 12 sets of 2 reps at 50%
Week 2: 10 sets of 2 reps at 55%
Week 3: 8 sets of 2 reps at 60%

Then, on week 4, **wave back down to 50% and start another 3-week wave.**

As fighters you should keep your rest periods short, anywhere from 30 to 45 seconds. With these short rest periods the box squat workout is also a form of lactic acid tolerance training.

Just as on your max effort day workout, follow your speed day box squat workout with 3 or 4 assistance exercises.

How To Choose Assistance Exercises

Once you've finished your core lift, say the Box Squat, perform 3 to 4 assistance exercises. Do assistance exercises immediately following your main lift on both your max effort and dynamic effort days.

You should choose your assistance exercises to accomplish three goals:

1. To achieve balanced, all-round development. Muscle imbalances are a major cause of injury, so work to eliminate them.

2. To work any weaknesses and bring them up to the level of your strengths.

3. To strengthen small flaws in your techniques. Many techniques fail because certain muscle groups are too weak to perform the desired movement. Before discarding a given technique, make sure you've strengthened the appropriate muscle groups. Also, you can perform the movements of your technique, or a component part of your technique, against resistance. You will find example of specific exercises to improve your techniques in this book in section 2.

Accommodating Resistance

Use chains or bands, or both together, on both your max effort day and dynamic effort day workouts. Wave the amount of band tension or the weight of the chains up for 3 weeks. Then reduce the tension on the fourth week and begin another 3-week wave.

Using Chains: Attach heavy chains to each end of the barbell. Using box squats as an example, lower the bar and sit back on the box. As you reach the bottom position the chains will pile up on the floor, thus reducing the bar weight. The weight will feel much lighter and will allow you to explode upward with maximum drive and speed. But as you rise up past your sticking point and reach what would normally be the strongest part of the lift, more of the chain comes off the floor. This adds weight to the bar in the portion of the lift where deceleration normally occurs, thus forcing you to continue driving with maximum force and speed. The chains, in other words, accommodate the weight to your weakest and strongest part of the lift.

Using Bands: Bands also accommodate resistance in that the tension is much less in the bottom position and increases steadily as you drive up past your sticking point to complete the lift. But bands have another added advantage: they create an **over-speed eccentric**. In other words, the bands will slingshot you back down faster than the speed of gravity itself. This activates your stretch reflex and creates greater kinetic energy in your tendons, ligaments, and muscles. This kinetic energy, which can be stored for up to 2 seconds, can be mobilized to help you achieve much greater starting and accelerating strength.

This type of training, when combined with the specific drills and exercises described in this book, will translate into tremendous explosive power on your throws, takedowns, and kicks.

Static Overcome By Dynamic Work & Relaxed Overcome By Dynamic Work

Static refers to isometric work, muscle contraction without movement. The dynamic work, as you know, involves movement. Box Squats provide both static-overcome-by-dynamic, and relaxed-overcome-by-dynamic work. These methods develop both absolute strength and explosive speed strength. When sitting back on the box in the box squat, for example, you momentarily relax the legs, hip flexors and glutes, while maintaining tension (static work) in the lower back and abs. Then you explode upward (dynamic work) with maximum force and speed. As you can see, the box squat provides both types of work.

Variety On Dynamic Day (Speed Day)

On box squats we vary the height of the box from just below parallel to as high as a quarter squat position. We also rotate the type of bar we use from a regular Olympic bar to the safety squat bar to a cambered bar. Sometimes we also use a front squat harness. All of these have a different feel and work you differently. We also stand on foam for some of our workouts which provides more muscle work. You can also put foam on the box. From week to week we wave the weight of the chains or band tension. All of these variations will more fully develop you, prevent accommodation, and keep you from going stale.

Other Exercises On Dynamic Day

When practicing grappling based martial arts you will invariably encounter times when your back or shoulders are sore, or even injured. Rather than halt all progress on your lower

body strength and speed, try to work around the affected area.

We often substitute the Plyo Swing (a.k.a. Virtual Force Swing), an apparatus Louie Simmons took from an old Soviet design and improved upon. It looks like a huge leg press machine, but the seat swings freely. You push off with your legs, and as you swing back down your feet contact forcefully with the platform.

This **"shock"** creates kinetic energy that can be used to generate maximum force and speed. The Plyo Swing utilizes both weight and bands. Again, the bands slingshot you down much faster than gravity. This creates an **over-speed eccentric** and thereby increases kinetic energy. The Plyo Swing will make your lower body very strong and fast.

The only downside to the Virtual Force Swing is that it, like all good equipment, is very expensive. At the time of this writing you can purchase one from www.westside-barbell.com for $2,799.00 plus $400 shipping and handling.
Unless you have a booster club to help you with fund raising projects, this may be out of your budget. Well don't worry, there are some other methods you can use on dynamic day that don't cost anything…jump training for example.

Jump Training

Although we often do jump training before or after our max effort workout and dynamic workouts, we occasionally eliminate the box squats and focus solely on some very concentrated jump training like that described in this book. The following section will describe jump training in more detail.

Percentage Training With Box Jumps

Our jump training is based on percentages and reps taken from Prilepin's Table, just as we do with our max effort work.

Prilepin's Table: Number of reps for percentage training.

(Prilepin's Table was based on the training of Soviet Olympic Weight Lifters)

Percent	Reps per Set	Optimal	Range
55 – 65	3 - 6	24	18 - 30
70 – 75	3 - 6	18	12- 24
80 – 85	2 - 4	17	10 - 20
Above 90	1 - 2	7	4 – 10

Note: In his research, Louie Simmons has adjusted the number of 90% and over lifts to 3 – 5 lifts. This is because the special exercises his power lifters use are much heavier than those of the Olympic lifts used in Prilepin's research.

Lets say, for example, that your best box jump is 36 inches. 75% would be 27 inches. 80% would be approximately 29 inches. 85% would be approximately 31 inches. According to Prilepin's Table, if you are working at between 80 – 85 % of your max, the reps per set should be between 2 – 4, and the optimal numbers of lifts (or jumps) per workout is 17. The range is between 10 – 20 jumps per workout. So on a day when you are eliminating the box squat, for example, you may want to go on the high end of the range—20 reps.

On a day when you are fatigued from the previous night's practice, or have a hard practice scheduled that night, it would be better to execute only 10 jumps which is the low end of the range. But whenever possible, it is best to schedule your jumps and other speed training for days when you are rested.

TRAIN TO BE FAST: ACCOMMODATING RESISTANCE

On both Monday (Max Effort Day) and Friday (Dynamic, or Speed Day), we often use "Accommodating Resistance" through the use of chains and bands. By attaching a heavy chain to each end of the barbell, the resistance on the bar is lessened as you lower the bar and is increased as you raise it.

In the Box Squat for example, as you lower down into the bottom position the chains pile up on the floor, reducing the bar weight considerably. At the upward position, you have the weight of the barbell itself plus the full weight of the chains. This allows you to explode upward out of the bottom position. As you drive up past the sticking point and reach what would otherwise be the easiest part of the lift, more of the chain comes off the floor and that adds a significant weight to the bar. Put another way, the chains accommodate the weight to your weaker and stronger parts of the lift.

Bands perform much the same thing, although they also pull you back down like a slingshot. This creates an overspeed eccentric, which activates your stretch reflex and creates kinetic energy in your muscles, tendons and ligaments, thereby adding to your speed and strength. Also, as you rise up out of a Box Squat for example, the bands stretch and add a great deal of resistance in the lockout portion of the lift. In other words, the bands also provide accommodating resistance in that they accommodate themselves to the weakest and strongest portions of your lift.

CARDIO TRAINING

The basis of all fitness training is having a strong aerobic foundation. There's no way around it; if you want to be a successful fighter or grappler, you better have gas in the tank, and not just enough gas to finish, but enough gas to run the other guy over. The authors often quote the great football coach Vince Lombardi when he said, "Fatigue makes cowards of us all." Without a strong heart, lungs and circulatory system, you'll never excel at any combat sport or martial art. It's just that simple.

To develop a good aerobic base or cardio endurance, choose an activity such as running, biking or any other steady-paced moderate exercise that keeps your heart rate at approximately 130 to 150 beats per minute. The general population's resting heart rate is about 70 to 80 beats per minute, but this is really an individual thing and no 2 people are exactly alike. It depends on your age, fitness level, sex, diet, heredity, where you live and other factors. Because of this, our figure of 130 to 150 beats per minute is also a general number.

Another great workout you can use for cardio endurance is to actually randori (free practice, live sparring) or do a lot of groundfighting randori. In Section 2, you will see some information on grappling yourself into shape. Let's face it, the best way to train for a fight is to practice fighting. However, when doing this, it's important that you and your training partners are all on the same wavelength. In other words, be sure to train with partners who understand how to maintain a steady pace. Too often, rolling on the mat ends up being a contest or match with both grapplers making it too competitive. Remember, it's training. You train in a gym and fight in an arena. Don't leave your fight in the gym. There's a time for butting heads, but not when you need to keep grappling for 30 to 60 minutes continuously.

Think of this as free form drilling. Just keep rolling. If your partner gets a good position for a submission, make him earn it but give it to him. Again, just keep rolling. A good rule to follow is that, regardless of what type of cardio work you're doing, train at a pace that you can smile while doing it. No kidding; smile. Bryan Potter calls this "smiling randori". If you can smile during the workout, it's at a steady, controlled pace. Now remember, we're talking about general cardio training. There is a time to step it up and work intensely during randori, sparring or live grappling. And there are, of course, different goals during the various phases of training, but here we're talking about building up a cardio base.

Monitor your heart rate more precisely by figuring your maximum heart rate (220 minus your age) and then keep your heart rate in a target zone of between 60% to 85% of your maximum heart rate. Another way of monitoring your heart rate which isn't quite as precise, but is pretty good, is to keep your training at a pace at which you can hold a conversation…or smile.

TECHNICAL TIP: Keep your training time in the weightroom short and sweet. Your workouts on Monday and Friday should be serious and to the point. Keep them to about 45 minutes to 1 hour and certainly no longer than an hour. During the rest of the week, you're working your muscles with freehand and body weight exercises, performing various types of circuits, and spending a lot of time in the dojo or on the mat. When you get to the weight room, warm up, train hard and then get on with life.

RUNNING: STILL NOT OUT OF STYLE

With the many new cardio machines on the market, running seems to have gotten a bad name. Sure, running is hard on you, and it's not always a nice day either. Either way, it's not as comfortable as being inside in an air-conditioned gym. There is no doubt that you will get a fantastic workout on a treadmill, elliptical machine or any of the many other excellent machines available, and in fact, you should use them to build your cardio base. However, even with all the new technology of training, the hard-core approach that running gives you simply can't be duplicated. Running outside hardens not only your body, but hardens your fighting spirit as well.

Don't get us wrong. Training in a controlled climate allows you to put out more concentrated effort. As coaches, we prefer to train our athletes in on-mat workouts in dojos or gyms where it's not too hot or too cold. Controlling the climate does, indeed, allow you as an athlete to train harder and sustain that training level longer; thus, getting more out of your training. Also, if the weather conditions outside are too bad for a good hard run, use the treadmill, indoor track at the community center or some other method to get in your cardio workout.

The bottom line is that to excel at grappling or fighting, you must have a strong cardio base as your foundation. Running is only one of many ways to build that foundation, but one that had been tested over time and proven effective. However, if you're injured or have some valid reason for not running, then don't run. The ideas is to increase your cardio capacity and strength and if, for some reason, running isn't beneficial, don't do it. You're training for fighting or grappling, and not running. Don't get so addicted to running that it cuts into other areas of your training. Running is simply one tool that helps build the machine and that machine is you.

There are a lot of ways to run. Change up your running routine to keep it fresh and avoid staleness. Here are some ideas that might help in your training.

Shot Put and Sprint

Go out for your run and carry a 10-pound shot (like they use in the shot put). As you run at a steady pace, toss the shot back and forth in each hand. Then, when you decide it's the right time, stop and chuck it out like a shot putter does. After doing that, sprint as fast as possible to where it landed and chuck it out again and once more sprint to where it landed. Do this for a set of 10 throws, and then start the routine over by running at moderate pace and tossing it back and forth in your hands. Continue this for a far as you want to run. If you don't have a round metal shot, use a 15-pound river stone. Throwing a rock is every bit as good as throwing a metal shot.

Throw and Chase

The Throw and Chase is similar to the Shot Put and Sprint, but instead of a shot, simply take along a football, baseball or some similar object when you go out for a run. Every so often, stop and throw the ball as far as possible, and then sprint to where it lands. Continue this for as long as you want to run. This is a fun way to break up the monotony of running.

Soccer Run

Take a soccer ball and kick it along as you run. Kick far, kick short, kick at angles, but keep running and keep kicking. Believe it or not, you'll fool yourself into running farther that you thought you expected and get a good run in.

Partner Catch and Run

Run with a partner and take a ball. Basically, your partner will throw the ball and you'll go out to catch it. When you catch it, your partner will run out for the pass or catch and you'll throw it to him. You'll continue this for as long as you want to run.

Farmer's Walk

This isn't running; it's walking. Do not, repeat, do not run... walk. If you run when doing this, you might injure yourself. The Farmer's Walk is very simple. You carry a heavy object in each hand and walk as far as possible. The Farmer's Walk can be used for both cardio training and strength training, depending on the amount of weight you carry and the distance covered. When training for cardio, carry a dumb-bell or kettlebell in each hand that weighs from 10 to 40 pounds, depending on your physical size, goals and fitness level. Generally, a 160-pound male athlete can carry a 25-pound dumb-bell in each hand when doing this workout.

Start walking at a brisk pace (but not a run or even a jog) with a dumb-bell in each hand. Walk as far as you can before setting the pair of dumb-bells down on the ground. Take a rest as needed, and then pick the dumb-bells back up and start walking again. Keep doing this for a long and far as you want to walk. Uh huh, it sounds easy, but try it. Your goal is to walk at least a mile before having to put the dumb-bells down. Once you walk a mile, add more weight and carry heavier dumb-bells. Your cardio not only improves, but your grip strength is improved immensely! The Farmer's Walk works your entire body, and targets your shoulders and traps like you won't believe.

PVC Tube Carry

This workout is similar to the Farmer's Walk. Instead of carrying a dumb-bell or kettlebell in each hand, carry a PVC tube filled with water (sand is okay too, but water sloshes around more and is more difficult to carry). Get a piece of PVC about 36 inches long and about 4" in diameter (or smaller, depending on the size of your hands). Cap up one end and fill the pipe with water, and then cap up the other end. You now have a good carrying implement. When you carry it, hold it any way you want, but start out by walking and holding the pipe in front of you and holding it with your hands. It's best if you walk briskly and use this implement in the same way you did the weights in the Farmer's Walk. What makes this tough is the water sloshing around in the PVC tube.

A variation of this exercise is to make a pair of PVC tubes filled with water and carry one in each hand as you walk. This is a variation of the Farmer's Walk and offers you a great workout.

Carry Something Heavy or Tow Something

Anytime you carry something heavy, it makes you work harder. Carry a heavy stone, a duffel bag, beer keg or barrel. Fill the beer keg or barrel with water so that it sloshes around and makes the workload more difficult. Again, don't run; walk when carrying heavy objects.

A good way to get in some cardio training is to pull or tow a moderately heavy sled. Towing a heavy sled is more of a strength building exercise, but towing a sled loaded with only moderate weight and pulling it for a mile will give you a seriously hard cardio workout. If you don't have a sled, tow a big tire. You don't have to get a 400-pound tire like they use in a strongman contest, but towing a heavy truck tire across the grass or around a track will work your butt off. Don't make this a daily routine, but use this type of training to break up the monotony of your regular running routine.

VARIOUS CIRCUIT TRAINING ROUTINES USING YOUR OWN BODY WEIGHT

If you want to develop a high level of fitness in muscular endurance, performing circuits using the weight of your own body will help a great deal. Doing high repetition body weight exercises enables your body to adapt to this training by developing miles of tiny blood vessels called capillaries. These capillaries serve as an oxygen transport system to your muscles and also serve to remove lactic and pyruvic acid; products that produce fatigue. This enables your muscles to work more efficiently.

Be creative and develop your own circuit training routines, but the ones included in the following pages are time-tested and recommended by the authors.

THE SHINGITAI SIX PACK

This is a great program for fighters and grapplers of all kinds and was discussed earlier in this section as a good example of what we mean when we talk about specific circuit training. When done as a circuit, it works the muscles you must develop to sustain and absorb the punishment of fighting. As with all circuits, do an exercise, then move on to the next exercise. Start off with doing 1 round, then, as you get stronger and better conditioned, work up to doing 5 rounds through the circuit. This is a tough routine and when you do the advanced level, is a circuit that takes a good bit of time to perform.

NECK BRIDGE
Hold the bridge up to 1-minute when starting, then as you progress, hold the bridge 2 minutes, and when advanced, hold the bridge 3 minutes or longer.

HINDU SQUAT
When starting out do as many reps as possible in 1 minute. As you progress, do as many reps as possible in 2 minutes, then on to 3 minutes, then 4 minutes, and finally to as many reps as possible for 5 minutes.

GLUTE HAM RAISES
When starting out do as many raises as possible in 1 minute. Then as you progress, do as many reps as possible in 2 minutes, and when advanced do as many reps as possible in 3 minutes.

SIT UPS
Do as many reps as possible in 1 minute when starting. Then work your way up to doing as many reps as possible, increasing by 1-minute increments, until you reach an advanced level at which you will do as many reps as possible in 5 minutes.

PUSH UPS
Follow the same routine of progression as with the Sit Ups. Take rest breaks as needed, but try to keep them short. Your goal is to get as many reps as possible in the designated time period.

PULL UPS (PALM OUT)
Follow the same routine of progression as with the Glute Ham Raises. Take rest breaks as needed, but keep them short. Again, the idea is to get as many reps as possible in the designated time period.

THE SHINGITAI BUILDING BLOCK CIRCUITS

Keeping in mind that Shin (Mental Toughness, Fighting Heart), Gi (Applied Technical Skill) and Tai (Physical Fitness, the Body) are all dependant upon each other to form a complete fighter or martial arts athlete, so the exercises in these circuits use a wide array of training methods and equipment. These circuits progress in both difficulty and the use of equipment, as well as in the actual skill of performing the exercises as they become more difficult.

There are 3 circuits in this series, each a bit harder than the last, and stacked one upon the other like building blocks. Use these circuits in place of weight training during a training cycle or specific period of training for an event. As you become fitter and stronger and are no longer challenged by one circuit, move on to the next circuit in this series. They provide a lot of different movements and will definitely keep you from becoming bored with your training routine.

It's important to properly warm up and do some stretching before performing these circuits. It's equally important to cool down and do some light stretches after completing each circuit.

> **TECHNICAL TIP:** The best workout routine is the one that works for you. Remember, however, to change your training exercises or routines from time to time to keep from going stale both physically and mentally. Also, if you don't try new training routines or programs, you won't learn and you won't improve. Over the course of your career, you will use a variety of training routines, so make it a point to learn something (either positive or negative) from every one of them. Don't hesitate to alter, improve or change what you see on these pages to make your training the most effective and efficient for your circumstances.

THE SHINGITAI TYRO CIRCUIT

The Shingitai Tyro Circuit is an effective way to develop muscular fitness, as well as cardio fitness for combat sports.

Perform as many repetitions as possible in 30 seconds on every exercise. Go through the entire circuit 1 to 3 times, depending on your goals and level of fitness. When initially performing this circuit, rest as long as needed between exercises. As your fitness level improves, reduce the amount of time you rest between exercises and eventually, move from on exercise to the next without any rest. Rest up to 3 minutes after completing a round through the entire circuit. As you adapt and your level of fitness improves, reduce the amount of time you rest between each round. Remember to rotate the order you perform the exercises from time to time. When you complete your circuit, cool down by walking with deep breathing for several minutes, followed by some light stretching. When this circuit is no longer challenging to you, proceed to the next level of circuit training.

1. HINDU SQUATS
2. PUSH UPS
3. CRUNCHES
4. SIT OUTS
5. BREGMAN HOPPING DRILL
6. HINDU PUSH UPS
7. PULL UPS
8. BENCH DIPS
9. FRONT BARBELL PRESSES (NO WEIGHT ON BAR)
10. GLUTE HAM RAISES

THE SHINGITAI COMPOUND CIRCUIT

This circuit is a step up from the previous one and incorporates some additional equipment. Perform as many repetitions as possible in 45 seconds on every exercise. Go through the entire circuit 2 to 3 times and rest 1 minute between circuits. Move from one exercise to the next as quickly as possible. When this circuit is no longer challenging to you, proceed to the next level of circuit training.

1. HINDU PUSH UPS
2. HINDU SQUATS
3. DANEK TWISTS
4. EXERCISE BALL DUMB-BELL PRESS
5. GLUTE HAM RAISES
6. GYM GRAPPLER TWISTS
7. UCHIKOMI WITH STRETCH BAND
8. BREGMAN HOPPING DRILL
9. FRONT BARBELL PRESS WITH ELASTIC BAND (NO WEIGHT ON BAR)
10. LUNGES WHILE HOLDING A DUMB-BELL OR KETTLEBELL IN EACH HAND
11. DUMB-BELL SHOULDERS:
    • FRONT RAISES: 12 REPS
    • SIDE RAISES: 12 REPS
    • BENT-OVER SIDE RAISES: 12 REPS
12. JUMP ROPE

THE SHINGITAI COMPOUND CIRCUIT

This circuit is more difficult because of the 1-minute duration of each exercise, as well as the use of harder exercises and a variety of equipment. Go through the entire circuit 3 to 4 times with a 1-minute rest after each complete circuit. This gives you 36 to 48 minutes of actual work. Advanced trainees can eliminate the rest after each circuit to increase the difficulty of this routine. As you near a major event or fight, cut back on the number of rounds in the circuit allowing you to increase the intensity. If you feel nauseated or faint during the routine, stop at that point and make it a point to do more the next workout.

1. KETTLEBELL CRAB WALK
2. DANEK (RUSSIAN) TWISTS
3. PLYOMETRIC BOX JUMPS (HIGH BOX)
4. BALL PLANK HIP TWISTS
5. PULL UPS USING TOWEL
6. MOUNTAIN CLIMBERS
7. CHAIR PUSH UPS
8. PLYOMETRIC WEIGHT JUMPS
9. BAND PUSH UPS IN RACK
10. GLUTE HAM RAISES
11. BREGMAN HOPPING DRILL W/BAND ON ANKLES
12. SHADOWBOXING (USE PUNCHES, KICKS, SWEEPS)

BREAD AND BUTTER BARBELL WORKOUT

This routine is a good one for "total body" training and is recommended for a person new to strength and conditioning or to anyone who wants a rock solid barbell workout. In other words, it includes working the legs, core, back, shoulders, neck and chest and arms in one workout. Its foundation is good, solid barbell training.

When author Steve Scott was a young man and soaking up all he could in weightrooms and gyms in and around the Kansas City area, he trained with a variety of bodybuilders, powerlifters, Olympic-style weightlifters and strongmen. One of those men was a strong man named Cary Glass. He was an experienced powerlifter and was Steve's supervisor at the community center where they worked and was, for several years, a great training partner and lifting coach. Cary believed that nothing could beat a good, solid barbell workout for real strength development. This routine is good, solid work and will give you overall development. There's nothing fancy about it, but it will make you strong. Do this routine every week for 3 weeks of each month and then take the fourth week off. Then, start fresh the first week of the next month and repeat the program. You will work out in the weight room 3 times a week.

Follow this barbell routine every Monday, Thursday and Saturday. Work on your flexibility on the days you aren't in the gym. If you can't work out on Monday, Thursday and Saturday because of your training time on the mat, try to follow this routine on the days you aren't working out full blast on the mat. If you have to work out on this barbell routine Tuesday, Friday and Sunday, then do it. Make sure you have at least a couple of days rest between each day in the gym. If you're starting out as a novice lifter, this is an ideal way to develop good, solid strength. Also, if you've been around weight gyms for a long time and simply want a good routine that hits the major muscle groups, this is the routine for you.

You'll know when to move up in weight when you can easily do the final 3 or 4 repetitions of the final set of the exercise. In other words, if you are doing the barbell curl and can handle the last few reps of your last set with relative ease, then add 5 or 10 more pounds so that the last 3 or 4 reps of that final set are hard, but possible to do safely. Eventually, after several months, add another set, so if you were doing 3 sets, move to 4 sets. After you've been doing this routine for 6 months or so, then go to 5 sets.

This routine follows the tried and true formula of working large muscles first. Do the exercises in the order listed.

MONDAY AND THURSDAY

BREATHING SQUAT
Perform 1 set of 20 repetitions. In between each rep, take 2 deep breaths. Take your time doing this lift. Don't rush through it. It's hard work, so take your time, do the exercise in good, strict form and let it do its magic on you. The goal is to load the bar with what you weigh. If you weigh 200 pounds, load the bar with 200. If you are new to training and can't use your body weight, use poundage that you can safely perform 20 reps with. Your legs, lower back, and hips will make remarkable gains, but this lift also helps you develop a strong, big rib cage and chest. Taking the deep, full breaths in between each repetition will make you work hard. Unrack the bar, take 2 deep breaths, and then start to squat. Rather than increase sets or reps for the Breathing Squat, add more weight. Add weight gradually and safely.

BREAD AND BUTTER BARBELL WORKOUT (CONT.)

When you are able to perform the last 3 or 4 repetitions with energy to spare, that's the time to add more weight to the bar. Perform the squat by using a good, straight back and perform a full squat. When you hit bottom, don't bounce back up, as bouncing is hard on your knees and lower back. Don't hold your breath when performing each squat. Breathe normally as necessary, inhaling on the way down and exhaling on the way up. The "breathing" in the Breathing Squat is done by taking 2 deep, full breaths in between each rep. Finish the squat, take 2 breaths, and then go for the next rep!

OVERHEAD PRESS

Perform 3 sets of 10 repetitions if you are new to doing this lift. Eventually, as you get stronger, your goal should be to perform 5 sets of 6 repetitions.

HIGH PULLS

Doing High Pulls will add strength and size to your body. This is an excellent exercise for your trapezius, upper back, shoulders, upper pectoral area and arms. If you want a strong neck, this is your foundation exercise to achieve it.

BARBELL TRICEPS CURLS

This is a great exercise for triceps, shoulders, upper back and forearms. Use a straight Olympic bar for this movement. The long bar, along with the fact that it's straight works a lot of stabilizer muscles.

BARBELL BICEPS CURLS

The king of biceps exercises is the Barbell Curl. Use an Olympic bar for this exercise. In addition to working your biceps, using a long, straight Olympic bar works all the stabilizer muscles as well. This is also a fantastic exercise for the development of strong forearms, which gives you a stronger grip. This exercise is also excellent for strengthening your elbow joints, which you need in any form of grappling.

DANEK TWISTS

Use a barbell plate that you can safely handle for 3 sets of 15 repetitions, and then move on to 25 repetitions. When you can handle that weight at 25 reps, then move to 4 sets of 25 reps at that weight, and then on to 5 sets of 25 reps at that weight. This exercise is also called the Russian Twist.

SATURDAY

DEADLIFT

Don't go for real heavy deadlifts when doing this routine. Use moderate to fairly heavy weight where you can do about 6 to 10 reps in each set. Perform 3 sets of 6 to 10 to start, and then move to 4 sets of 6 to 10, then on to 5 sets of 6 to 10. Use controlled, good lifting form when doing the deadlift. This is excellent for lower back development, but really works just about every muscle in your body. You will develop a strong grip and a good set of traps if you do this exercise on a regular basis.

BENCH PRESS

The Bench Press is a good upper body strength developer, but since the late 1960s, too many people have relied on it as the only way to achieve upper body strength and development. Doing the Overhead Press with a barbell develops greater strength. But then, a lot of guys like big "man boobs," and performing the Bench Press on a regular basis will give them to you.

UPRIGHT ROWING

Stick to using a higher rep count on this exercise. Start out with 3 sets of 10, then move to 4 sets of 10 and eventually move on to 5 sets of 10. This is an excellent upper body developer, and focuses in on your trapezius, shoulders and upper back.

DANEK TWISTS

As you did on the other days, use a barbell plate that you can safely handle for 3 sets of 15 repetitions, and then move on to 25 repetitions. When you can handle that weight at 25 reps, then move to 4 sets of 25 reps at that weight, and then on to 5 sets of 25 reps at that weight. The Danek Twists is the primary core exercise in this workout routine, so make it a point to do it every workout. Use it as the last exercise in your routine.

THE "I HATE YOU" ROUTINE

This isn't the most scientific workout ever invented, but it's one that you'll definitely remember. More than one athlete has uttered the phrase that gave this workout its name. Basically, it consists of 2 giant sets with 1 set of Breathing Squats between them. For our purposes, a "giant set" is a group of 4 or more exercises done immediately after each other with no rest between sets, and they can be any 4 you wish. You perform 1 set of 10 reps on each of the 4 exercises without rest between each set. After you perform a Giant Set, rest about 2 minutes, then hit your second round of your giant set. When you complete your initial giant set, rest about 2 minutes, and then perform 1 set of 20 repetitions on the Breathing Squat. Rest about 2 minutes after your Breathing Squat, and then take on your second giant set, consisting of 4 exercises performed in the same way you did your first giant set. It's grouped into 3 parts and looks like this:

- Giant Set
- Breathing Squats
- Giant Set

A personal preference is to do the initial giant set of dumb-bell exercises, followed by the Breathing Squat, and then going to the second giant set consisting of barbell exercises. However, you can use any exercises you wish in your 2 giant sets, just make sure you do that set of Breathing Squats in the middle of them. It's the Breathing Squat sandwiched in the middle, in combination with the intensity of the giant sets that makes this a hard workout.

This routine is a good one. Do it once a week as a substitute for one of your regular workouts on that particular day. For instance, do this routine on a Wednesday instead of what you would normally do on a Wednesday. Use weight as heavy as possible and still get 10 reps in. Use weight that will push you hard, but make sure to use good, strict form on all of the exercises. Don't cheat or swing the dumb-bells or barbells. Here it is in a nutshell:

Perform a Giant Set. Do 1 set of 10 reps on each exercise and immediately move to the next exercise without rest.

- Alternating Dumb-Bell Press
- Dumb-Bell Pullovers
- Seated Dumb-Bell Concentration Curls
- Seated Dumb-Bell Triceps Extensions

Rest about 3 minutes.

Perform 1 set of 20 Breathing Squats at your body weight.

Take 2 deep breaths before your 1st rep and then take 2 deep breaths between each of your 20 reps.

Rest about 3 minutes.

Perform a second Giant Set. Do 1 set of 10 reps on each exercise and immediately move to the next exercise without rest.

- Barbell Bench Press (Medium to Narrow Grip)
- Barbell High Pulls
- Barbell Triceps Curls
- Barbell Biceps Curls

Try this routine once in a while for a good, hard workout. You're right; there's no core or abdominal work in it, but it's still a great routine as a change of pace and will certainly help build your strength.

> **TECHNICAL TIP: Check in Section Two for photos and explanations of how to perform all the exercises described in this section.**

KICKBOXING OR BOXING STRENGTH ROUTINE

If your specialty is punching and kicking, this routine will add power to your punches. This is a good program for MMA fighters who want to increase their striking power. While there's a lot to be said for the statement "punchers are born, not made" there's also a lot to be said for the fact that strong people hit hard too.

Punching and kicking power comes from a solid foundation and a strong set of hips and strong legs so this routine includes plenty of explosive power training. It travels from the bottom of your foot through your legs, then up through your body and into your shoulder and arm, then to your fist to the point on your opponent's body where you hit him. Also, a strong back directly translates to a hard punch. As a striker, you need good, solid core strength for hip movement and rotation when throwing a punch or kick, as well as the ability to absorb punishment. You also need the strength to hold your gloved hands up for an extended number of rounds in a fight with your shoulders, arms and upper back. If your neck is strong, it will help absorb the punishment you take to your head, so this routine includes training for your traps and neck as well.

Perform this routine on 2 days per week with at least 2 to 3 days between each workout. We're listing them as on Monday and Thursday, but you can use any days of the week you wish as long as you have enough rest between the days. **Important: Use enough weight so that the last 3 or 4 repetitions in the last set are difficult but not impossible. When the last 3 or 4 reps become easier, move up in weight by about 5 to 10 pounds.** Check Section 2 for the photographs and explanations of each exercise.

MONDAY

Perform 3 sets of 10 repetitions on each exercise unless otherwise noted.

1. LEG PRESS MACHINE
2. LEG PRESS POP UPS Use lighter weight than in the Leg Press.
3. BELT SQUATS Perform 3 sets of 6 reps and use heavy weight.
4. HYPEREXTENSIONS (FRONT) Perform 3 sets of 25 reps.
5. HYPEREXTENSIONS (SIDE) Perform 3 sets of 25 reps.
6. HANGING LEG RAISES TO CURL UP
7. BENCH DIPS Perform 3 sets of as many reps as possible per set.
8. PULL UPS (PALMS OUT) Perform 3 sets of as many reps as possible per set.
9. DIPS Perform 3 sets of as many reps as possible per set.
10. BARBELL HIGH PULLS
11. DUMB-BELL PULLOVERS
12. SEATED DUMB-BELL BICEPS CONCENTRATION CURLS
13. BARBELL OR DUMB-BELL SHRUGS
14. BARBELL FRONT PRESS (Use 20 or 25 pound barbell-no weight on it.) 2 sets of 50 reps.

THURSDAY

Perform 3 sets of 10 repetitions on each exercise unless otherwise noted.

1. PLYOMETRIC SHORT BOX JUMP Perform 3 sets of 6 reps.
2. PLYOMETRIC HIGH BOX JUMP Perform 3 sets of 6 reps.
3. CABLE MACHINE LEG KICKS
4. EXERCISE BALL PLANK HIP TWISTS
5. MEDICINE BALL TWISTS Perform 4 sets of 25 reps.
6. STIFF LEG DEADLIFT
7. GYM GRAPPLER ROTATIONS
8. EXERCISE BALL OVERHEAD DUMB-BELL PRESS
9. ONE ARM DUMB-BELL BENT OVER ROWS
10. SEATED TRICEPS BARBELL CURLS
11. BARBELL BICEPS CURLS
12. DUMB-BELL PUNCH ALTERNATING
13. STRETCH BAND NECK RESISTANCE (FRONT, BACK AND BOTH SIDES)
14. 1BARBELL FRONT PRESS (Use 20 or 25 pound barbell-no weight on it.) 2 sets of 50 reps.

Be sure to warm-up and cool-down (including stretching) before and after this routine. If you're still sore from working out after 2 to 3 days, then wait until you're not sore anymore. About 3 to 4 weeks before your fight, use lighter weight on all exercises and if you're using body weight on some exercises, perform fewer repetitions. Drop training in the weightroom about 2 weeks before your fight.

PLAY CARDS

A great way to break up the monotony of training is to play cards in the gym. Get a deck of cards, and take out the Jokers. Shuffle the deck of cards. You can do this alone, but it's a lot more fun when you do it with one or more training partners.

Okay, the cards are ready to go, so here's how this routine works. Instead of doing a set of your normal number of repetitions, take a card off the top of the deck and do the number of reps that corresponds to that card. For instance, if you draw the 8 of Diamonds, you do 8 reps. Face cards always count for 10 reps and aces always count for 11 reps.

Instead of doing 5 sets of 10 on a particular exercise, you may do 1 set of 11, 1 set of 3, 1 set of 7, and 1 set of 10, depending on what cards you draw.

You can do this on the mat or almost anywhere. When you're going live or doing randori, play cards. Each round of Randori corresponds to the card you draw. If you draw a 5 of Clubs, you go 5 minutes. If you draw the 10 of Hearts, you go 10 minutes. You can do this with Uchikomi drills as well. If you draw the 7 of Spades, you perform 7 fit ins, if you draw the King of Hearts, you do 10 fit ins. You get the idea.

This breaks up the monotony of training, but don't do it too often. This type of workout provides for a good break when you think you're getting stale from training.

ONE LIFT DAYS

Every so often you might want to devote one entire workout to a specific exercise. Talk to some of your training partners and decide that on a specific date you can get together to do nothing but that particular exercise on that day and get intense doing it. You can do this once in a while, once a month or even once a week. For several years, a small group of us got together for "Man Tit Monday". All we did every Monday was the Bench Press. There were usually about 4 or 5 of us and we did as many hard, heavy sets and reps on the Bench Press we could each Monday. We did that for about 2 or 3 years on a steady basis. Sure, the Bench Press isn't one of the lifts recommended highly in this book, but it provided a break from our normal training routine and we had a lot of fun on the days we got together. Something else we did was to select a particular day and make it a Squat Marathon. We would perform as many sets and reps of Squats as we could (then spend the next couple of weeks recovering from it!) that day.

For many years, we could get together for what we called the "Dumpster Olympics". We trained in the basement weight room of a community center and would haul the barbells, dumb-bells, kettlebells, lifting stones and anything else we could outside in an area where the dumpster was located. We didn't do it to hang around a stinking dumpster, but it was the only place where we could haul the weights and equipment outside, and training outside on a nice day was a welcome break for us, so we used that area. We often had friendly lifting contests in a variety of lifts, from 1-Hand Dumb-Bell Presses or Snatches to Stonelifting contests. We also had our barrel and our beer keg filled with sand out there and would often do some heavy training lifting them out by that old dumpster.

A big part of anyone's long-term training is doing things like this. Remember that working out in the gym is something that you should enjoy. Having a "Man Tit Monday" or "Squat Marathon" is a great addition to your long-term training experiences. This may not be the most scientific lifting or training advice, and we certainly don't recommend it if you are in a training cycle or preparing for a fight or tournament, but it provided some excellent training and made all of us stronger men for having done it.

THE RUSSIAN DUMB-BELL SHOULDER ROUTINE

During the 1980s, a couple of athletes who trained with author John Saylor at the U.S. Olympic Training Center Judo Squad brought back a trough training routine they learned while competing in the Tblisi Cup in Georgia, when it was part of the old Soviet Union. This workout works the entire shoulder girdle and is a good one.

Pick up a pair of dumb-bells that you can perform 8 to 12 repetitions with (on each arm). Perform the following exercises in one continuous set. Don't put the dumb-bells down between exercises; go straight to the next exercise. Depending on your goals, need and fitness level, perform 1 to 3 sets. (Check Section 2 for photos and full explanations of how to perform each exercise.) In addition to developing strength in your shoulders, this workout builds terrific endurance and strength in your hands and forearms. Working your muscles from a variety of angles is important for all grapplers and fighters and routines like this offer this type of variety.

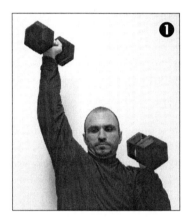

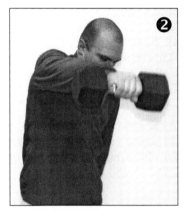

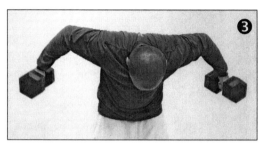

DUMB-BELL BENT-OVER SIDE RAISES
Bend forward at your waist and with a dumb-bell in each hand, held at arm's length under your chest, simultaneously raise the dumb-bells out away from your body in a reverse flying motion.

ALTERNATING OVERHEAD DUMB-BELL PRESS
Alternately press the dumb-bell overhead for the desired number of reps.

ALTERNATING DUMB-BELL FORWARD PRESS
With a slight bend in your elbow, alternately raise the dumb-bell straight forward to the point just above your head.

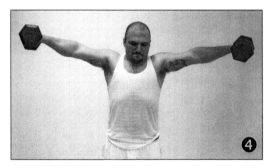

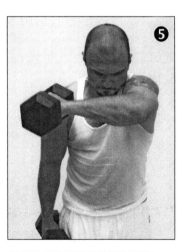

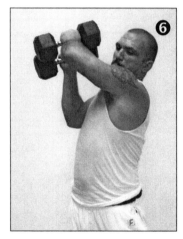

DUMB-BELL SIDE RAISES
With a slight bend in your elbows and with both dumb-bells held in front of your body, simultaneously raise the dumb-bells to the side.

ALTERNATING DUMB-BELL CROSS-BODY CURLS
Swing the dumb-bell across your body up to your opposite shoulder.

DUMB-BELL JUDO SWING AND PULL
Take a step to one side as though you are taking the first step into a forward throw. With the momentum this step creates, swing both dumb-bells up toward your face as if you are pulling an opponent in for a forward throw.

THE 5-MINUTE DUMB-BELL DRILL

Back in the 1970s, author John Saylor started doing the "5 Minute Dumb-Bell Drill" and got great results from doing it. It's really pretty simple really and not as formal as the Russian Dumb-Bell Shoulder Routine, but like all good workouts, entails a lot of hard work. Take a pair of dumb-bells, (John used 50 to 60 pounders) and perform a variety of continuous exercises you like in any order you wish. The objective is to keep the dumb-bell moving and not put them down until a specified time limit is up. Since John was training for judo and the length of a judo match was 5 minutes, he performed two or three 5-minute rounds of this drill. It's pretty informal, but it's an intense upper body workout. If you stay on the 5-Minute Dumb-Bell Drill twice a week for more than 3 weeks or so, you'll go stale. When this happens, switch to another circuit training routine, and continue doing your body weight exercises on the in-between days.

Here are some tips to make the 5-Minute Dumb-Bell Drill work for you:

1. Choose a pair of dumb-bells that have a combined weight of 1/3 to 1/2 your body weight.

2. Since the weight of the dumb-bells will be heavy, perform any leverage type exercise (such as Forward Raises, Bent Over Raise, etc.) first while you are still fresh. After getting them out of the way, perform exercises that work larger muscle groups, such as Bent-Over Rowing, Alternate Curls, Presses, etc. Remember, just keep the dumb-bells moving.

3. This drill will most likely be too long to start with, so initially, perform this drill for a time period you can do and keep good form. If your match time is 5 minutes, make it your goal to perform a drill for 5 straight minutes while keeping the dumb-bells moving. Eventually, you will improve to where you can perform two 5-minute rounds, and then three 5-minute rounds.

4. It's helpful to write down a circuit of dumb-bell exercises on a piece of paper, chalkboard or anywhere you can take a quick look at during the routine as reference. You may write out 10 different exercises or only 4 or 5, but the important thing is to continually do them and keep the dumb-bells moving for the entire time period.

TECHNICAL TIP: Training with dumb-bells or kettlebells provides you with an opportunity to train a lot of muscle groups at a variety of angles and positions. Training with these implements works the many small stabilizer muscles in your body as well as larger muscle groups. Use dumb-bells or kettlebells on a regular basis and you will experience a significant increase in your functional strength.

THE MOTHER OF ALL SETS

Jim Marshman, a good friend of both authors and a top coach in St. Petersburg, Florida, developed this routine after observing John Saylor run his athletes through the 5-Minute Dumb-Bell Drill at the Olympic Training Center. Jim liked the idea and took it home with him to train his team. After a while, Jim decided the routine needed some more structure. He found that when his athletes reached a certain fatigue level, they had trouble deciding what exercise to perform next. He was also concerned they might not work opposing muscle groups enough, so he developed the MOTHER OF ALL SETS.

Warning: This routine is tough. Do not, repeat, do not, try to perform this routine until you have achieved a very good level of fitness. If you have any medical conditions or problems, especially heart problems or high blood pressure, do not perform this routine.

Use Dumb-Bells. Choose a pair of dumb-bells with the combined weight between 1/3 to 1/2 of your body weight. Warm up with 50 to 100 Hindu Squats, depending on your level of fitness. Perform the routine in the order listed below. Check Section 2 for a complete explanation of each exercise.

This routine is a continuous set of 6 exercises consisting of the following:

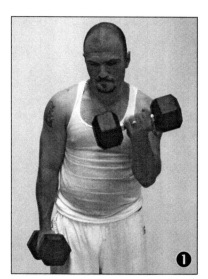

BICEPS CURLS (ALTERNATING OR TOGETHER)
Mike curls the dumb-bell making sure not to cheat by swinging the weight.

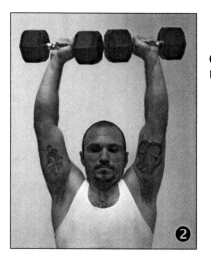

OVERHEAD PRESS (ALTERNATING OR TOGETHER)
Use a standard overhead press in this exercise.

THE MOTHER OF ALL SETS (CONT.)

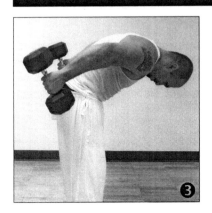

TRICEPS KICKBACKS

Mike makes sure not to jerk or swing the dumb-bells as he performs the kickback movement.

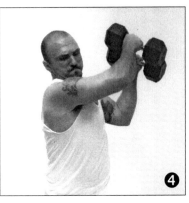

JUDO DUMB-BELL SWING AND PULL (ALTERNATE SIDES)

The Judo Swing exercise is a great all-around dumb-bell exercise, working your entire upper body, including your core.

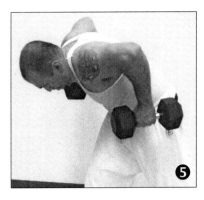

BENT OVER ROWING (TOGETHER)

Don't jerk the weights up when doing this exercise.

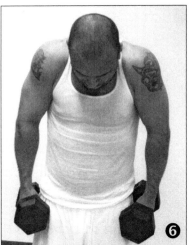

SHRUGS (TOGETHER)

When performing the Shrug, be sure to roll your shoulders to get maximum effect

One set of the Mother of All Sets consists in doing each of the above-listed 6 exercises with 10 reps, then 8 reps, then 6 reps and finally 4 reps without stopping. Put the dumb-bells down and then perform 50 to 100 Hindu Squats. **You have now completed one set of the Mother of All Sets.**

Rest 2 to 5 minutes or until your heart rate returns to about 120 beats per minute before starting the next set. As you progress, you will work up to 4 to 5 complete sets. Each set should take around 5 minutes to complete.

This routine develops serious muscular endurance and a good bit of strength as well. There's never been anybody who's done this routine for any length of time and gotten arm weary in a fight. When you train like this, you'll have a clear advantage over more conventionally trained fighters or grapplers. You'll be as tough in the last minute of the fight as you were in the first. Doing workouts like this is hard on you, but it's better to suffer in training than in an actual fight or match.

GARAGE GRAPPLER ON-MAT WORKOUT ROUTINE

This routine isn't a strength workout or specific fitness routine, but one that you can follow or use as a pattern for workouts of your own on the mat.

Not everyone trains in a large club or gym. Many of you reading this book are what are known as "garage grapplers." In other words, you and some of your buddies get together and work out in a garage, basement or other place and have put together some money to get a decent mat. In cases like this, there may be only 4 or 5 of you training together, so you have to make the most out of your time together and get the best workout possible. Quite a few great grapplers and fighters are garage grapplers. If you know how to train effectively, you can, and will, get some great workouts with only a few people on the mat. What is necessary is structured training. Follow a schedule that allows you to warm up and stretch properly, drill on skills and techniques, perform fitness drills, set aside time to roll, go live or randori, and then have an effective cool-down. Don't just show up, swing your arms around in the air as a warm up and then beat the snot out of each other. The training routine listed here is a good example of training effectively with efficient use of time and energy while on the mat. For a complete explanation of the drills and exercises listed here, check in Section 2.

Let's say you and your 3 training partners get together 3 times per week at the garage of one of the guys. You have limited mat space; say something like 20 feet wide by 30 feet long. All of you train regularly on both cardio and strength on the days you're not on the mat and you're in good shape throughout most of the year. Your primary interest is submission grappling and some of you compete in sport judo and sambo as well. Okay, we laid the scenario for the sample training routine to follow.

WARM UP AND STRETCH

BREAKFALLS AND TUMBLING
Do about 5 minutes of breakfalls and tumbling.

SHRIMP ACROSS THE MAT
Perform the Shrimp drill across the mat and back, doing at least 50 shrimping movements.

PARTNER SIT UPS OR CRUNCHES
Each partner performs 2 sets of 50 reps.

STRETCH
Functionally stretch for about 5 to 7 minutes, making sure you are completely stretched out and ready to train.

PARTNER GOOD MORNINGS
Each grappler does 1 set of 10 reps.

PARTNER SIT UPS
Each grappler does 1 set of 50 reps.

PARTNER PICK UP AND CARRY DRILL
Each partner does 2 sets of carrying his partner across the mat.

RODEO RIDE DRILL
Each partner performs two 30-second rounds with total cooperation from his partner.

SPINNING JUJI DRILL
Each grappler does 10 sets of 4, with total cooperation from his partner.

GUARD PASSING DRILL
Each partner performs 3 sets of 10 reps of his favorite guard pass on each side (60 total) with no resistance from his partner.

BREAKDOWN DRILL
Each partner performs 3 sets of 10 reps of his favorite breakdown (from all fours to the back) on each side (60 total).

BRIDGE AND ROLL DRILL
Each grappler does 1 set of 10 reps with total cooperation and then performs 2 or 3 rounds of escaping from a hold-down with 100% effort from both grapplers.

GRIP FIGHTING (IF TRAINING IN A GI)
PUMMELING (IF TRAINING WITHOUT A GI)
Perform a 1-minute round with everyone on the mat or perform at least 5 or 6 rounds.

UCHIKOMI (FIT INS FOR THROWS)
Each grappler performs 10 sets of 10 reps.

THROW ON CRASH PADS
Every athlete performs at least 50 full throws, and if time permits, 100 full throws.

GARAGE GRAPPLER ON-MAT WORKOUT ROUTINE

RANDORI, GOING LIVE OR ROLLING

Each athlete goes 5 3-minute rounds in groundfighting Randori, and then goes 5 3-minute rounds starting standing Randori.

COOL DOWN AND LIGHT STRETCH

Everyone Shrimps back and across the mat once, then does a light stretch to finish the workout. Allow your body to stop sweating before leaving the dojo or gym.

This workout actually breaks down to 4 specific parts:
1. Warm Up and Stretch
2. Drill Training for both Fitness and Skill
3. Randori or Going Live
4. Cool Down

We didn't include any time for working on new moves in this workout, but if you want, you can include this phase of training right after your Drill Training and before Randori.

Sure, it will take you a while to finish this, usually about 2 hours. It's time well spent and you'll be tired, sore and bruised when you go home, and that means you had a good workout!

SOME FINAL THOUGHTS ON SECTION ONE

This first section of the book focused on why (and how) effective training works. If you're like the authors, you most likely will want to know why and how something works. Then you'll be better able to make it work. Also presented in this section was the importance of functional stretching as well as some different routines to make your training more interesting, more difficult and more effective. You can develop your own training routines or programs based on what event you're training for, your goals, your fitness level and any other factors. Use your imagination and develop your own training routines. You'll find that, over the course of time, you will use many different workout routines. Some will be more effective than others, and the best way to find out what works best is to try a lot of them and, most important, keep on training. The next section of the book presents a great many different exercises, drills, lifts and movements that you can use when putting together an effective, coherent and efficient training program.

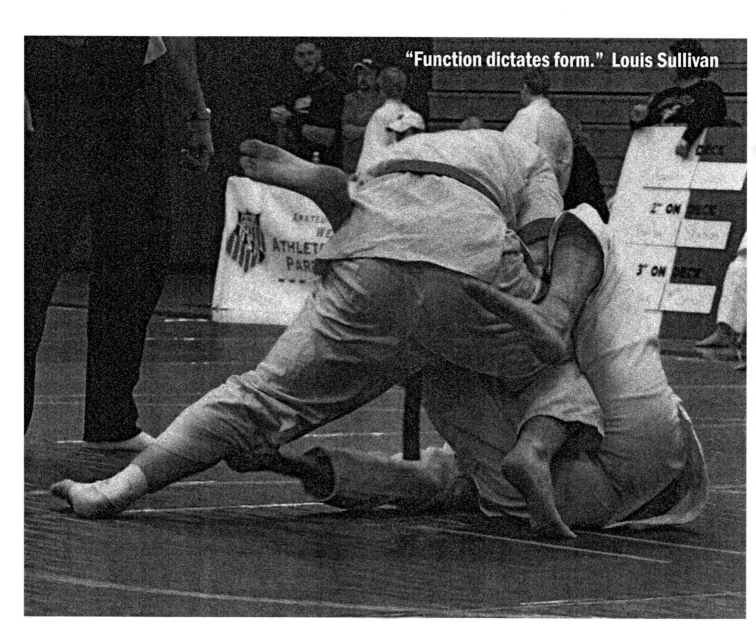

"Function dictates form." Louis Sullivan

SECTION TWO
EXERCISES & DRILLS: HOW THEY HELP YOU WIN ON THE MAT

• • • "It's not what you can do before you're tired, but after that counts." Chris Clugston

WHAT'S IN SECTION TWO:

Part 1: Exercises and Drills on the Mat, With or Without a Partner
Part 2: Freehand Exercises and Drills off the Mat, With or Without a Partner
Part 3: Barbell Training and Gym Equipment
Part 4: Dumb-bells and Kettlebells
Part 5: "It's So Old Fashioned, It's Cool" Training
Part 6: Exercise Ball Training
Part 7: Medicine Ball Training
Part 8: Plyometrics, Jumping, Hopping and Explosive Power Training
Part 9: Agility Ladder, Stair Training, Balance Board and Obstacles

AN OVERVIEW OF WHAT SECTION TWO IS ABOUT

This section's main purpose is to present a variety of exercises, drills, movements, games or other physical activities that you can use in your training. In addition to that, we will show why and how these specific exercises work and how they translate to winning performances on the mat. We may show a specific exercise using a medicine ball, and then show a specific situation or technical application of how the strength developed from using that medicine ball actually works. Obviously, there will be more than only one application of how working with that medicine ball can help you win on the mat, but you will see that it has value and there's a definite reason for doing that particular exercise or drill.

Each and every exercise presented in this section works muscles specific to your needs as a fighter or grappler. Specific training methods and exercises will help you develop into a well-rounded fighter, provided you have already built an adequate base through general and directed exercises and training methods. When you think of specific exercises, think of them in the following way:

1. These exercises require the same energy systems as those required in your specific event (a judo match, MMA fight, or any event). This is known as Metabolic Specificity.

2. You will use the same muscle groups as those required in a match or fight. This is called Muscle Group Specificity.

3. These exercises and drills mimic the movement patterns of your techniques. This is called Movement Pattern Specificity.

When an exercise or training method includes all of the above characteristics, it's a specific exercise. Of course, the most specific training for a fighter or a grappler is the fight itself, but if all you do is fight, you will never develop your potential in your skills from a technical standpoint. That simply means that if you want to be the best fighter or grappler you can possibly be, you need to train as smart as you do hard.

Remember that most of the following exercises in this section won't, by themselves, develop you into a well-rounded grappler or fighter. That's not their purpose. Use these drills, exercises and games in a total program of fitness training and development. You won't become a well-rounded grappler or fighter if you only do a few of these exercises. During your career as an athlete, try to use as many of these exercises as possible in your overall development. Specific exercises are designed to strengthen and develop only those energy systems, muscle groups and movement patterns of the specific purposes for which they are useful. Make sure you include general and directed exercises, drills and training methods in your overall training program. In other words, make certain your body is physically prepared to work hard on these exercises, drills and games included in this section.

There are a lot of exercises for you to choose from, and they're categorized in how we like to train with them. Use this section as a good reference guide. Mix and match different exercises, drills and movements to develop your own training routines or circuits; but remember what we said earlier...make sure you are physically able to perform them and get the most out of them. In some cases, we offer specific, time proven routines for a particular drill or exercise that we, or others, have used. Take what is shown here and don't hesitate to change anything to fit your needs.

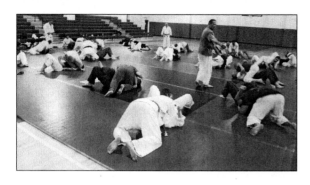

SECTION TWO: PART 1: EXERCISES AND DRILLS YOU CAN DO ON THE MAT, WITH OR WITHOUT A PARTNER

● ● ● "The best piece of training equipment in any dojo is another human being." Harry Parker

TRAINING ON THE MAT

The reason you're reading this book is to increase your knowledge of what it takes to be more efficient on the mat grappling with or fighting an opponent. There are a lot of exercises, drills and games you can do on the mat, with or without a training partner. The bottom line in training for any type of grappling or fighting is that the best training you can get is to actually get on the mat and train. How hard and how smart you train, both on and off the mat, determines your success. This photo shows John Saylor teaching a group of grapplers to move fluidly from hold to hold at his spring training camp in Perrysville, Ohio.

This part of Section Two is bigger than the other parts. The following exercises, drills and mat games can be done with or without a partner on the mat. While the main focus of working on the mat is usually working on drills, skills and going live or doing randori, don't forget to spend some time on your fitness and conditioning. Often, these mat drills and exercises get double-duty; they serve as both excellent fitness drills and skill drills and positively impact your conditioning and skill development. We all know that we have limited time to work on the mat each week, so use your mat time intelligently and efficiently. You can use these exercises and drills as a good warm-up prior to stretching or use an excellent conditioning and fitness drills anytime during your on-mat workout. These exercises are great "finishers" as well. Use them to finish your workout to get that last percentage of effort from your body before cooling down and going home.

A good training formula to follow for most workouts is:

1. Warm-up your body with some exercises, drills or games. These exercises literally warm your muscles up for the next phase of your workout, which is:

2. Functional Stretching.

3. Drill Training. Work on drills to increase your skill, fitness and other areas of your ability and fitness. This included groundfighting drills, throwing and takedowns drills on the crash mats as well as Uchikomi drills.

4. Work on new skills. Take some time to work on new moves and improve your skill level.

5. Open Training. Call it randori, going live or rolling, but try to get some time in for this phase of training.

For more ideas on drills and exercises you can use on the mat, read DRILLS FOR GRAPPLERS by Steve Scott and published by Turtle Press.

TRAINING TIP: For most people, training time on the mat is limited. We all have families, jobs and obligations in life that always, somehow, seem to "get in the way" of our mat time. Mat time is precious, and as a result, we need to use it wisely. This first part of Section Two presents some exercises, drills and games that you can use when on the mat to get the most out of your time on it. Many of these exercises can be used off the mat as well. A lot of these drills and exercises not only develop your physical fitness, but they also can improve your skill level from a technical perspective.

CARTWHEELS, TUMBLING AND BREAKFALLS

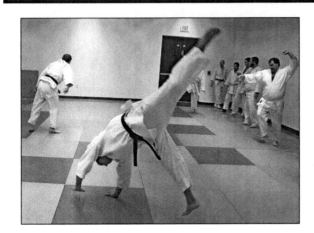

As part of your initial warm-up, make sure you do a good amount of breakfalls and tumbling. Cartwheels and round offs also provide great agility and coordination training. Perform breakfalls, cartwheels and round offs down and back the length of your mat several times before your workout.

PULLING IN ON AN OPPONENT

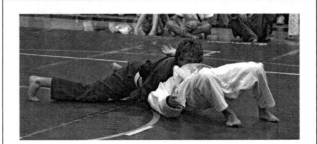

PULLING IN ON AN OPPONENT WHEN PINNING HIM USES THE SAME MUSCLES AS PULLING YOURSELF ALONG THE MAT

Pinning an opponent requires that you control him with your entire body and this drill emphasizes the muscles that lock an opponent down and not let him up. This pin at the junior nationals shows why it's important to develop the strength to control your opponent. Winning is the result of effective training.

MAT SWIMMING

This is a good exercise before stretching. This gives your upper body a good workout and develops your shoulders, triceps, upper back and pectorals.

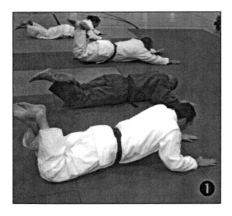

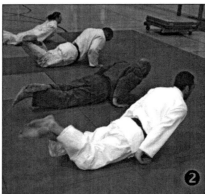

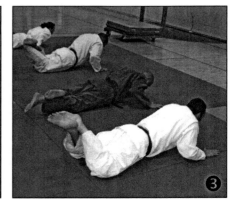

The athletes lie on their fronts, bend their knees and hook their ankles to keep from using them in this exercise.

The athletes reach out with their hands and pull themselves forward.

Repeat this sequence to complete the drill. "Swim" from one side of the mat to the other.

BUTT SCOOTS

This is a great warm-up before stretching. This exercise works your core, triceps, shoulders and pectorals. A good drill is to do Mat Swimming to one side of the mat and Butt Scoots back.

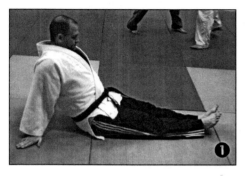

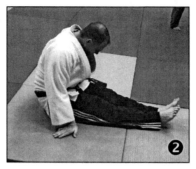

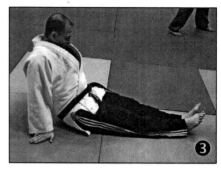

Bryan sits on the mat with his legs extended as shown and reaches back with both hands.

Bryan pulls himself backward as shown.

Bryan repeats the movement. This exercise works the core area and upper body very well and is a good, general exercise to use before your stretch out.

BUTT SCOOT WITH LEGS UP

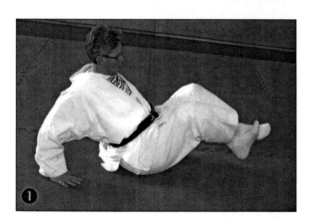

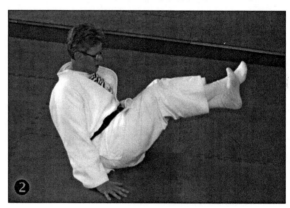

Sandi makes this exercise more difficult by hooking her ankles together and lifting her feet off the mat.

This variation works the core and it also gives you more work in the shoulders and upper back.

SHRIMPING

An exercise that should be done every workout is Shrimping. Different people may have different names for it, but no matter what you call it, it's an important exercise. Being able to shrimp is a fundamentally important skill in fighting from the guard or anytime you are on your back, hips or backside. This is also a great core exercise. It is often used as a warm-up before stretching. Shrimp from one side of the mat to the other.

One of the primary exercises every grappler should do is Shrimping. This is a tremendous core workout and is a skill used in every grappling sport known to mankind.

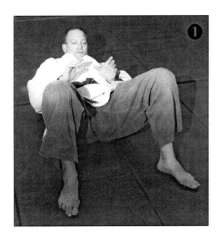

Bryan starts by lying on his back as shown.

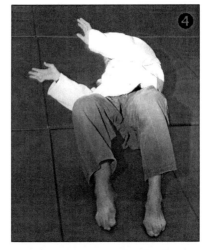

Bryan turns onto his left side and hip and draws his feet in close, making sure to keep solid contact on the mat with both feet. Look at how Bryan curls up reminiscent of a shrimp.

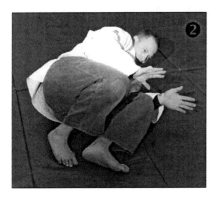

Bryan pushes off the mat with both feet, extending them, and scoots his body backward

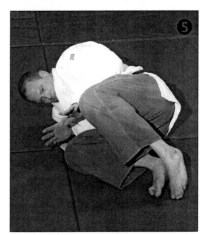

Bryan quickly flips over to his right side to repeat the shrimping exercise on that side.

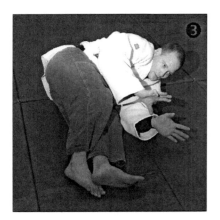

Bryan repeats the shrimping exercise on his right side.

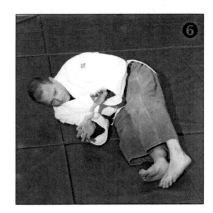

Bryan pushes with his feet against the mat and repeats the shrimp movement.

SHRIMP DRILLS BEFORE A WORKOUT

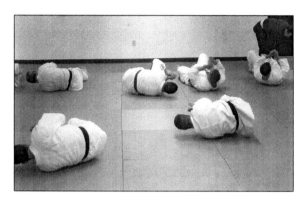

The guys are shrimping as one of the initial warm-ups done every practice or workout.

SHRIMP USING BELT (PARTNER ON MAT)

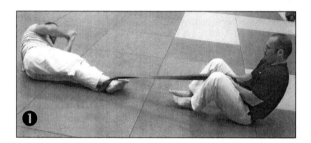

To make this shrimp drill a bit harder, Chris sits on the mat.

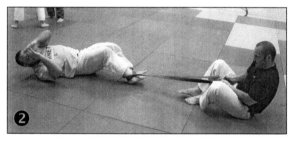

As Jake shrimps in the direction of his head, Chris moves along the mat following Jake.

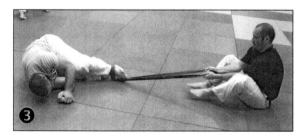

Jake will shrimp across the mat, and Chris will switch positions with him and perform this drill across the mat the other direction.

SHRIMP USING STRETCH BAND

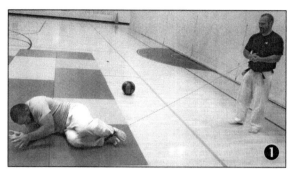

Jake performs shrimping with a stretch cable tied around his ankles.

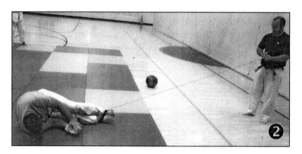

Chris holds the cable and follows along behind Jake with the band stretched. This gives extra resistance to the shrimp exercise.

SHRIMP USING BELT (PARTNER STANDING)

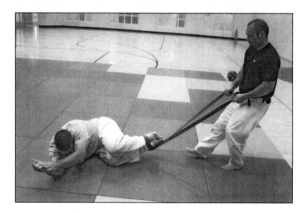

Jake has a judo belt tied looped or tied around his ankles as he shrimps. Chris holds each end of the belt and follows along behind Jake to provide resistance.

SHRIMP WITH MEDICINE BALL

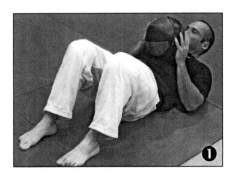

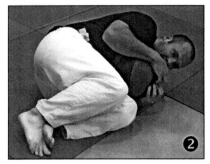

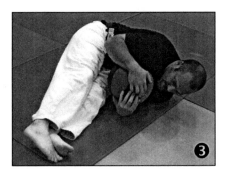

Add some more work to the shrimp exercise by holding a medicine ball and doing it.

Chris makes it a points to hug the ball tightly to his torso as he performs the shrimp.

Shrimp across the mat and back as a good warm-up before stretching or as a good finish after a hard workout.

WHY SHRIMPING IS IMPORTANT

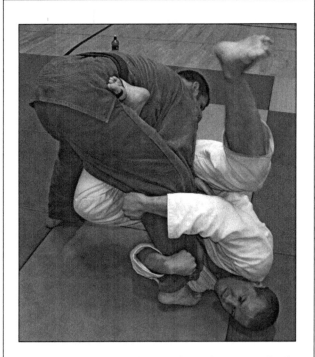

Here's shrimping in action. Being able to move freely and with control from the buttocks or back position is vital to every grappler. Mike is on his side fighting Eric from the guard position using his skills of shrimping effectively.

SHRIMPING TO GET THE ADVANTAGE

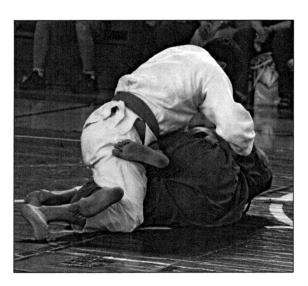

IF YOU SHRIMP WELL, YOU CAN MOVE TO ALMOST ANY POSITION TO GET THE ADVANTAGE OVER AN OPPONENT

Mobility is a key factor in using the guard, and shrimping develops the skill, agility and strength necessary to do it. Jarrod Fobes is one of the best leglock technicians around and his ability to move freely and lace his opponent's leg from the guard position stems directly from hours of practice in the basic movement of shrimping.

PARTNER NECK PUSH UPS

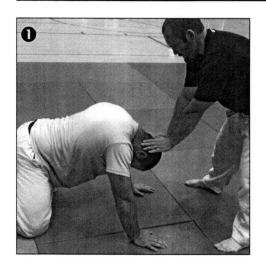

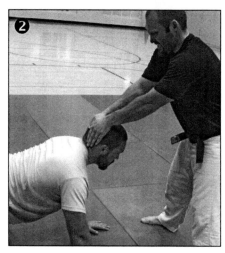

1. Neck and trap strength are vital to any grappling sport. Jake is on all fours and Chris has both, or one hand, on Jake's head as shown. Jake raises his head up.

2. Chris provides some moderate resistance, making the exercise difficult enough so that 10 repetitions are enough.

PARTNER FOOT SNAPS

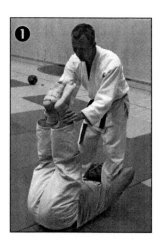

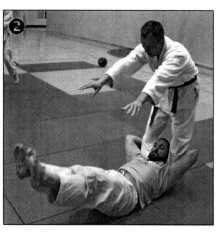

1. A good, old drill that really works your core, hips and legs is the Foot Snap Drill. Jake is on his back with his feet in the air as shown and holding onto Mike's ankles. Mike grabs Jake's feet.

2. Mike pushes hard on Jake's feet as shown. Jake will bring them back to the starting position as soon as his feet touch the mat

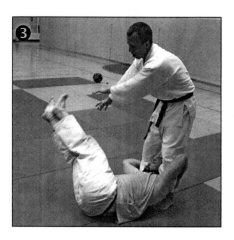

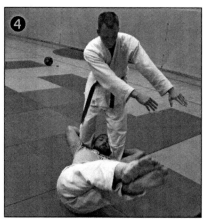

3. Mike can vary this exercise by snapping Jake's feet to the right.

4. When Jake brings his feet back up to the starting position, Mike snaps Jake's foot to the left. Repeat this for 10 reps, then switch places.

PARTNER ROLL AROUND DRILL

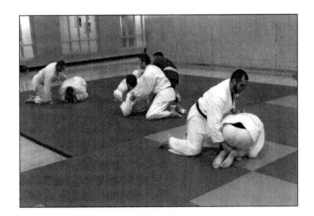

The guys are rolling each other around the mat as a warm up before stretching.

This is a good warm-up before stretching and a lot of fun. One grappler rolls up really tight and round and his partner rolls him around, all over the mat. It's a little tougher for the grappler that rolls his partner to not stand and stay on his knees.

RODEO RIDE DON'T LET HIM GET UP DRILL

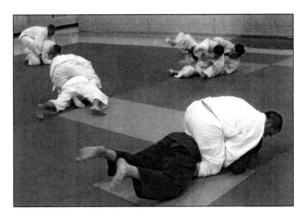

Get your partner in a rodeo ride, making sure your legs are dug in deep for control. The bottom grappler tries to get up and the top grappler won't let him. Not only does this develop your skill in this important position, it's also a tough workout.

PARTNER PULL

This is a great drill for developing strength in gripping and the upper body. You can do it flat on your front, in a seated (or even kneeling) position, and standing. Each grappler pulls as hard as possible, keeping good form and balance for 30-second rounds.

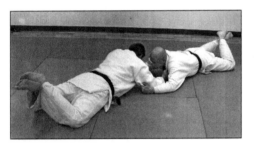

This variation of the exercise has the grapplers lying on their fronts and holding each other's lapels and sleeves. This is a great exercise for grip strength and upper body strength.

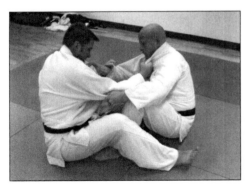

A good variation is for both grapplers to be seated (or on their knees) and pull on each other.

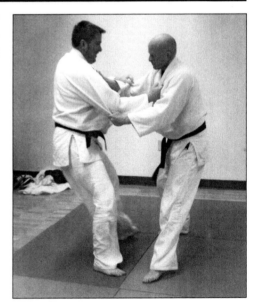

Doing this exercise standing is also a good workout. The athletes can either do the drill moving around or stay in one place on the mat. The important thing is for both grapplers to maintain good, erect posture to get the most out of this exercise.

PUSH-PULL DRILL

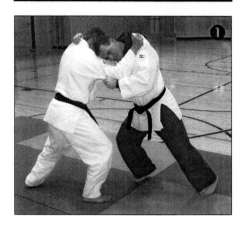

Bryan and Drew grab onto each other and at the coach's signal of "push" will push hard on each other, making sure to maintain good body posture.

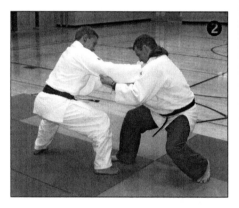

When the coach signals "pull", the athletes immediately pull on each other. The coach will signal either "push" or "pull" at uneven time intervals. Do this for about 30 to 45 seconds as a good warm-up.

PARTNER SIDE HOPPING

This is an excellent plyometric exercise you can do on the mat. One grappler balls up tight while the other hops over him from side to side. Do this in drills of 30-second rounds and to make it harder, hop as high as possible each jump. This will slow the tempo of the drill down, thus enabling you to generate more explosive power on each rep. In this variation, do 5 or 6 hops, then switch.

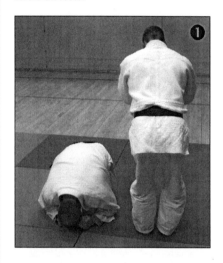

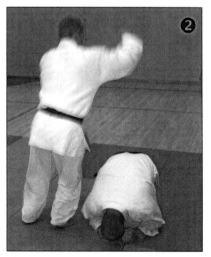

Drew hops over Bryan sideways with as much explosive power as possible. Do this exercise in 30-second rounds. To make it harder, Drew will hop as high as possible each time (slowing down the tempo of the drill) and emphasize more explosive power with each hop. Perform 5 or 6 hops, then switch roles.

QUICK SIDE HOPPING

This is a slight variation of the Side Hopping exercise. One grappler sits with his legs extended and his partner hops side to side over them.

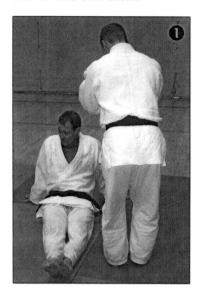

Drew hops sideways over Bryan's extended legs, doing as many hops as possible in 30 seconds.

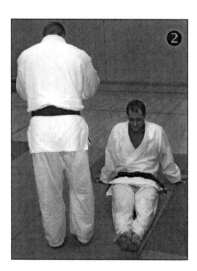

This drill helps develop "quick feet" for lower body coordination as well as explosive power. Use this exercise for younger athletes to help them develop lower body control, speed and power.

PARTNER LEGS SPREAD QUICK SIDE HOPS

This is a variation of the Side Quick Hops. The bottom grappler widens his legs so that the top grappler has to hop in between them to add to the work.

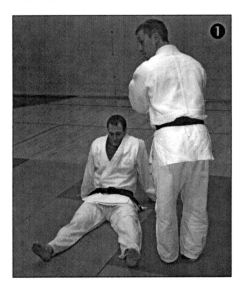

Bryan is sitting on the mat with his legs extend and wide.

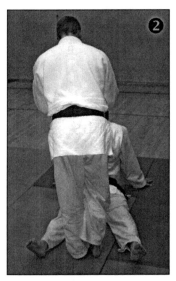

Bryan is sitting on the mat with his legs extend and wide.

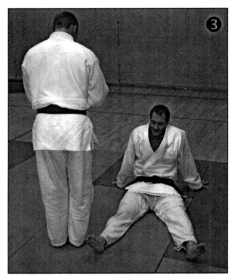

Drew does as many side hops as possible in a 30-second round. As with many of these exercises, this is a good warm-up before stretching or a great way to cool down or finish a workout.

OBSTACLE JUMPS

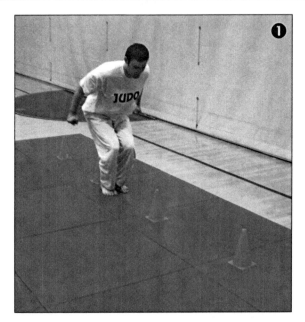

Derrick jumps over any obstacle you wish to put on the mat. In this case, we're using cones. Make the obstacles as big or small as you wish. Obviously, the larger or taller the obstacle, the more plyometric effect it will have.

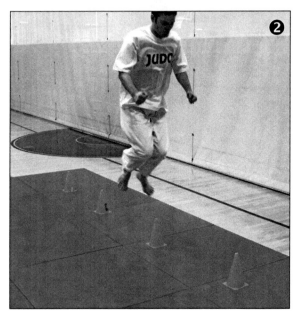

Make every effort to make each jump as effectively as possible. Don't use poor form simply to get the drill over with.

OBSTACLE SIDE HOPS

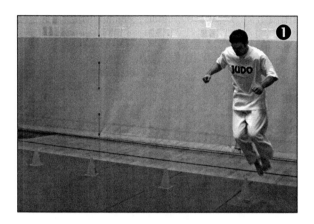 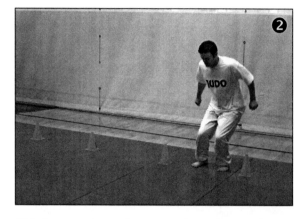

Derrick is hopping sideways over cones in this photo, but you can use any obstacle you wish.

This is a good exercise to use from time to time to break up the monotony of training. Using cones, agility ladders, exercise balls or any piece of equipment can really help in breaking the everyday routine of your on-mat workouts.

BELT JUMPS

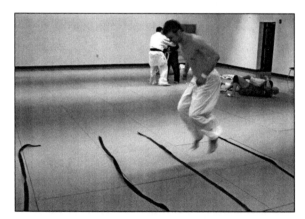

Derrick jumps over belts placed at uneven distances. This drill is a good plyometric drill as a cool-down after a hard workout.

AGILITY BELT HOPPING

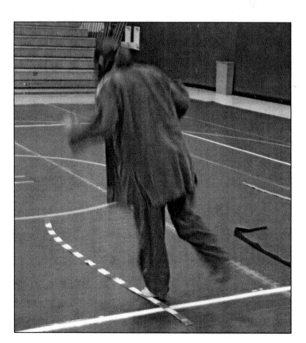

AnnMaria can do this on 1 leg or on both legs. She hops down the length of her belt stretched on the mat. This is a good agility drill that helps strengthen the support leg.

CLIMB THE TREE DRILL

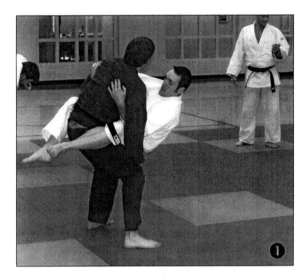

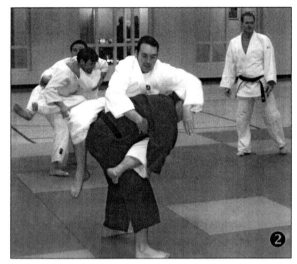

Jarrod stands in a strong, balanced position. Chas jumps on Jarrod and climbs all around him. The idea is for Chas to climb all the way around Jarrod's body without falling on the mat.

This is a good workout for both grapplers. The grappler doing the climbing is really getting a good agility and total body workout. The grappler serving as the "tree" has a total body workout as well, but is required to use more strength. Have each athlete go several rounds of climbing the tree with each other every so often as a change of pace in training.

HOW CLIMBING ALL OVER SOMEONE WORKS

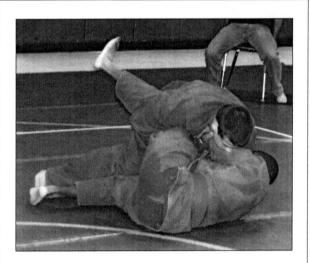

Being able to get hold and climb all over an opponent, going from one point of control to the next, results in breaking your opponent down and beating him. National AAU Champion Dillon Brink gets his opponent onto his back with a far arm-near leg breakdown on his way to pinning him.

CRAWL GET-AWAY GAME

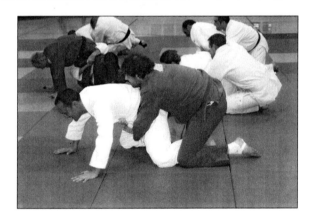

Shannon is doing his best to keep Chad from crawling forward in this great warm-up game. This is an all-around fitness drill that is a good warm-up before stretching. Have the group team up with one grappler on his hands and knees. The teams get on one side of the mat. The goal is for the grappler on hands and knees to crawl to the other side of the mat. His partner must try to pull him back and not let him crawl forward.

CIRCLE GAME

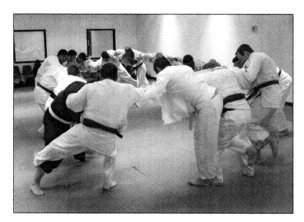

Have the group get in a circle and grab each other's jacket lapels. The idea is to foot sweep, trip or take everyone else to the mat. When any part of an athlete's body other than the bottom of his feet hit the mat, he's out. The remaining athletes grab each other again and resume the game. Go until only 2 people are left. This is a great warm-up game.

TOE TAP GAME

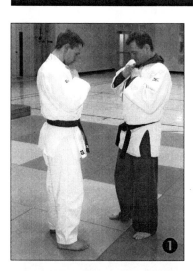

This is a good, quick cardio workout and a great agility drill. Face each other with your hands at your chest so you won't use them. One athlete is the attacker and the other is the defender.

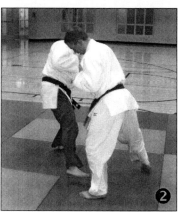

Bryan tries to touch Drew's feet as many times as possible in 30 seconds. Drew must do his best to keep Bryan from tapping his feet. Drew shouldn't turn his back on Bryan to keep this drill going well. This is a good drill to work on foot speed for foot sweeps or entering into throws.

SUMO

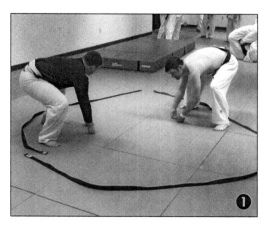

Form a sumo ring judo belts and play some sumo. This is a fun game to break the monotony of training.

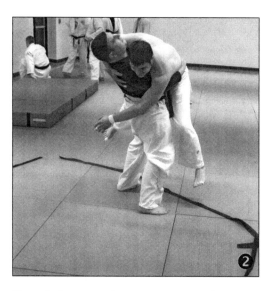

You win in sumo when your opponent is put out of the ring or any part of his body other than the bottom of his feet touch the mat.

CONDITIONING FOR COMBAT SPORTS

SIT ON HIS CHEST

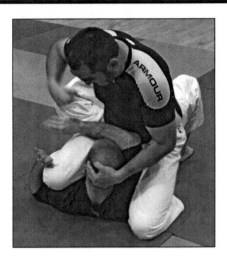

This is a good drill for the top and bottom grapplers. Basically one grappler sits on his partner's chest or stomach in the mount position and the bottom grappler tries to get him off.

Brian sits on Jorge's chest, providing weight. Jorge will bridge or arch up, and do his best to get Brian off of him. Takes turns bridging each other off or do it in timed drills. You can take this a step further and have the top grappler provide resistance of varying levels.

PUMMELING AND HAND FIGHTING

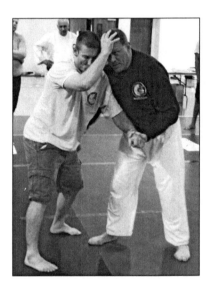

For no gi grapplers and MMA fighters, pummeling is the equivalent of grip fighting for grapplers who use jackets. Hard rounds of pummeling and hand fighting are necessary for total body strength, endurance and developing a strong grip. This drill teaches you to pursue your opponent and dominate him. Good, hard pummeling, hand fighting and grip fighting teach you to stalk your opponent, control him and dominate him, and if you can do this, you will win.

GRIP FIGHTING DRILL

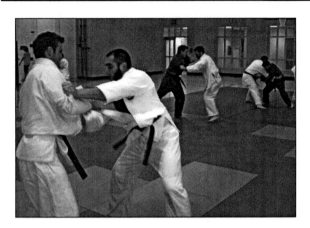

ALSO CALLED GRIP RANDORI OR GRIP FENCING. THE BEST WAY TO DEVELOP A STRONG GRIP IS TO GRIP FIGHT A LOT!

We have a number of exercises in this book for developing grip strength, but the best way to develop grip strength is to do a lot of grip fighting drills. Doing a lot of rounds of Grip Randori with many different partners on a regular basis will give you a very strong grip and develop your skills in grip fighting. Every workout, and we mean EVERY workout, we do grip-fighting randori. The idea in this drill is to dominate your partner and continually get the better grip and dominate him. He will do the same to you. We tell our athletes that this is randori without the throws, takedowns or groundfighting. You must beat him with your grip. Perform about 5 1-minute rounds with a new partner every round. Remember, don't try to throw your partner; beat him with your grip! This drill also helps you develop your tactics of controlling your opponent with the grip you intend to throw him with. If this drill is done with intensity, it is a tough one. If you want to develop an aggressive, no-nonsense style and not be afraid to get hold of an opponent, this drill is a must for every workout.

CONTROL THE GRIP AND CONTROL YOUR OPPONENT

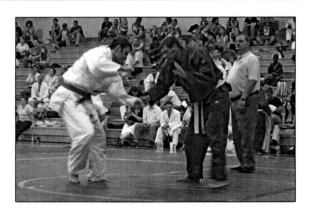

National AAU Judo Champion Kelvin Knisely dominates his opponent with strong, aggressive grip fighting. Before you throw your opponent, you have to get hold of him!

PULL DOWN HIS HEAD DRILL

There are a lot of gripping and pummeling drills and this is one of them. Both grapplers get a head and arm grip and try to pull the other's head down to the mat. Both grapplers can attempt to pull each other's head down at the same time or have one grappler be the aggressor and try to pull his partner's head down while his partner resists. For more information on gripping drills, refer to DRILLS FOR GRAPPLERS, published by Turtle Press.

In addition to the good, old-fashioned, hard work of doing pummeling drills at high intensity, a rugged drill to develop the pummeling and gripping power, as well as general body strength for grappling is the Power Pummeling Drill.

POWER PUMMELING DRILL

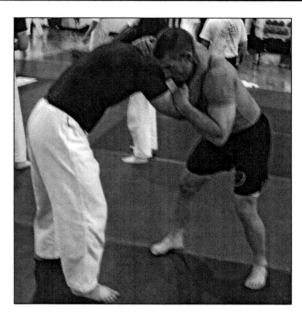

Both grapplers stand in place and do not move their feet while attempting to get the better advantage in a pummeling match. This forces the upper body to work hard, especially at the waist, hips and core. Believe it or not, it's hard on the legs as well.

MUAY THAI CLINCH PUMMELING

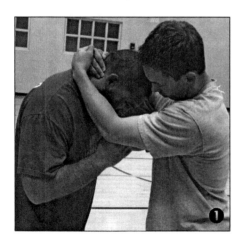

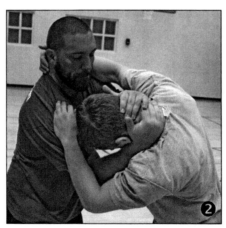

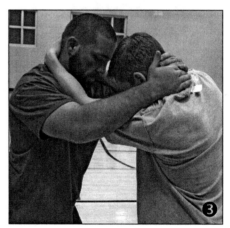

Drew has Jake in a Muay Thai clinch and Jake will hand fight to get his own clinch. Drew attempts to pull Jake's head down for control and Jake must work to establish a better tie-up. You and your partner can work with varying degrees of resistance.

Jake "swims" his hands up through Drew's clinch to establish his own tie-up. Jake pulls Drew's head down to establish control.

The guys keep pummeling and attempting to control the tie-up. Perform this drill in 30-second rounds, or any time limit rounds you wish.

RODEO RIDE GAME

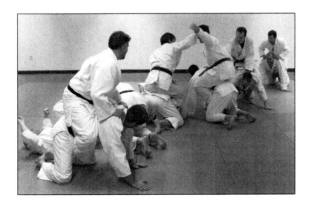

The athletes team up and one is the horse and the other is the rider. Riders try to pull other riders off their horses. The last rider and horse team left wins. This is a really good warm-up before stretching. The muscles of the legs and hips are emphasized in this exercise as well as all the stabilizer muscles needed to have an effective rodeo ride.

This drill is a lot of fun, even for adults and not just for kids. Remember, it's okay to actually have fun and enjoy yourself while training. There are enough times when training on the mat is far from fun, so take the opportunity from time to time to do a drill like this to lighten things up and still get a good workout.

PARTNER PUSH-UPS

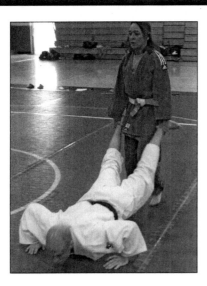

Push-ups are one of the best exercises ever invented and taken for granted by most athletes. AnnMaria is holding Kelly's ankles as he does push-ups. This is a terrific upper body workout. As with most of these exercises, we recommend the athletes do this drill in 30-second rounds, doing as many repetitions as possible in each round.

WHY THE RODEO RIDE DRILL WORKS

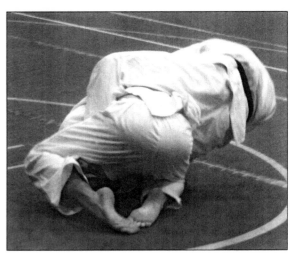

The top grappler in this photo has his legs hooked in tightly on his opponent and working in his choke. Good leg control in the rodeo ride is the result of good technical training, but the foundation is a solid lower body, hip, glute and core strength. This comes from lots of time working in the gym, working from this position both in technical and skill drills, but also in fitness drills and training.

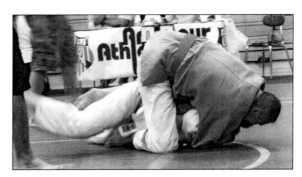

The rodeo ride is an important skill in any type of grappling or MMA. Strong legs and hips and developing the stabilizers necessary to ride an opponent are important in having a good rodeo ride. Jeff Owens has his hooks in tight and is controlling his opponent in this freestyle judo match.

PARTNER CRUNCHES (SEATED)

This is an outstanding core developer and can be used before or after a workout.

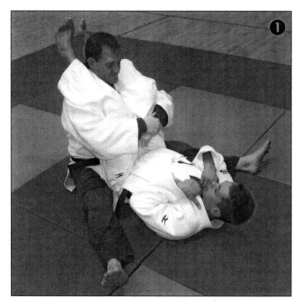

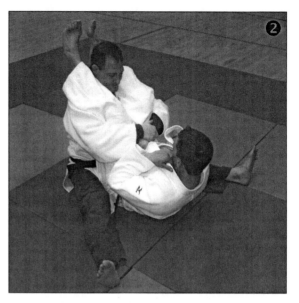

Drew is on his back as shown with Bryan holding onto his legs for support.

Drew crunches up. If doing this as a group, do this in sets of 30-second rounds. Each athlete does as many repetitions as possible in 30 seconds. Usually 1 to 3 rounds per athlete is enough during a workout.

PARTNER CRUNCHES (STANDING)

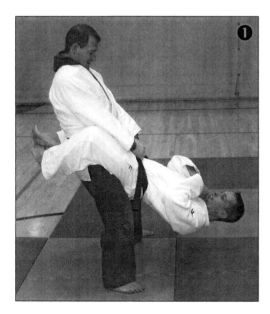

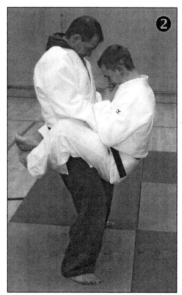

Take the crunches up a level and do this exercise standing. This way, both athletes benefit. Bryan is holding Drew and getting a good total body workout doing so, while Drew really keys in on his core muscles.

Bryan is standing and holding Drew as Drew hooks his legs around Bryan's waist.

As with the seated variation of this exercise, do this drill in 30-second rounds with the athlete doing as many repetitions as possible in the 30 seconds.

PARTNER ON ALL FOURS SIT UPS (FACING FRONT)

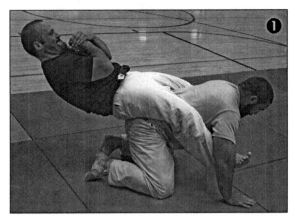

This is good way for both athletes to get a workout doing sit-ups. Chris hooks his feet under the armpits of Jake.

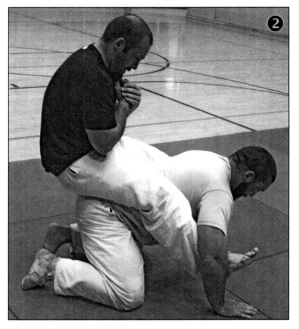

Chris sits up and will repeat this for a set number of reps or in a timed drill. Jake gets of good workout also by holding Chris up in this all fours position.

PARTNER ALL FOURS SIT UP (FACING REAR)

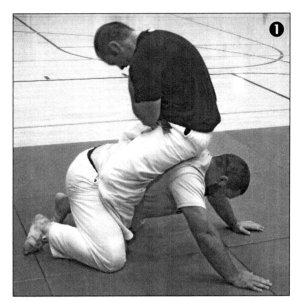

Chris can do this sit-up drill in this way by hooking his feet in Jake's hips as shown.

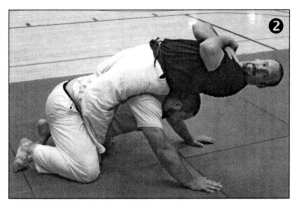

Chris can lean back really far and Jake can get an added workout by using his head and neck to push Chris back up.

PARTNER GOOD MORNINGS

The core area, and in this case, the muscles in the lower back, are vital and worked in this exercise. Many athletes tend to ignore the lower back, opting for the "washboard ab" look. Having a strong back is instrumental in picking up your opponent in any direction. Additionally, just about every body part is worked in this exercise.

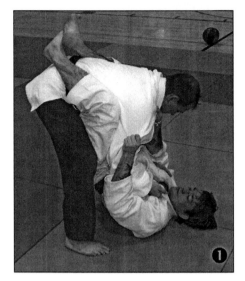 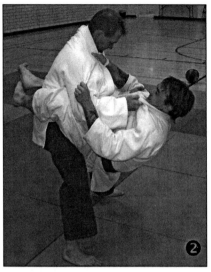 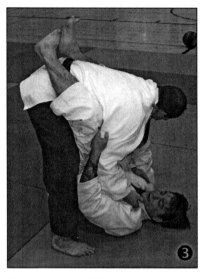

Bryan is standing over Nikolay, who is lying on his back with his legs hooked around Bryan's waist. Bryan holds onto Nikolay's jacket. If Nikolay didn't have a jacket on, Bryan could hook his hands and arms under Nikolay's armpits to lift him.

Bryan makes it a point to have his knees slightly bent. We want you to work your lower back, but also to use good lifting form when doing this exercise. Bryan picks Nikolay up off the mat, arches up and straightens up as he stands.

Bryan lowers Nikolay to the mat, making sure to ease him down and not drop him. Do this exercise in 30-second rounds with as many repetitions as possible in each round. This is a fantastic "finisher" to a workout.

HERE'S WHY YOU DO GOOD MORNINGS

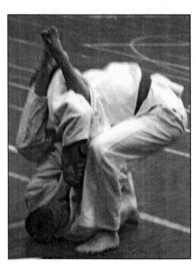

The standing grappler (LEFT) is about to pick the bottom man up off the mat to negate the armlock (or even a choke such as a Triangle Choke). In judo, sambo and many styles of jujitsu and grappling, picking your opponent off the mat gets the referee to call for a break in the action. In grappling sports where there is no break in the action if you pick your opponent up, it's even more important to have the strength to hoist him off the mat and shake him loose from you.

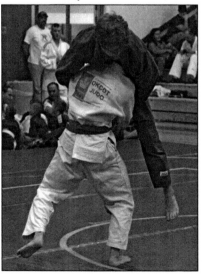

Pick up throws like this one (RIGHT) require a lot of technique, but the foundation of that technique is a strong body. Anytime you throw or take down an opponent, you need a strong lower back, hips and core. All the muscles in your body are linked together like a chain. Working the muscles of the core, which definitely includes your lower back, will serve you well in many situations on the mat. Don't let your lower back be your weak link.

PARTNER HOP & CRAWL (OVER AND UNDER DRILL)

This exercise is good for explosive power in jumping and is a good cardio workout as well. As with many exercises in this section, this is a good way to warm up before stretching, but it can also be a great "finisher" after a hard workout. Do this drill in sets of 30-second rounds with the athlete doing as many repetitions as possible in each round.

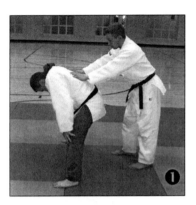

Bryan is bending at the waist as Drew prepares to jump over him.

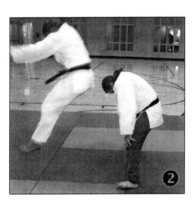

Drew jumps over Bryan.

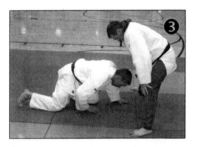

When he lands, Drew gets on his hands and knees and crawls through Bryan's legs.

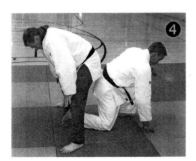

Drew finishes this repetition and will immediately do another.

PARTNER PLYOMETRIC JUMPS

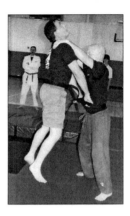

Explosive power from the legs and hips are important to throws, takedowns and ground-fighting. Not only that, you generate a lot of power for punching from these areas as well. Brian is holding onto John's belt and doing as many jumps as possible in 30 seconds. You can also do this in sets of 10 repetitions with each grappler doing a specific number of sets.

EXPLOSIVE POWER IN FORWARD THROWS

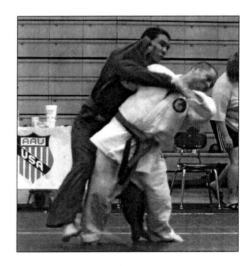

EXPLOSIVE POWER IN FORWARD THROWS COMES FROM PLYOMETRIC TRAINING

David Fortin's use of plyometric training helped him use this Shoulder Throw effectively. A strong foundation is needed for explosive power in a throwing technique.

PARTNER PICK UPS

Many throws and takedowns rely on a solid base and core strength. Using this drill can dramatically improve your strength level.

1. Bryan shoots under Nikolay, making sure to use good form and not bend over at his waist.

2. Bryan picks Nikolay up. Do this in sets of 10 repetitions each or in a timed drill. One good variation of this drill is to have a crash pad nearby and Bryan will do 10 Partner Pick Ups, then throw Nikolay onto the crash pad on pick up number 11.

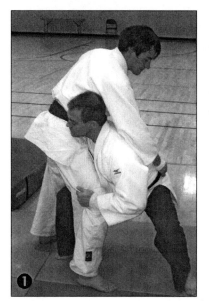

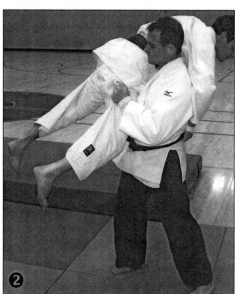

PARTNER WHEELBARROW WALK

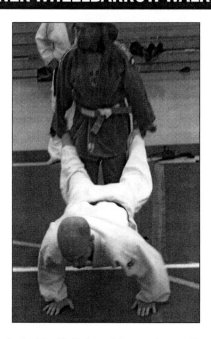

AnnMaria holds Kelly's ankles as he walks forward on his hands. You can change this drill so that Kelly walks backward while AnnMaria holds his ankles and walks backward. Kelly can walk sideways, go around in circles or walk on his hands in any direction to add more work to this exercise. This is an excellent exercise to work the shoulders, triceps, upper back and pectoral areas, but it's also a great exercise to work the smaller stabilizer muscles as well.

PARTNER PICK UP AND WALK

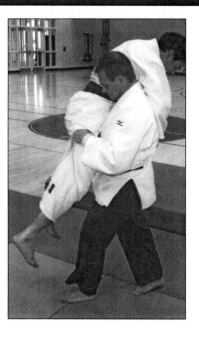

A good variation to add control to the entire movement is for Bryan to pick Nikolay up and walk forward with him. Bryan can also vary the drill by walking around in different directions. You never know if the guy you're trying to pick up and throw will fight like crazy and you have to walk a few steps to gain more control of him. This exercise helps prepare you for this situation.

PARTNER PICK UP WITH RESISTANCE

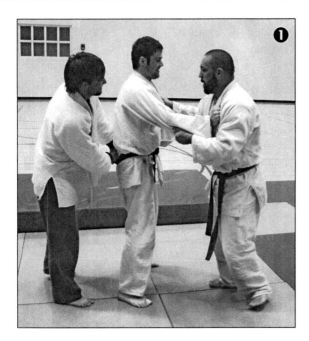

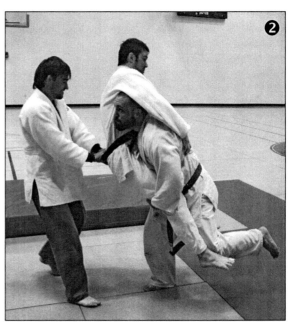

Jake is ready to lower his level and shoot in to pick Derrick up in a double leg throw. Nikolay is holding Derrick's belt.

Jake shoots in and picks Derrick up as far as he can. Nikolay holds onto Derrick's belt to add resistance and keep Jake from lifting him too high.

DEVELOP PICK UP POWER AND DRIVE

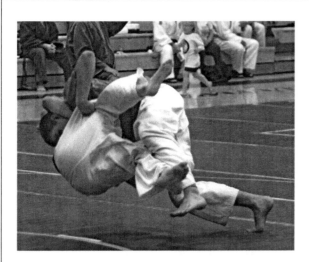

Throwing your opponent to the mat with control and force is developed by hard work in the gym and on the mat. This double leg scored maximum points in a freestyle judo match.

WHY PICK UP DRILLS WORK

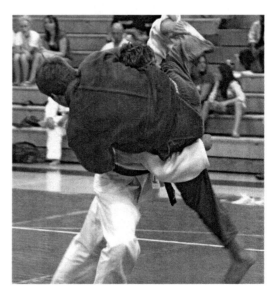

Here's why doing a lot of pick up drills work. This photo was taken at a national judo championship and shows how you can slam your opponent to the mat if you have trained yourself to do it. You can see how this athlete picked up his opponent and to gain more control and to add power to the throw, he is moving forward. Excellent training habits get excellent results.

PARTNER BUCK DRILL

1. Matt has his right arm hooked around Jake's head much the same way he would do a head and arm throw. Jake uses his hands and arms to grab around Matt's hips. It's important for Jake to have his head jammed onto the front of Matt's right shoulder for maximum control. Jake squats as low as he wishes to start the drill.

2. Jake arches up and "bucks" Matt up in the air. Jake can vary this exercise by walking forward a few steps with Matt up in the air for more control. Do 10 repetitions each or in a timed drill of 30 seconds for each athlete.

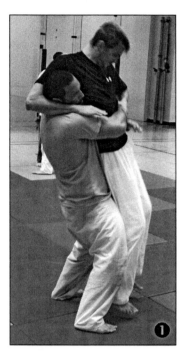

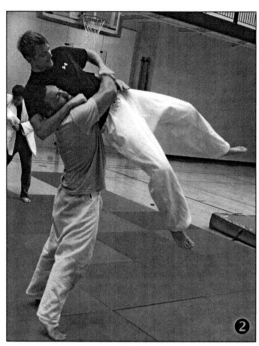

WHY THE BUCK DRILL WORKS

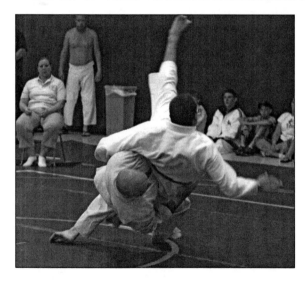

Big Will Cook throws his opponent to the mat with force and control. Call it what you want, the Suplex, Supple, Soufflé, Ura Nage, Belly-to-Belly, or the Buck, lifting your opponent up and slamming him back to the mat is a great throw. Whether it's used in MMA, judo, wrestling, sambo or any sport, this is a powerful throw. Lots of hours working on his core, hips and legs resulted in this powerful throw. The Buck Drill helped prepare Will to be able to do this throw when it counted at the judo nationals.

PARTNER PICK UP AND WALK (SCOOP HOLD)

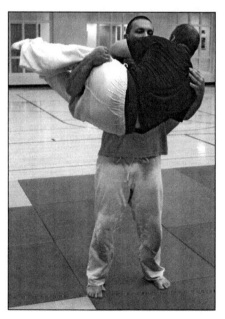

Jake picks Chris up as shown and takes him for a walk across the mat. In all carrying exercises, make sure you walk slowly and deliberately and never run. Safety is important in training.

BEAR HUG CARRY

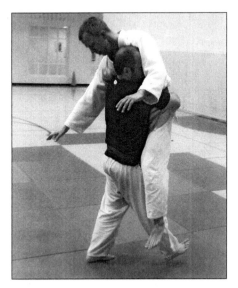

Chris gets Mike in a bear hug, picks him up and walks him across the mat.

FIREMAN'S CARRY WALK

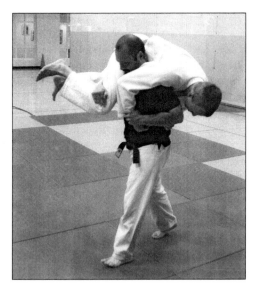

Load your partner up in a Fireman's Carry across your shoulders and walk across the mat.

FIREMAN'S CARRY SQUATS

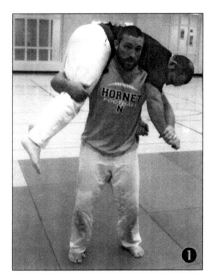

❶

Jake loads Chris up onto his shoulders as shown.

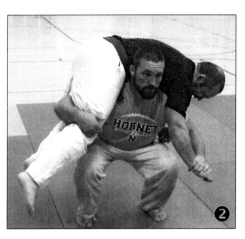

❷

Jake does a slow, deliberate squat, making sure not to bounce when he reaches the bottom of the squat.

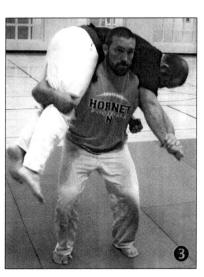

❸

Jake finishes the squat. Each athlete can do 10 or more reps as a good finish to a hard workout.

PARTNER SQUATS USING SCOOP HOLD

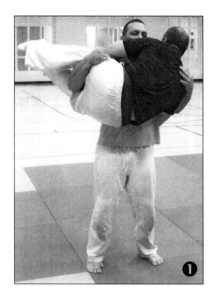

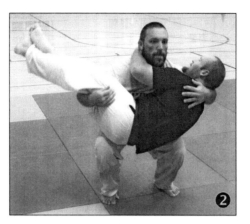

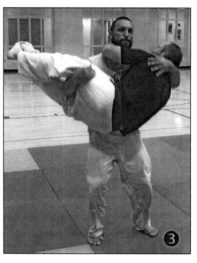

Jake picks up Chris as shown.

Jake does a good full squat with control. Don't bounce when squatting.

Jake finishes the squat. Do a set of 10 or more each as a good cool-down after a hard workout.

THE FIREMAN'S CARRY PAYS OFF ON THE MAT

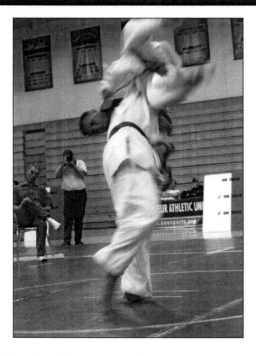

HAVING THE STRENGTH TO DO THE FIREMAN'S CARRY PAYS OFF ON THE MAT

It takes a lot of both strength and skill to throw an opponent like this. Scott Brink uses the Fireman's Carry with good results.

PICK UP THROWS REQUIRE SKILL AND STRENGTH

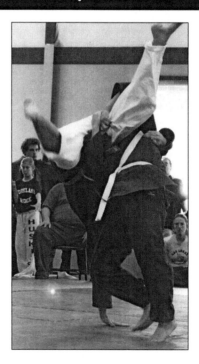

Picking up and carrying your training partner simulates doing the same thing you do to an opponent. This pick up throw in a freestyle judo match shows that hard training pays off.

BREGMAN HOP (UCHI MATA HOPPING DRILL)

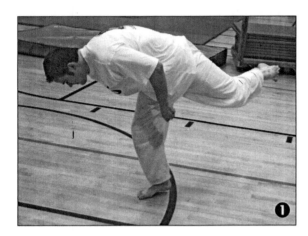

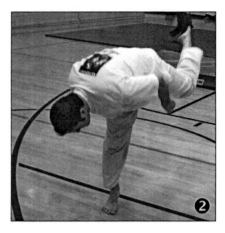

Jim Bregman, one of the greatest judo athletes ever from the United States, used this series of drills to make his Uchi Mata (Inner Thigh) throw one of the best in the business. Derrick is balancing on his right leg with his left leg extended backward, making sure to have his toe pointed. Derrick leans forward.

Derrick hops around in a full circle maintaining balance and control of his movement. Doing this simulates the throwing action of the Inner Thigh throw. This exercise helps develop all the stabilizer muscles in your legs and well as the agility, coordination and control necessary to execute skilled throwing techniques.

USE HANDS AS SUPPORT WHEN STARTING

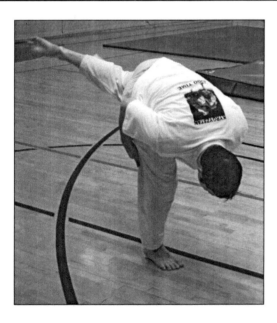

USE HANDS AS SUPPORT WHEN STARTING, BUT NOT LATER

When you start this drill, you can grab your base leg for support, but as you get better at balancing yourself, avoid grabbing your leg with your hands.

HOPPING ON THE BALL OF YOUR FOOT

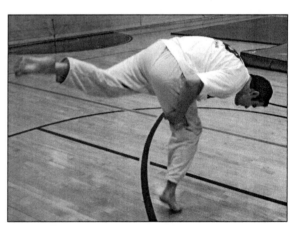

You can make this drill more difficult by hopping around on the ball of your supporting foot as shown here. Grab your leg when you first perform this drill to maintain your balance, but as you get better, avoid grabbing your leg.

TECHNICAL TIP: You can use and perform many of the drills and exercises shown in this part of the book off the mat as well as when on the mat.

BREGMAN LEG REAPS (UCHI MATA THROW DRILL USING A SUPPORT)

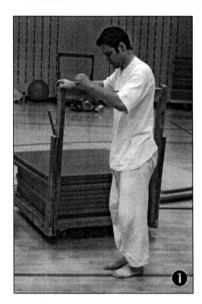 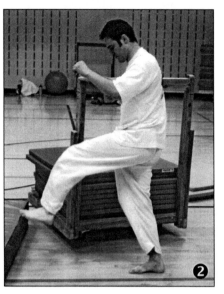

A good way to practice reaping or sweeping and to develop the muscles needed to have powerful leg sweeps is to do this drill as often as possible.

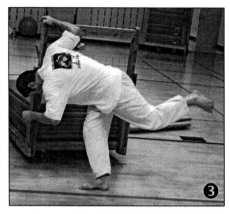

Derrick holds onto a support.

Derrick swings his left leg forward, making sure to point his toe for control.

Derrick reaps or sweeps his left leg back in the same motion he uses to throw an opponent.

BREGMAN HOPPING FORWARD ALONG A WALL

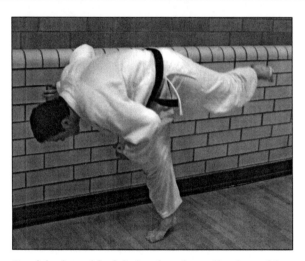

Derrick places his right hand on the wall to brace himself as he does the Bregman Hopping Drill. Derrick hops forward along the line of the wall on his right leg. He will hop back the other way holding onto the wall with his left hand and hopping on his left leg.

BREGMAN DRILL VARIATION

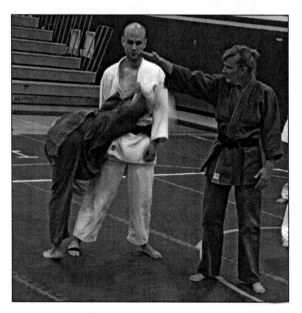

World Judo Champion AnnMaria (Burns) DeMars shows how you can use this leg reaping drill on the mat with partners. AnnMaria is holding onto Kelly for support while Sharon holds her hand up about shoulder level to serve as a target for AnnMaria's foot. AnnMaria holds onto Kelly's jacket as she reaps her right leg up high to touch Sharon's outstretched hand with her right foot.

BREGMAN HOPPING DRILL AND THROW WITH UCHI MATA (INNER THIGH THROW)

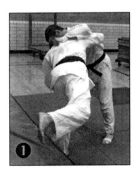 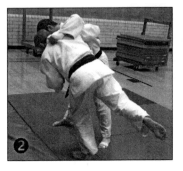 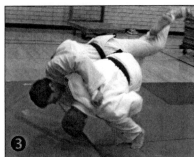 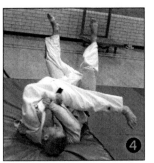

Drew is balanced on his left leg as he holds onto Derrick. Notice the crash mat at the bottom left of the photo. Drew's right leg is up off the mat.

Drew hops to his right (toward Derrick) on his left foot. Drew is moving into position to throw Derrick with Uchi Mata (Inner Thigh Throw).

Drew continues to hop on his left foot and leg toward Derrick and fits into position to throw Derrick.

Drew throws Derrick onto the crash mat. This drill really helps any grappler who is developing his Uchi Mata. Balance, coordination and agility are developed, as well as leg strength in supporting the hopping action.

This is a more advanced hopping and throwing drill.

HERE'S WHY THE BREGMAN DRILL WORKS

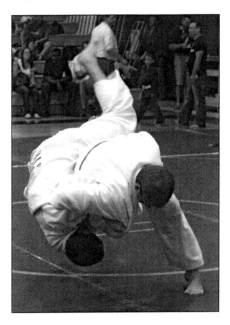

The Inner Thigh Throw (called Uchi Mata in judo) is one of the most widely used throwing techniques of all time. Scott Brink drills his opponent to the mat with a spectacular throw. Look at how his left leg is driving off the mat with the full power of the throw driving his opponent over. The hopping drills that U.S. Olympic Medallist Jim Bregman first made popular develop control and balance necessary for world-class performance in the Uchi Mata.

BACK VIEW OF WHY THE BREGMAN DRILL WORKS

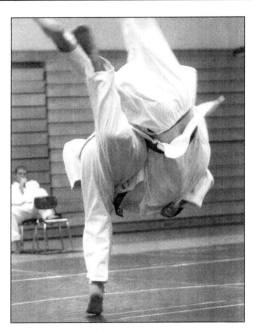

Mike Thomas caught his opponent with this spectacular throw and shows the balance and power of his Harai Goshi (Sweeping Hip Throw). Look at how Mike's left foot is balanced on the mat and generating tremendous power into the action of the throw. The Bregman Hopping Drill series develops the physical skills needed for a variety of throws (not only Uchi Mata) that require you to balance and support your entire body weight (and that of your opponent) and slam him to the mat.

PARTNER KICK PUSH DRILL (FRONT)

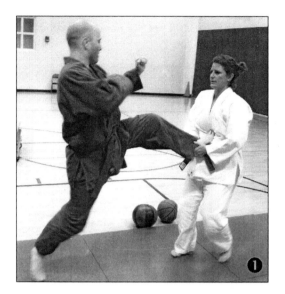 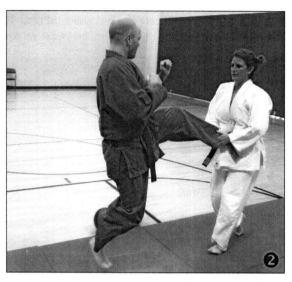

A good exercise to develop more power into your kicking is to place your foot against your partner's midsection and push forward as Brian is doing in this photo with Steph.

As Brian hops forward, pushing, Steph moves backward so Brian must continue to hop forward.

PARTNER KICK PUSH DRILL (SIDE)

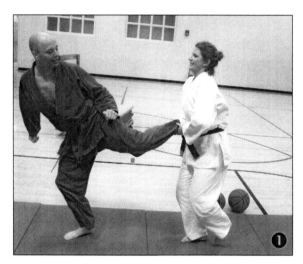 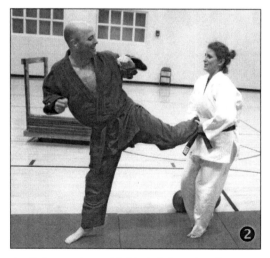

Brian works on his side kick by placing his left foot onto Steph's midsection as shown.

As Brian pushes with his left foot, Steph moves backward, forcing Brian to hop toward her. This is a great balance and coordination drill and is good for leg strength on the support leg.

UCHIKOMI (FIT INS) THE KING OF SKILL DEVELOPMENT FOR THROWING

This is an excellent exercise for skill development and cardio training. Pronounced "oo-chee-ko-mee" this drill is one of the oldest used in judo and jujitsu. This is a repetitive drill for the development of throwing techniques. Uchikomi has been used for years to develop throwing skills.

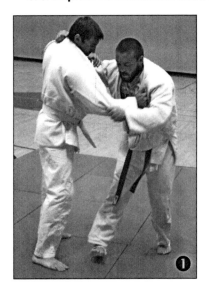

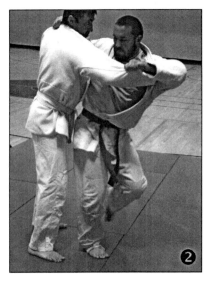

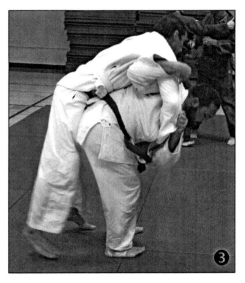

Basically, you are practicing your throws without actually throwing your partner. The goal is to fit your body into position each time using good form. Each time you fit in and come right back out, that is a repetition.

Jake uses his hands to pull and control Roy as he fits his body into place for a forward throwing technique.

Jake fits in using the 1-Arm Shoulder Throw (Ippon Seoi Nage). Jake will immediately come out of this and hit in again with another fit-in.

TECHNICAL TIP: Your goal is to perform one Uchikomi per second, but more importantly, use good, mechanically correct form and technique when doing your Uchikomi drills. Doing the actual throw is easy; the hard part is getting into the correct position instinctively every time.

MOVE AROUND THE MAT DRILL

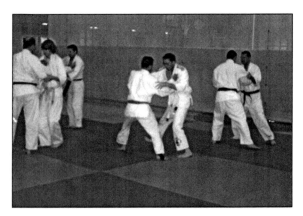

You and your partner move around the mat with each other. This is a good warm-up drill before stretching and helps you learn good movement on the mat. You can move in straight lines or randomly around the mat. You can cooperate with each other or offer resistance.

BUTSUKARI (FOOT SPEED) DRILLS TO IMPROVE THROWING

One of the best exercises or drills to use for improving your foot speed when throwing an opponent is the "Butsukari." Pronounced "boot-soo-kar-ee" this is an old drill used for many years in judo and is the fore-runner of the Uchikomi. In fact, many judo people consider them to be one in the same, but the Butsukari focuses more on foot speed than the Uchikomi drill.

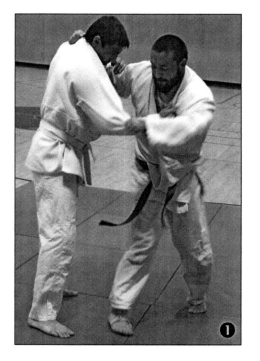

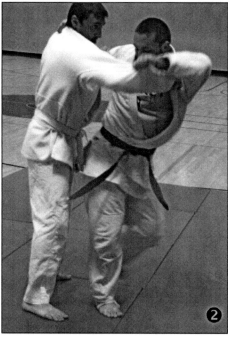

1. Doing Butsukari improves, not only your foot speed but also greatly assists your coordination skills in precise foot placement for throwing techniques.

2. Jake steps in, making sure his footwork is precise as he pulls Roy's right sleeve with his left hand.

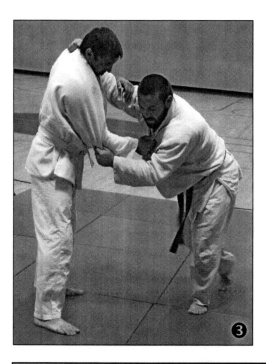

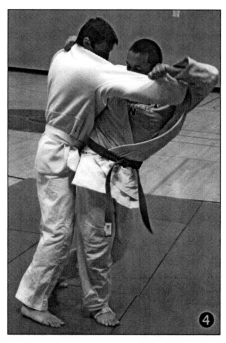

3. Jake jumps out and will start again.

4. Jake continues with another Butsukari. While some consider this drill "old fashioned" it's an effective drill and is a mainstay of elite judo and sambo athletes all over the world.

TECHNICAL TIP: The Butsukari drill is an excellent way to develop both coordination and foot speed. It also teaches you to pull your opponent to you with control and explosive power so that you will throw him more easily. Sometimes called a "Half Uchikomi" this drill produces positive results in foot speed and coordination.

UCHIKOMI DRILL TRAINING

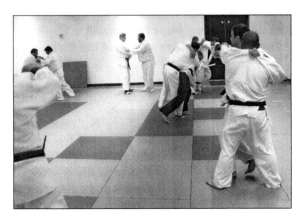

This shows the group doing an Uchikomi drill. Uchikomi training is similar to shadow boxing for fighters. It's a fantastic way to develop the many complex skills necessary to throw an opponent. The hardest part of any throwing technique is actually getting into the best position to do the throw and Uchikomi training helps tremendously. It's an old drill, but one that has proven its value.

TIMED UCHIKOMI
Do as many good, skillful fit-ins in a specified time limit. Another good way of doing this is to pyramid the time limit. Start with each partner doing as many fit-ins as possible in 30 seconds, and then go a 20-second round, followed by a 10 second round. It may not sound like much time, but it's harder than it sounds. You can always increase the time as you improve.

I DO 10, YOU DO 10
You can do 10 fit-ins, and then your partner does his 10. If 10 are too easy, do 25, 50 or any number you wish.

STATIC UCHIKOMI
A good way to develop the fine points of a throw is to do your fit-ins with your opponent standing still. Since your partner isn't resisting, your eventual goal should be to get in 1 Uchikomi per second.

INTERVAL STATIC UCHIKOMI TRAINING ROUTINE
When author John Saylor was the Head Coach for the Judo Squad at the U.S. Olympic Training Center, he developed this Interval Training Static Uchikomi routine for his athletes. Remember, elite athletes in Colorado Springs, Colorado at high altitude did this routine. It's a gut buster.
    Set 1: 4 rounds of 1-minute Static Uchikomi with 1 minute rest between rounds.
    Rest 2 minutes or wait until your heart beat returns to 120 before starting next set.
    Set 2: 8 rounds of 30-second Static Uchikomi with 30 seconds rest between rounds.
    Rest 2 minutes or wait until your heart beat returns to 120 before starting next set.
    Set 3: 10 rounds of 15-second Static Uchikomi with 15 seconds rest between rounds.
    Rest 2 minutes or wait until you heart beat returns to 120 before starting next set.
    Set 4: 6 rounds of 15 second Static Uchikomi with 15 seconds rest between rounds.

MOVING UCHIKOMI
Static Uchikomi drills are excellent for developing basic skills and entries into throwing technique, as well as for endurance training. However, not many (if any) opponents you encounter will stand still for you and let your throw them. By using Moving Uchikomi drills, you will develop the "feel" for how to attack a moving opponent, and when performed in interval training style, will also develop excellent cardio endurance. You and your partner can move in any pattern you wish: a straight line forward and back, move laterally, move about in a circle, or in a random pattern around the mat. The idea is to get in a lot of fitting practice.

INTERVAL MOVING UCHIKOMI TRAINING
Pick a throw and then move around the mat attacking your partner throughout timed rounds. Since you're moving and setting your partner up between attacks, your heart rate won't climb as high as it did when you did the Interval Static Uchikomi drill. However, this is a tough drill, so make sure you're in good enough shape to tackle it.
    Set 1: 4 rounds of 1-minute Moving Uchikomi with 1 minute rest between rounds.
    Rest 2 minutes or wait until your heart beat returns to 120 before starting next set.
    Set 2: 8 rounds of 30 seconds Moving Uchikomi with 30 seconds rest between rounds.
    Rest 2 minutes or wait until your heart beat returns to 120 before starting next set.
    Set 3: 10 rounds of 15 seconds of Moving Uchikomi with 15 seconds rest between rounds.
    Rest 2 minutes or wait until your heart beat returns to 120 before starting next set.
    Set 4: 6 rounds of 15 seconds of Moving Uchikomi with 15 seconds rest between rounds.

MOVING UCHIKOMI COMBINATION THROW DRILL
A good variation of this drill is rather than attacking with a single throw, string a series of throws together in a combination ad you move your partner around the mat.

CIRCLE UCHIKOMI DRILL

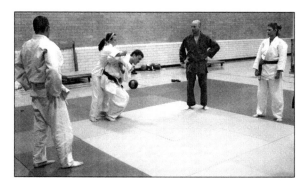

A good way to vary your Uchikomi training is to have your training partners get into a circle, and then do 10 fit-ins on each person. As one person finishes, the next person will start. You can also have your coach or a training partner time each person for a specified time period and do as many Uchikomi as possible per person. You can also do this with everyone standing in a line. How you put variety into your training is only limited to everyone's imagination.

GYM UCHIKOMI

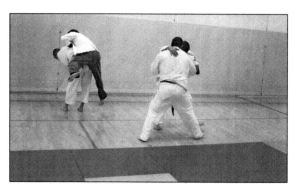

If you have limited mat space but access to a big gym, this drill is excellent. Perform Uchikomi on the gym floor moving up and down the length of the floor. This provides everyone with a lot of fit ins and since you're not doing this drill on a mat, and you don't want to accidentally throw your partner on the floor, it forces you to be more precise and careful in doing the actual technique.

TAKE ON THE LINE GROUNDFIGHTING UCHIKOMI

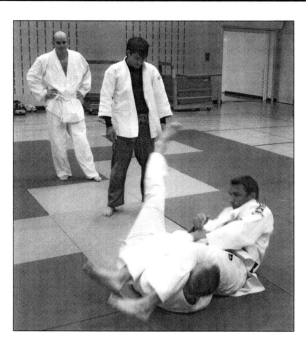

Here's a good drill for groundfighting. Select a skill such as the Spinning Juji Gatame as shown here and have each athlete take on the line as Roy is doing. You can do this as a timed drill where each athlete does as many reps as possible or have each athlete do a specified number of reps. This is a great drill when there are only a few athletes on the mat and it offers excellent cardio training in addition to the skill training.

GROUNDFIGHTING UCHIKOMI (FIT IN PRACTICE)

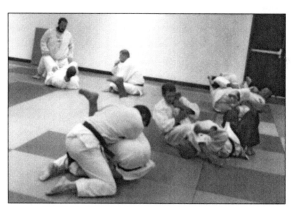

A lot of people think that Uchikomi or repetition exercises only apply to throws, but you can do them in groundfighting as well. Basically, you do a move for a specified number of repetitions, and then it's your partner's turn. To develop good skills, cooperate with each other. One grappler does 5 reps, and then his partner does 5 reps. You can also do a timed drill so that one grappler does as many good fit ins as possible (say, for instance, a spinning Juji Gatame) in 30 seconds. Then, his partner will do as many as possible in 30 seconds. You can vary levels of resistance, but it's best done with 100% cooperation from both athletes so both of you benefit from the skill development and the good cardio workout it provides.

PARTNER 3-MAN HOOK AND DRIVE DRILL

3-Man Uchikomi Drill

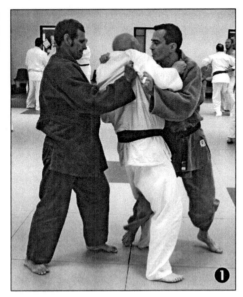

Also called a "sandwich" drill. Poor Kevin is in the middle, while Kelvin holds him up as Kirk hooks in with an Inside Hook or Major Inner Reap Throw. Kirk uses his right leg to hook the inside of Kevin's left leg. (An Outside Hook or Major Outer Reap Throw can also be used in this drill. Kirk will simply use his right leg to hook the outside of Kevin's right leg.)

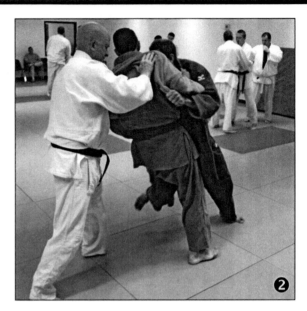

The group has switched positions and Kelvin hooks with his right leg and drives full blast into Kirk, in the middle. Kevin's job is to hold Kirk up and keep from getting thrown. Kelvin hooks in hard and holds this for a 3-count using this drill as an isometric drill to increase the power into the throw. This drill is effective because it's based on Isometric principles. Isometric holds will build tremendous strength in the sticking point of your throwing attack. Often, a fighter enters his throw really well, but fails to throw his opponent because of a weak finish. This drill develops a great amount of drive in the hips and legs, as well as in the rotational muscles of your core and torso, which are vitally important in all forward throws. Depending on your goals and fitness level, perform 1 to 3 sets of 5 reps with a 3-second hold on each rep.

WHY THE HOOK AND DRIVE DRILL WORKS

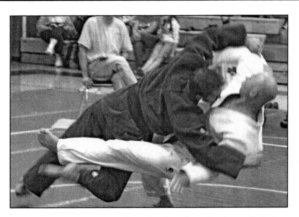

Here's a great example of why the Hook and Drive Drill works in a national tournament. Drew Hills is using the O Uchi Gari (Major Inner Reap) throw with good effect.

HOW THE HOLD AND RELEASE DRILL WORKS

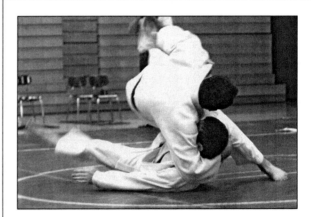

Look at the way Mark Lozano has thrown his opponent to the mat. This explosive drive puts his opponent flat on his back with tremendous force. The isometric action of the Hold and Release Drill translates into positive results for you!

PARTNER HOLD AND RELEASE DRILL (SEATED)

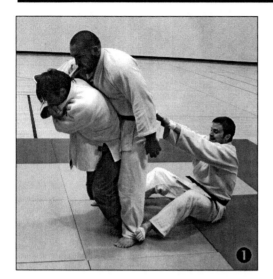

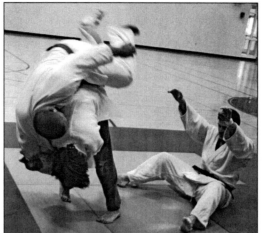

**3-Man Uchikomi
Static Overcome
by Dynamic Work**

This is another isometric drill for throwing that is very effective. This is similar to the 3-Man Hook and Drive Drill, with the exception being after the attacker hand struggle for 3 seconds, the spotter will let go of the middle athlete and let the attacker to complete the throw onto a crash pad. Nikolay fits in with a Shoulder Throw with Jake in the middle and Derrick holding Jake. Derrick has his feet placed on the back of Jake's feet at Jake's heels as shown and uses both hands to hold Jake's belt.

Derrick counts to 3 and lets go of Jake's belt. Nikolay throws Jake hard to the mat. Make sure you have a crash pad located immediately in front of the grapplers for safety. Derrick makes sure to roll back as he lets go of Jake's belt to avoid getting kicked by Jake's feet. What you are doing in this drill is similar to the effect of weight releasers in powerlifting. When using weight releasers, for instance on the Squat, the lifter goes down into the Squat with maximal weight. When he hits the bottom of the Squat, the weight releasers remove a large amount of weight and the lifter can now explode up out of the bottom position. This develops tremendous speed and power.

PARTNER 3-MAN HOOK AND DRIVE DRILL

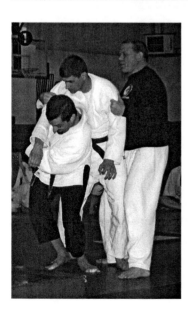

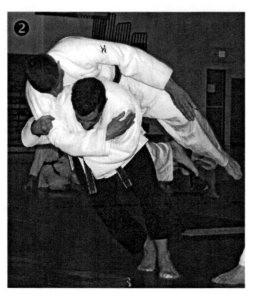

1. John is holding onto Scott (in the middle) while Jim fits into a shoulder throw. Jim starts to pull hard and begin his throw. John increases the resistance by pulling back on Scott. This is the same drill as the previous one, except that John is standing and holding onto Scott.

2. John lets go of Scott and quickly steps back. Jim throws Scott with more force than he would in a regular throwing drill. Getting thrown this hard isn't pleasant. For everyone's safety, use crash pads in these hard throwing drills. These isometric drills are very effective, but they're not pleasant. Use them early in your training cycle when you are working on skill training and drilling.

CRASH PAD THROWING

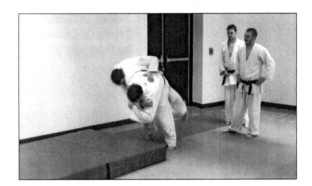

You get a tremendous workout and can do a lot more full throws with your training partners when you use a crash mat. Be careful to position your body and your partner's body so that you will throw him on the crash pad. Using crash pads develops your instinct and skill in following through and slamming your opponent hard onto the mat, then following through to a groundfighting technique. If you throw a good fighter, you must take the throw straight to the mat and finish him. Use your imagination and invent drills to improve your throwing and takedown skills. Try to work up to performing 100 full throws every practice onto the crash pads.

If you want to develop strength in your throws, use heavier partners to throw onto the crash pads. If you want to develop explosive speed, use lighter partners. Since crash pad training really keys in on strength and explosive power (and not primarily endurance), perform 5 sets with a longer recovery period between sets. The number of sets you perform per workout will depend on what other things you need to accomplish during that workout, as well as your fitness level. Usually, to start out, try to get in at least 25 or so full throws on the crash pad and work your way to 100 per workout. Remember, if you're training for an upcoming tournament or are in a training cycle for a major event, do some of your throws with partners in your same weight class to get the feel of how someone your own body weight feels on a consistent basis. This photo shows the guys taking on the line, throwing each athlete in line. You can also use a timed drill where each grappler does as many good throws as possible in a specified time.

THROW YOUR JACKET DRILL

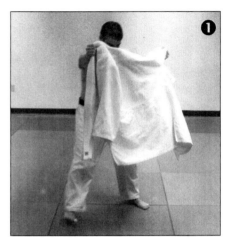

This is a good warm-up before stretching, but it's often used as a cool-down or as a finish to a workout. Basically, Derrick grabs his jacket and throws it around the mat, pretending there is an opponent in that jacket.

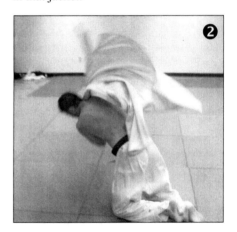

Derrick throws his jacket around. This is one opponent you should never lose to!

TECHNICAL TIP: Here's the reason why 3-Man Uchikomi Drills work, based on research. The 3-Man Uchikomi drills we've shown are all what are called Contrast Methods. When you've trained against the weight and resistance of two men (as done in a 3-man drill), it's a lot easier to throw just one!

With the Contrast Method, the contrast between the maximal weight as the lifter lowers into the squat and reduced weight as he drives back up to the top makes the weight feel light. Another example of this Contrast Method is a baseball player swinging a weighted ball bat before his turn at the plate. When the extra weight is removed, the bat feels light in his hands and he can swing the bat much faster.

Abundance or Surplus as a Factor in Throwing: Earlier in this book, we talked about the idea of creating an abundance or surplus in the various qualities needed for success in grappling, fighting or any martial art (or any event or activity). You want to have more strength, endurance, speed, flexibility and mental toughness than you actually need. This is the point of 3-Man Uchikomi Drills; you are developing an abundance of strength—even more than needed—in critical positions of a throwing technique. ONLY THROUGH ABUNDANCE OR SURPLUS CAN YOU OBTAIN RELIABILITY OF PERFORMANCE IN ANY FIGHTING SKILL.

HOFFMAN DRILLS
**DRILLS YOU CAN USE TO STRENGTHEN THE DIFFERENT PARTS OF
YOUR THROWING TECHNIQUES AND DEVELOP SPECIFIC ENDURANCE**

The following 4 drills were initially developed by Wolfgang Hoffman, 1964 Olympic Silver Medal Winner and later, the German National Judo Coach. He had his athletes exercise to failure but we've given set time limits to each exercise so that you don't hold back. The idea is to prefatigue a certain part of the body and then perform the technique.

These special drills are excellent for you to strengthen some part of your technique while at the same time serving as a form of lactic acid tolerance training. You do this by prefatiguing a part of our body and then link a technique that relies on that body part. Some people believe that all you need to do is to strengthen a technique is to simply practice that technique in its entirety. While this has some benefits, it won't solve the problem you have in some weak part of your technique. For an example, if your O Soto Gari (Major Outer Reap Throw) doesn't work when you need it to because your supporting (driving) leg gives out before you complete the throw, you need to develop the muscles in that leg to get the job done.

> **TECHNICAL TIP:** To strengthen any weak links in your arsenal of skills, you can use drills and exercises to solve problems. In many cases, drills can help you increase your fitness levels and skill levels at the same time. If you only practice the whole technique and not key in on the weak parts of it, you'll never solve any problems you may have. Remember, every skill or technique you do is a series of movements, all connected to each other. The stronger each movement is, the stronger the entire technique is.

HOFFMAN DRILL #1: PARTNER JUMP SQUATS AND THROW DRILL

This exercise is designed to develop explosive power from your legs that is necessary for all forward throwing techniques where you drive off both your legs. Depending on the time limit you set, this drill also develops a high level of anaerobic endurance, and is a form of lactic acid tolerance training.

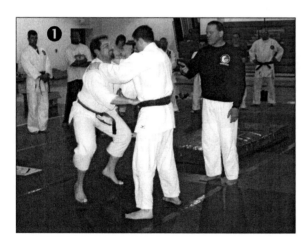

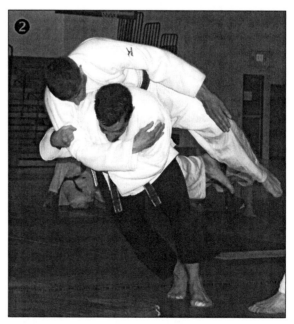

Jim faces Scott and grabs his belt with both hands. On John's signal, Jim performs jump squats for the specified time. Scott places his hands on Jim's shoulders and provides some resistance. As Jim reaches the top of his jump, Scott will push Jim back down with his hands. This causes an over-speed eccentric motion and kinetic energy will be stored in Jim's tendons, ligaments and soft tissue enabling him to explode back up to the next rep. Over-speed eccentrics are one of the best ways to develop explosive power. John will time Jim for 30 seconds, 45 seconds or 1 minute depending on Jim's fitness level and goals.

As soon as Jim finishes his jump squats, he immediately throws Scott with a forward throw that he drives with both of his legs. (Jim is using the Shoulder Throw in this photo.)

HOFFMAN DRILL #2: PARTNER PUSH UP AND GRIP FIGHT

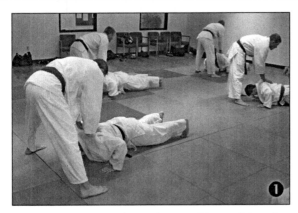 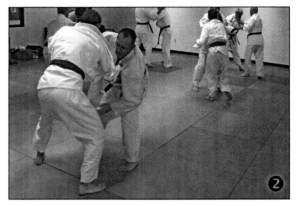

One partner drops to the push up position and the other provides resistance with his hands. Perform push-ups for a specified time limit. If you're new to this exercise, start with 15 seconds and work up to 30, then 45, and then 60 seconds. Chad is doing the push-ups and Aaron is standing.

When the time limit is up, Chad jumps up immediately, faces Aaron and starts grip fighting to get the dominant grip and position. If, after about 15 seconds, Chad isn't able to dominate Aaron in the grip fighting or get through his defense so that he can get in a throw or takedown, Chad will drop and do another set of push-ups. Repeat this sequence 5 times. Be sure to confine your techniques to an upper body situation.

HOFFMAN DRILL #3: PARTNER 1 LEG HOP & PUSH AND PERFORM A 1 LEG THROW

This is a good drill that strengthens your driving leg (your supporting leg) for 1-leg throws such a leg hooks, sweeps and throws like Uchi Mata (Inner Thigh Throw). This drill ties in really well with the Bregman Drills shown elsewhere in this part of the book.

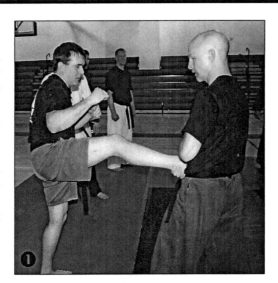 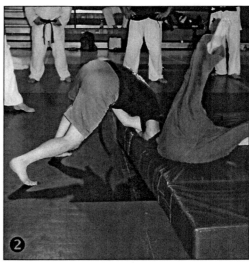

Brian's left leg is supporting him as he places his right foot in John's midsection. As John provides resistance, Brian pushes John across the mat until his supporting (driving) leg is fatigued. It's a good idea to put a time limit on Brian's hops and drive portion of this drill, so depending on your fitness level, drive your partner across the mat for 30 seconds, 45 seconds or 1 minute.

Immediately following the hops, Brian throws John onto the crash pad 5 times in a row. It's important for John to provide the right amount of resistance as Brian drives him across the mat. John will ease up if Brian's not moving forward, and if Brian's moving easily, John will add a little more resistance. The purpose of this drill is to pre-fatigue your driving leg with hops and then execute 5 1-leg throws where you drive off that same leg.

HOFFMAN DRILL #4: THROW YOUR PARTNER AND PICK HIM BACK UP

This drill develops overall body strength and endurance as well as grip strength, but the best thing is does for you is to develop your overall toughness. Perform this drill by doing 1 to 2 sets of 8 throws. You do 8 throws, and then your partner will do his 8 throws. Important: This is a tough drill for the guy getting thrown. Don't attempt this drill unless you and your partner have good skills in breakfalls!

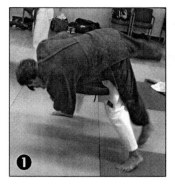 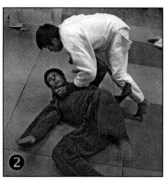 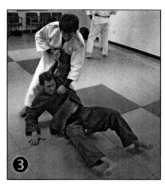 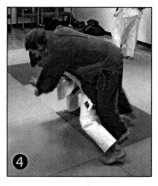

Alisher throws Kelvin to the mat.

Kelvin hits the mat with Alisher holding on with both hands.

Alisher drags Kelvin up off the mat to quickly throw him again.

Alisher throws Kelvin after pulling him up off the mat and will continue this until he has performed 8 throws.

STRETCH BAND RESISTANCE FOR UCHIKOMI

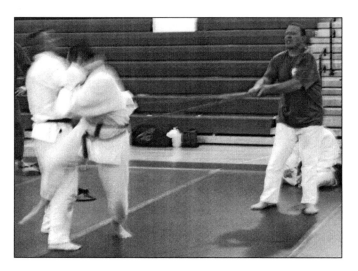

There are more Stretch Band Drills that can do on the mat later in this book.

Make your uchikomi practice for fit-ins for throwing tougher. John Saylor is holding one end of an elastic training band (but you could use a judo belt just as well) with the other end tied around the belt or waist of Jim. Mike is the target for the drill and John is far enough away from Jim to keep the band tight. **John has now increased the intensity of this 3-Man Uchikomi drill by using an elastic or stretch band.** Jim attacks with his uchikomi as shown in this photo and John provides enough tension in the band (or belt) to make Jim work harder when he attacks. This really helps in giving you more explosive power into your throwing or takedown attacks. There is more on band and cable training later in the book.

FIT IN, CARRY AND THROW DRILL

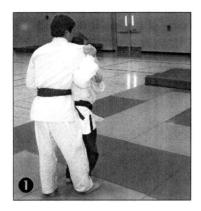
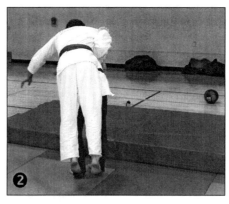
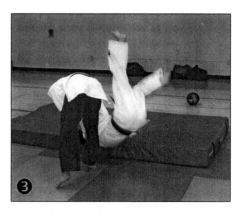

Bryan fits in for a Shoulder Throw (or any over-body throw) on one side of the mat.

Bryan loads Nikolay up and walks him across the mat to the crash pad.

Bryan throws Nikolay onto the crash pad. The pair runs back across the mat and Nikolay takes his turn.

RANDORI: THE BEST WAY TO GET INTO FIGHTING SHAPE IS TO PRACTICE FIGHTING

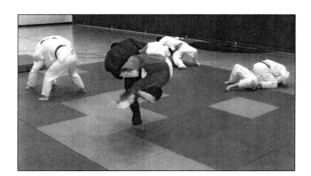

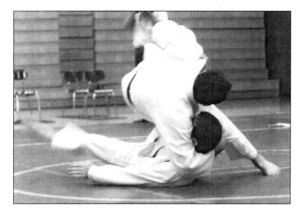

If you're training to be a fighter or a grappler and the best way to prepare yourself for fighting is to fight. However, there's a huge difference between training in a dojo or in a gym and an actual fight or match. The Japanese use the word "randori" to describe "free practice." In wrestling, it's called "going live" and in many MMA gyms, it's called "rolling." Call it what you want, it's not a fight; it's a workout. But, having said that, it's easily understood to be a practice match, with the emphasis on practice. If you go full blast, 100%, and caveman every time you roll with the other guys in the gym, you'll limit yourself to only using the moves you are good at and not be willing to try new things in a variety of situations.

Randori, going live or rolling in the gym or dojo should provide you and your training partners with a variety of situations and positions. Also, if you beat up on your training partners, you'll soon be without many training partners. Set the ground rules with your workout partner; sometimes you'll both go 100% and sometimes you'll both agree to go only 50%. Bryan Potter uses what he calls "smiling randori" from time to time. That's when you and your partner go just hard enough that you can manage to smile.

TECHNICAL TIP: Randori, Going Live or Rolling isn't a match; it's practice. There's a difference. It's a time to try new moves, tactics and other aspects of your sport. If you're working with someone who's not as good as you, don't beat him up. Instead, try different things, and allow him to try some things as well. Don't have your best fights in the gym or dojo; make sure they happen where it really counts.

GROUNDFIGHTNG RANDORI: GETTING INTO FIGHTING SHAPE

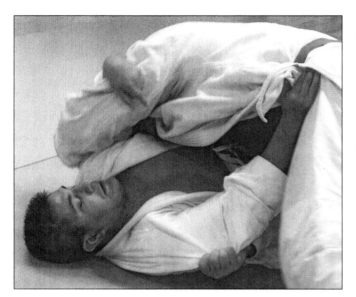

A terrific way to fight yourself into shape is to do lots of rounds of groundfighting randori. Terry and Jake are taking their training seriously in this round of groundfighting. Start in various positions that actually come up in a real match and start rolling. Going on the ground like this gives you no chance to slouch off. Go in timed rounds and use your imagination on how to make this training more interesting. Take on a new, fresh partner every minute, going 5 or more partners in a row. Go for 2-minute, 3-minute, 4-minute or 5-minute rounds to push yourself all the harder.

Caution: Don't simply show up, warm up and then fight for an hour. You can do this once in a while, but not all the time. A well-rounded workout is vital to your success. Simply showing up and fighting is not well rounded and won't yield positive results. You need to perform drills, work on your skill and technique and have structure to your training. If you want to win, train hard, but also train smart!

PARTNER BRIDGES (CHEST TO CHEST)

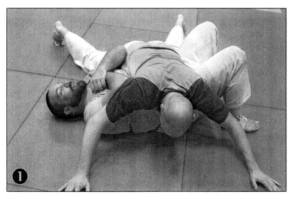

Ben lies across Jake as shown to provide weight. Jake is on his back ready to perform a bridge.

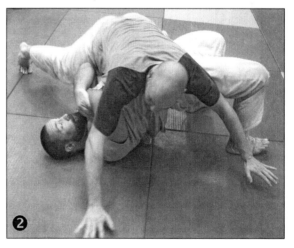

Jake bridges up for 10 repetitions, then will switch places with Ben. You can also do this drill for a specified time period, usually 30 seconds.

PARTNER HEAD AND ARM PIN BRIDGE

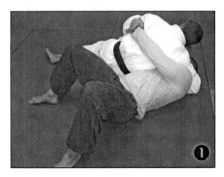 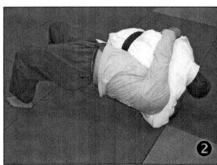 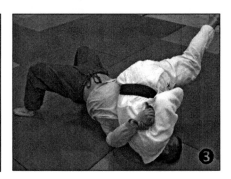

Drew is holding Bryan in a Head and Arm Pin (Kesa Gatame). Any pin or hold will do for this drill however.

Bryan bridges as shown.

As Bryan bridges, he quickly rolls Drew over his shoulder as shown. Bryan can roll Drew over, or ease onto his back to do another repetition. Do this drill in 30-second rounds or sets of 10 repetitions. Drew can offer varying degrees of resistance, but as a strength drill, it's recommend that Drew simply serve as "weight" for Bryan.

STEAL THE BALL DRILL FROM THE GUARD

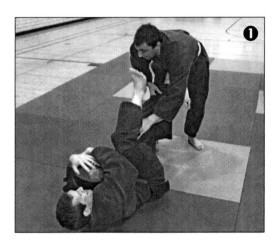 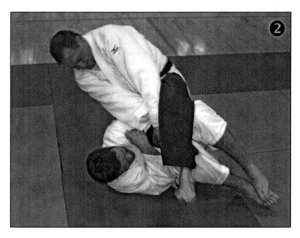

One athlete holds a ball (or anything for that matter, but a ball works best) as shown here. Don't hold the ball and roll over onto your front. Stay on your back or side as in the guard position. The top grappler's job is to take the ball away from his partner.

This is an active drill that works both athletes harder than you might think. This is primarily a core exercise, but it really works the entire body. When one grappler gets the ball away from his partner, they trade positions. You can also do this in timed rounds.

STEAL THE BALL FROM JUJI GATAME LEG PRESS

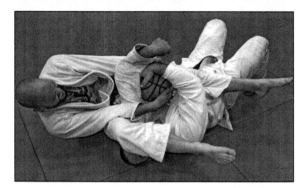

This is the same drill as the other one from the guard position, but Jake is on his back and Ben has him in a leg press position for Juji Gatame. Jake tries to keep the ball and Ben tries to get it away from him.

WHY STEAL THE BALL DRILL WORKS

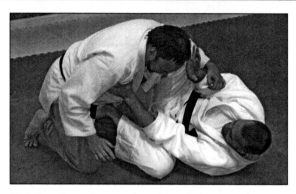

Fighting from the guard position is hard work, especially on your core area. Your abdominals, low back, glutes, legs and just about every other part of your body works hard in this position.

PRYING OPPONENT'S ARM FREE IN THE LEG PRESS

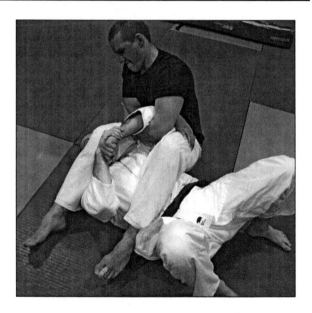

PRYING OPPONENT'S ARM FREE IN THE LEG PRESS POSITION TO APPLY JUJI GATAME

Jarrod is working hard to pull Brian's arms apart to secure Juji Gatame. Brian must keep his arms in close to his body and keep Jarrod from prying them apart. The Steal the Ball Drill is a good way for Brian to develop the strength to keep his arms in and defending against an armlock.

3-PERSON PIN ESCAPE DRILL

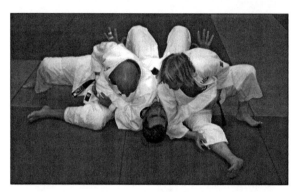

Two partners hold down the third partner in this tough drill. This is a great total body workout, including cardio. This variation shows the top 2 pinning the upper body.

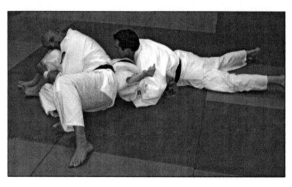

This variation is tougher and one partner holds the upper body while the other partner holds the lower body. This is a tough drill, but one that is a good addition to your training.

PARTNER THIGH SQUEEZE

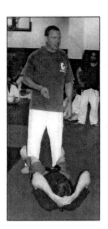

John stands between Brian's legs as Brian uses them to push in. John can stand with his legs close or far apart, forcing Brian to work the inner thighs and hip flexors.

WHY YOU NEED STRONG THIGHS, HIPS AND LEGS

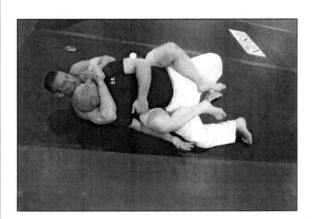

Mike had Scott in a strong rodeo ride, setting him up for a rear naked choke. Using your legs to control you opponent is a vital skill and having the strength and flexibility to use your lower body effectively is developed through effective drill training and exercises.

LEG PRESS FROM GUARD

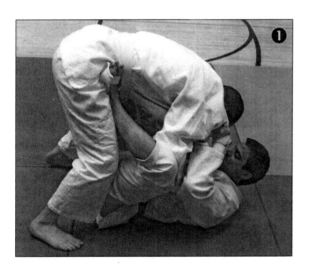

Derrick is on his back in the guard position with Nick above him as shown. Derrick has each foot jammed in each of Nick's hips.

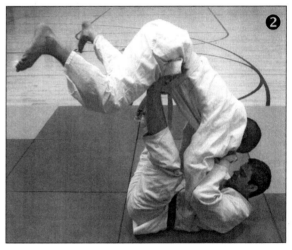

Derrick does a leg press as shown. This is a great leg strengthening exercise for fighting from the guard when doing sweeps and rollovers.

BUTTERFLY LEG PRESS FROM GUARD

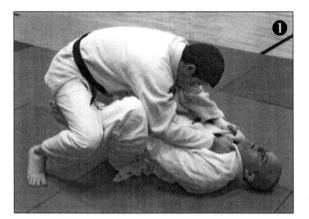

Nick is on his back with his shins jammed in each of Derrick's inner thighs as shown.

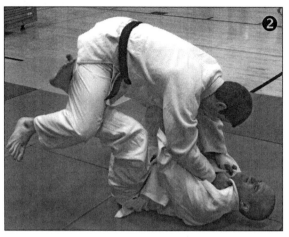

Nick does a leg press from this position. This is a tough exercise but really helps develop the leg and hip strength from this position for sweeps and fighting from the guard using your legs.

TRIANGLE CHOKE DEFENSE DRILL

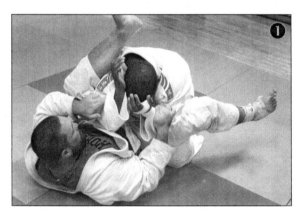

Jake, on the bottom, is trying to form a Triangle Choke on Andre. Andre's rolls his right shoulder in (like a boxer would) and he jams his right elbow into Jake's left leg preventing Jake from forming the triangle.

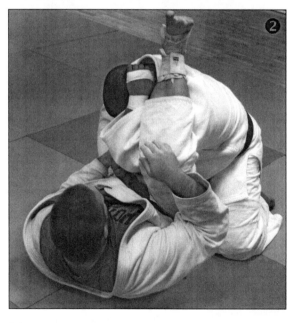

Jake immediately switches legs and moves his right leg up to start the triangle while Andre blocks that leg as well and blocks the triangle. This is a good workout and develops good skills for the Triangle Choke and how to block it form this position.

PARTNER JUJI GATAME ARM CURLS (1 ARM)

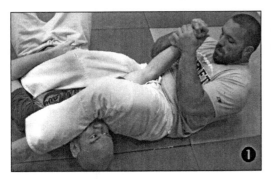 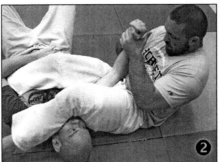 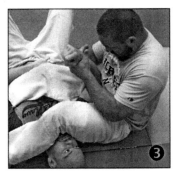

Ben is on his back with Jake on top of him in the Leg Press position. Jake is holding Ben's right arm as shown.

Ben uses his right arm to curl up and Jake offers no resistance other than the weight of his body.

Ben completes the curl with his arm and pulls Jake up. This is a good exercise for the entire arm. Ben will perform 10 reps and switch sides and do this drill with his left arm.

PARTNER JUJI GATAME ARM CURLS (BOTH ARMS)

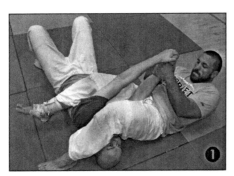 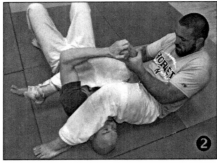 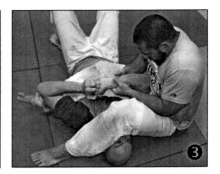

Ben is on his back with Jake holding him with the Leg Press. Ben uses his left hand to grab his right hand as shown.

Ben curls Jake up, with Jake offering no resistance other than the weight of his body.

Ben completes the curl using both arms. Do 10 reps per arm, then switch positions and let your partner do his.

WHY ARM AND SHOULDER STRENGTH IS IMPORTANT IF YOU'RE STUCK ON THE BOTTOM

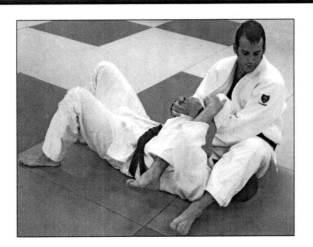

Kelvin is on the bad end of Josh's leg press position and has to protect his arm. Josh is pulling hard to pry Kelvin's arm free so he can stretch it out for the tap out. Kelvin's technical skills, along with some serious arm strength, are what it takes to get him out of this bad situation.

BELT TOWING

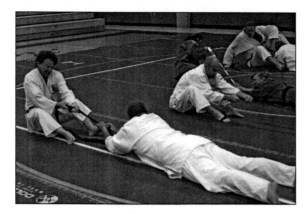

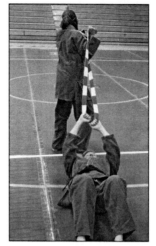

You can also hold your belt over your arm and shoulder in the same way you would use your arm and shoulder in a Shoulder Throw. Your partner lies on her back and holds onto your belt as you tow her across the mat.

Here's the basic variation of this towing drill. This is a tough workout and is good to use, once in a while, as a finisher after your on-mat training.

Sit on your rear end while your partner lays on his front as shown. Each of you grabs an end of your belt and you pull him backward across the mat. This group of coaches at a coach clinic got a good workout. This is a great drill as a warm-up before stretching and is excellent for upper back development.

TUG OF WAR (STANDING OR SEATED)

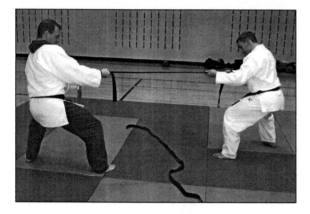

Use your belt as a rope and play tug of war. Use another belt or put a tapeline on the mat to use as a marker to cross over. When you pull your partner over the line, you win.

Any variation of this exercise is a benefit to your training. Play tug of war when you are seated on or the knees.

PLACE MORE STRESS ON YOURSELF IN TRAINING

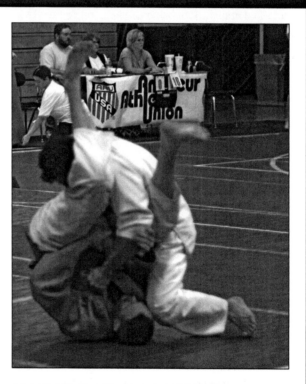

PLACE MORE STRESS ON YOURSELF IN TRAINING THAN YOUR OPPONENT WILL IN A MATCH
A result of your hard training is your attitude that no matter what any opponent throws at you in a match or fight, it can't possible be as tough as what you went through in preparation for that fight. Your success in a fight or in a tournament is the direct result of your efforts when training for that fight.

SECTION TWO: PART 2: FREEHAND EXERCISES OFF THE MAT

• • • "Do what you can with what you have where you are." Theodore Roosevelt

The purpose of "freehand" exercises is to use your own body weight. Often called "calisthenics" these exercises provide hard, honest work and should be included in every athlete's training program. This part of Section 2 presents some good freehand exercises for you to use as a reference. You might have a slight variation of how it's shown here, but a good push up is a good push up. Also, there are an almost infinite variety of ways to do these exercises, so play around with them and try to make them harder to do or adapt to your capabilities. While not every exercise ever invented is shown here, we highly recommend doing them.

Freehand exercises are great because they require no (or minimal) equipment, can be done when you're traveling and in a hotel room or can be done as a break from training in the weight room. Freehand exercises are the best way to start someone out in a strength program, especially kids. Lifting your body weight with control and balance is tough work and freehand exercises provide a strong foundation for any athlete.

A good way to perform Freehand Exercises is to decide how many sets you want to perform and then do as many reps as possible per set. In other words, set a goal of doing 10 sets of push-ups. Then, do as many reps as possible each set. You can also do these exercises in a specified time. For instance, do as many good Burpees as possible in 1 minute, then 2 minutes, and then 3 minutes. Another good workout you can do is to get some "quality time" when watching television. Instead of running to the refrigerator during a commercial, do as many Push Ups, Crunches, Burpees or other Freehand Exercise as possible during that commercial break. After an hour of watching the boob tube, you'll find that you got a decent little workout.

Add them to your regular workout routine as filler. Freehand exercises are versatile and useful for all athletes.

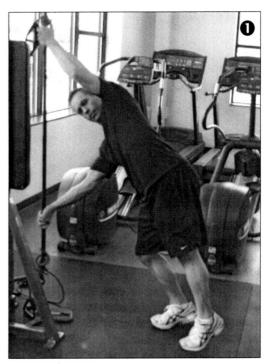

Starting with the toughest freehand exercise around, the Flagpole is a demonstration of serious strength and control of your body. The longer you can hold the position, the harder it is and the stronger you are. Drew starts this exercise by grabbing both hands on a vertical pole as shown.

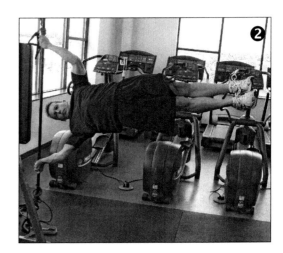

Drew completes the Flagpole by leaping up and holding his body out sideways using his arms as shown. Drew held this position for 12 seconds, demonstrating impressive strength and body control.

BURPEE (SQUAT THRUST)

The Burpee is an old standby and for good reason. It's a great exercise for cardio endurance, hip and leg strength and is generally, one of the best exercises you can do.

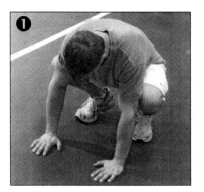

Drew squats down as shown.

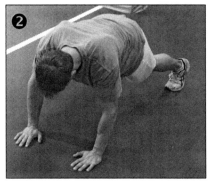

He shoots both his legs out straight behind him.

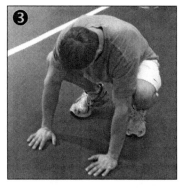

Drew brings his legs back under him in a squat.

DRIVING OFF THE LEG

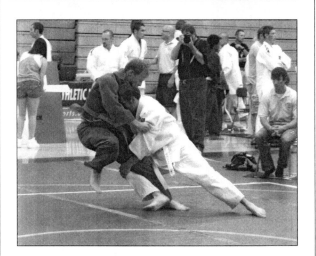

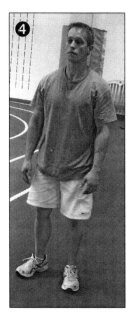

Drew finishes the exercise by standing up straight, ready to do another rep.

DRIVING OFF THE LEG TO THROW AN OPPONENT REQUIRES STRENGTH

Exercises like the Burpee or Mountain Climber develop the explosive strength necessary to throw opponents to the mat as Josh Henges is doing here at the AAU Grand Nationals.

MOUNTAIN CLIMBER

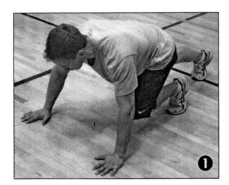

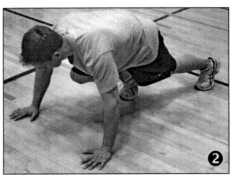

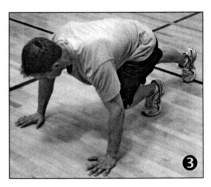

This is a good freehand cardio exercise. Do this in sets of 25 or 50, or in a specified time such as 30 seconds or 1 minute rounds. Drew starts with his left leg forward and right leg extended.

Drew moves his right foot forward and shoots his leg foot back as shown.

Drew continues this for the specified time or number of repetitions he chooses.

CRUNCHES (BENT KNEES)

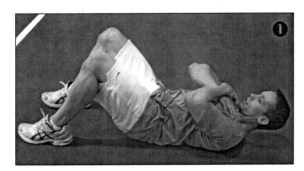

This isn't a sit up, but rather a "crunch" where you curl up and tighten your entire core. Some people place their hands behind their head when doing this (or any crunch or sit up) exercise. We recommend you place your hands across your chest as shown rather than behind your head or neck. When placing your hands behind your head, you tend to use them to help lift you up as your body crunches or curls up in this exercise.

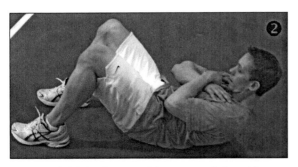

Drew curls his body us, making sure to tighten his core and abdominal muscles.

CRUNCHES (LEGS UP)

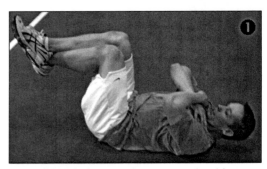

Drew lifts his legs as shown to make this exercise harder.

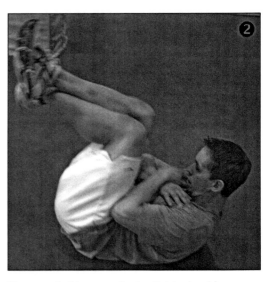

Drew curls his upper body, tightening his core.

SIT OUTS

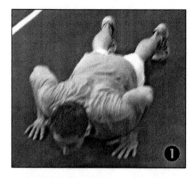

This is a good cardio workout, but is excellent for agility and coordination. An old drill from wrestling, it's really a good exercise that any athlete should use on a regular basis. Start this exercise in a push up position.

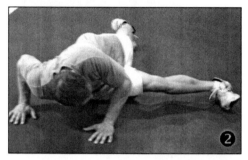

Drew shoots his right leg to his left as far as possible.

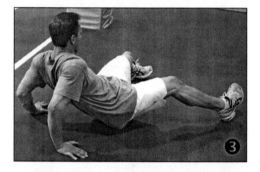

Drew turns to his left.

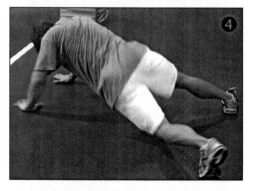

He then swings his left leg backward under his hips.

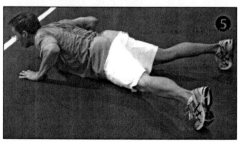

Drew finishes the rep in the push up position as shown.

PLANK

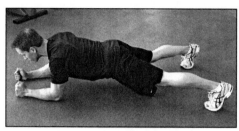

This exercise is a great exercise for your core muscles. It also doubles as a muscular endurance and balance movement. We'll have more on this exercise in the section featuring the Exercise Ball. Drew is balanced on his forearms as shown with legs fully extended and on his toes. He holds his body up and straight as a board (this is why it's called a "plank"). Hold this exercise for as long as possible with a minimum of at least 30 seconds. Do 5 sets of holding it as long as possible for a good workout.

PLANK WITH ARM RAISE

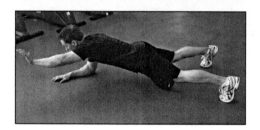

Make the plan harder by lifting one arm.

PLANK ARM & LEG RAISE

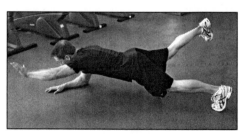

Make it even harder by lifting your left arm and right leg, then switch to your right arm and left leg.

PLANK TORSO STRETCH

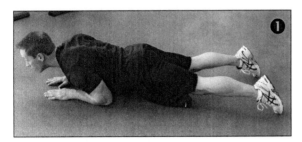

This is harder than it looks. Drew holds himself in a plank.

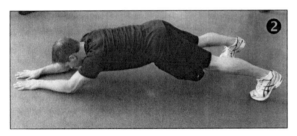

Drew moves both of his arms out in front of him as shown as he arches up slightly with his hips.

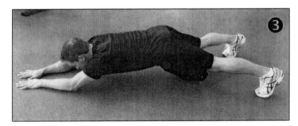

Drew is on his toes and as he moves his hands out as far as possible in front, he moves his feet back as far as possible.

PLANK HIP TURN

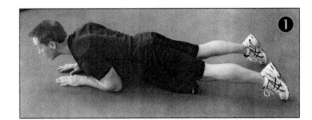

Drew holds himself in a plank.

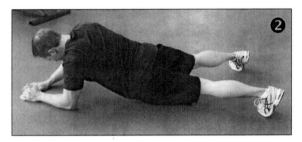

Drew turns to his right as shown, making sure not to touch his hip on the floor.

HIP AND LEG STRENGTH AT WORK ON THE MAT

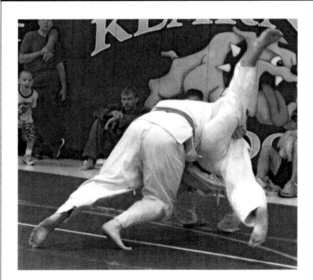

Whether it's on the mat or in a street fight, the ability to lift up your opponent and slam him down comes from strong hips and legs. The arms have the job of securing your opponent to your body as you execute the technique. When you have fully developed hips and legs you will have more weight centered in your lower body, making your body more stable in general. Your body is like a house; build it from the basement up.

HALF SIT OUTS (JUDO SIT OUTS)

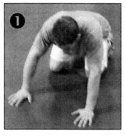 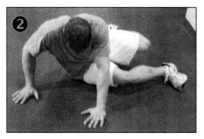 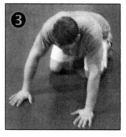 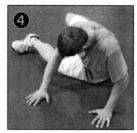

This is a good agility drill and a good cardio workout as well. Drew is on all fours.

Drew shoots his right leg through.

Drew then brings his right leg back and assumes the all fours position again.

He immediately shoots his left leg through. He repeats the sequence for as many reps as possible.

HINDU SQUAT

The Hindu Squat was a standard for the old-time Indian and Pakistani wrestlers such as the Great Gama, who is said to have performed as many as 4,000 repetitions of this exercise every day. He would include 1-leg squats and jumping squats as well. While there may be some controversy about the number of reps he did daily, there was never any doubt about the strength of Gama's lower body and it came from hard training. High repetition Hindu Squats build a strong lower body and overall endurance.

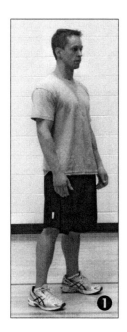 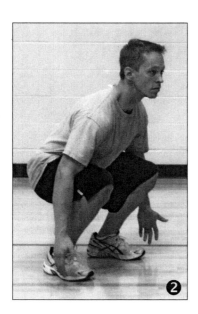 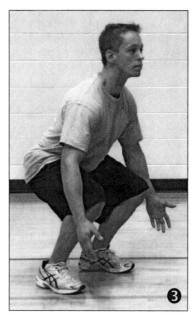 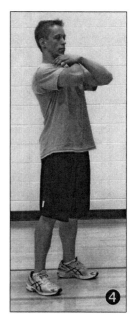

To do this exercise, stand with your legs under your hips, keeping your back straight.

Drew squats low as shown, making sure to keep his back straight and look forward. Drew scoops with his hands and arms. Drew does a full squat, making sure not to bounce back up from the bottom of the squat.

Drew scoops his hands and arms forward as he raises up from the squat.

Drew completes the Hindu Squat by crossing his hands in front of his chest.

SUMO OR MODIFIED HINDU SQUAT (WIDE STANCE)

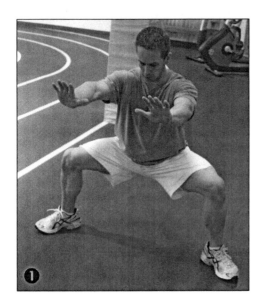

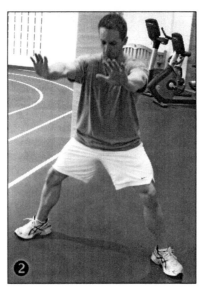

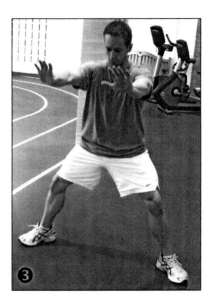

Drew is performing the Sumo Squat or Modified Hindu Squat. He is holding his arms out in front of him and has taken a wide stance with his feet pointing outward as shown. The Sumo Squat works your inner thighs really hard along with your hip flexors, quads and hamstrings.

Drew squats down as far as he can and then comes back up. Don't bounce on the Sumo Squat, but rather squat up and down with control. Like the Hindu Squats, perform Sumo Squats at a steady pace and make it your goal to perform 100 reps every 3 minutes.

Drew comes out of his Sumo Squat to finish the rep and will immediately start another one.

TECHNICAL TIP: The Hindu Squat is an excellent exercise for the development of leg and hip strength. When performing the Hindu Squat, make sure your knees are extended directly out in a straight line over your toes as you squat down. Initially, you may feel some soreness in your knees, but as your tendons and ligaments become stronger, this will disappear. Let your arms drag loosely at your sides and curl them up to your chest as you rise up out of the squat position. Perform the Hindu Squats at a steady pace and make it a goal to be able to do 100 reps every 3 minutes. Do as many as possible in a set, and work up to being able to perform as many as 500 reps in 1 set. You can do Hindu Squats as often as 5 days per week, although you don't need to perform 500 reps each workout. Allow for hard training days and easy training days when doing Hindu Squats.

GLUTE HAM RAISES

This is an outstanding exercise for strengthening the hamstrings, glutes, and to a lesser extent, the calves. One of the big reasons athletes sustain knee injuries is because they have much stronger quadriceps muscles (the muscles in the front of their upper legs) than they do hamstrings (the muscles in the back of the upper legs).

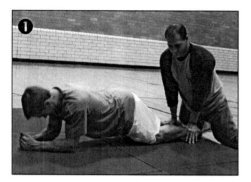

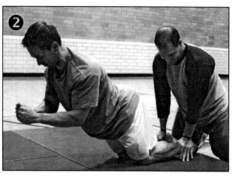

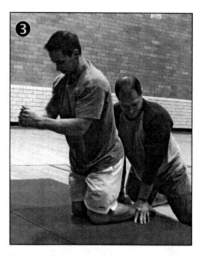

Bryan is holding Drew's lower legs and ankles with Drew laying on his front as shown.

Using his glute ham strength, Drew raises as shown.

Drew raises completely up to complete the rep, and will lower to start his next rep.

TECHNICAL TIP: Glute Ham Raises strengthen your hamstrings and glutes like no other exercise! This exercise will give you tremendous overall power and explosive strength in your lower body and lessen the chance of you sustaining knee injuries and hamstring pulls. Don't be fooled into thinking that you can substitute Leg Curls or Leg Extensions for the Glute Ham Raise. The Leg Curl only strengthens the belly of the muscle, and not the insertions that stabilize the joint. Once in a while, the Leg Curl can be useful for the sake of measuring your strength. If you can't leg curl at least 60% of what you can perform on the Leg Extension, you are vulnerable to hamstring and knee injuries.

PLOW PUSH UPS

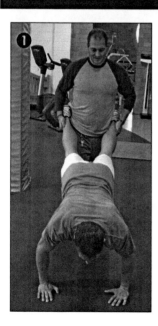

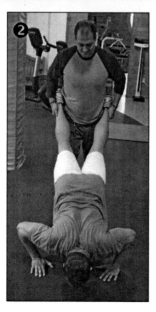

1. Bryan holds Drew's ankles and legs as shown. Drew is in the "up" position for a push up.

2. Drew performs a push up form this position. Do as many reps as possible in a specified time.

PLOW HOPS

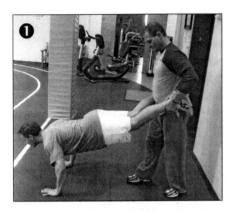

This is an excellent plyometric exercise for the upper body. Bryan is holding Drew's legs as shown. Drew is supporting himself with his hands.

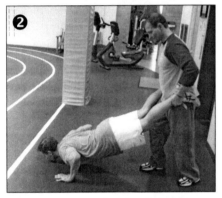

Drew lowers himself and gets ready to spring up with his hands and arms.

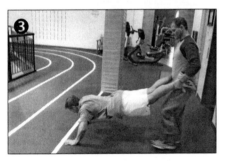

Drew springs up and as he does, he moves forward. Bryan follows along behind him holding Drew's ankles as shown.

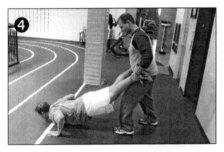

Drew readies himself for another rep.

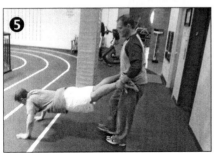

Drew springs up and propels himself forward again. Drew will perform 10 reps or can do this in a timed drill.

PLOW HAND WALK

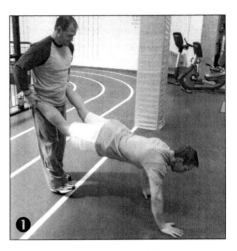

Similar to the Plow Hop, this exercise really works your shoulders, back, triceps, and core muscles. Bryan holds Drew's ankles and legs as shown.

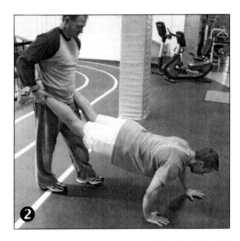

Drew walks forward on his hands. To make this tougher, Drew will walk sideways, turn in a circle or walk backward with Bryan holding his legs and following Drew wherever Drew walks.

PUSH UP

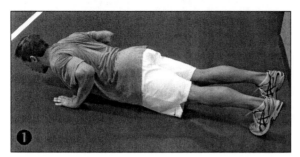

The good, old-fashioned Push Up is one of the best exercises ever invented! It works your entire body.

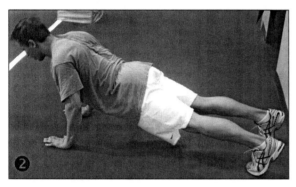

There are many variations of this old stand-by, so use them all and have fun doing them.

HIP STRENGTH AND FLEXIBILITY

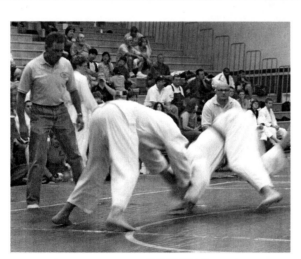

HIP STRENGTH AND FLEXIBILITY ARE KEYS TO WINNING ON THE MAT

The Hindu Push Ups are one of the exercises that develop your hips, legs and lower back, as well as your shoulders. You never know what position you will be in on the mat or in a fight, so do everything you can to prepare for anything that may happen.

HINDU PUSH UPS

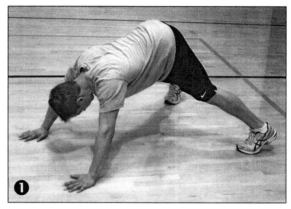

Drew places his hands and feet wide apart with his rear end up in the air as shown to start this exercise.

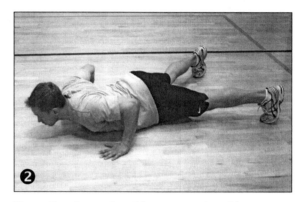

Drew dips forward making sure to drag his torso on the floor as he does.

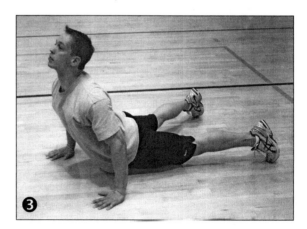

Drew arches up forward with his head as high as possible and his hips on the floor. He swings back up to start another rep. As with Push Ups, do in timed drills or a set number of reps.

CONDITIONING FOR COMBAT SPORTS

HEAD TO HEAD PUSH UP CHALLENGE

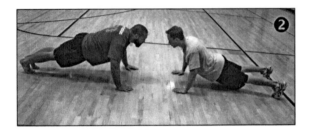

A fun way to train, either off or on the mat, is to go head to head with a training partner in a Push Up contest.

Look at each other and see who can do 50 or 100 push ups faster. You can also have someone keep time and see who does the most push ups in a specified time period.

HEAD TO HEAD HINDU PUSH UP CHALLENGE

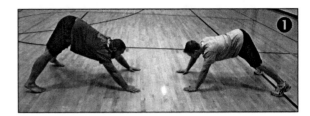

This is the same as the push up challenge, only using the Hindu Push Ups.

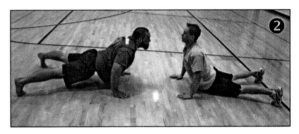

Make sure you are far enough away from each other so that you don't hit heads. This is a great way to get some extra training in.

POLE DANCING (PERFORM UCHIKOMI OR BUTSUKARI DRILLS ON A POLE)

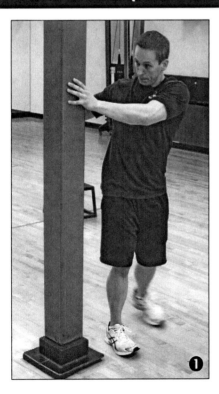
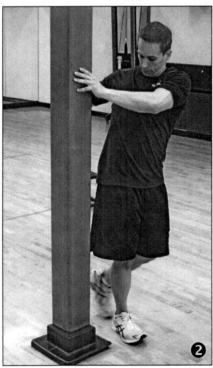

1. Foot speed drills for throwing can be done using a pole. Drew uses both hands to grab onto a pole.

2. Drew steps in with his fit ins in this excellent exercise you can do anywhere. Ask any old judo jock and he or she will tell you about doing thousands of these in the course of their careers.

WALL FIT-IN (UCHIKOMI OR BUTSUKARI) DRILL

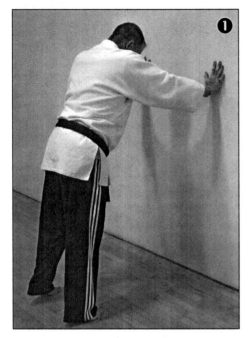

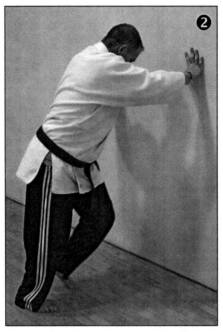

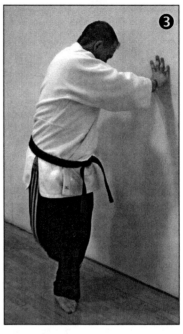

A good way to practice your footwork for a throw is to do Wall Fit Ins. Bryan extends his arms and leans against a wall. This is great for skill, but is outstanding as a cardio exercise.

Bryan's legs are placed far back and away from the wall so he can perform his fit ins with his feet.

Bryan completes a rep and will come out for another one. Do lots of these. Do 4 sets of 25, then 4 sets of 50, then 4 sets of 75, then 4 sets of 100 as you improve.

BREGMAN LEG REAP DRILL

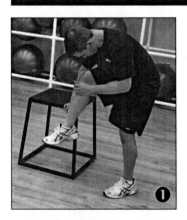

Similar to the exercise shown in Part 1, this drill is excellent for developing any reaping or hooking throw. It's also a good exercise for general fitness, even if you're not a grappler.

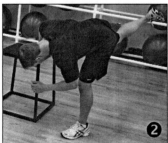

Perform this exercise as shown and do them in 4 sets of 25, adding more reps as you progress.

A STRONG LEG REAP

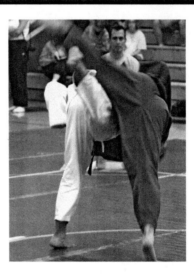

A STRONG LEG REAP IS NEEDED IN THROWS SUCH AS UCHI MATA (INNER THIGH THROW)

The powerful reaping or sweeping action of the leg is the major characteristic of effective and spectacular throws as Uchi Mata, Harai Goshi or O Soto Gari. Drills like the Bregman Leg Reap Drill enable you to develop the strength, flexibility, balance, agility and coordination to perform these throws on skilled, resisting opponents.

PARTNER SQUATS

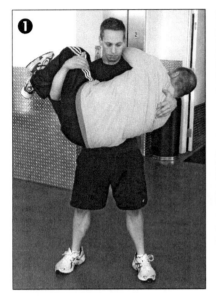 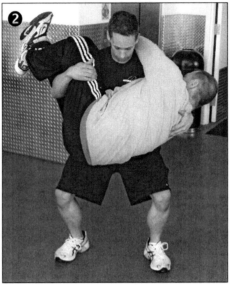

1. For a fun break from your normal training, grab a training partner, pick him up and do a set of squats.

2. Remember, you're holding another guy up, so make sure you perform a good, solid squat and don't drop him. That might make him mad!

SISSY SQUAT

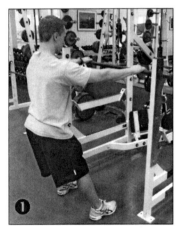 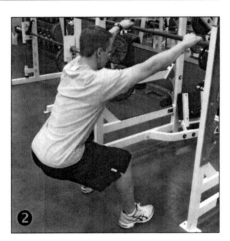

Maybe it's called a sissy squat, but it really isn't. This is a great squat using your own body weight. Drew holds onto a bar with both hands and places his feet on the floor under the bar as shown. Drew leans away from the bar with the weight in his buttocks.

Drew squats, making sure to lean away from the bar and placing his weight in his buttocks as he squats. Drew will perform a full squat, making sure not to bounce when he hits bottom. Perform this set in high repetitions, such as 25 to 50 per set. The Sissy Squat can be used as a good substitute for the days you may not feel up to working heavy on the Squat. This exercise is excellent for complete lower body and hip strength development.

STRENGTH

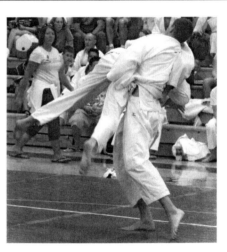

IT TAKES STRENGTH TO PICK UP AN OPPONENT AND THROW HIM

Sure, technical skill is extremely important, but to be able to perform skills like this at an elite level, you must have a solid foundation of strength first. Freehand exercises such as Partner Squats develop the strength needed to throw a resisting opponent. Throws like this Te Guruma (Hand Wheel Throw) are the result of functional training that includes Freehand Exercises.

SECTION TWO: PART 3: BARBELL AND GYM TRAINING

● ● ● **"Therefore, strengthen your feeble arms and weak knees." Hebrews 12:12**

Training in the gym is more than simply working out or getting stronger. Besides your dojo or area that you have your mat or floor where you practice your grappling or fighting skills, the weightroom is one of the most important spaces you occupy as an athlete. Often, you gravitate toward a place where you feel most comfortable and can get the type of workout that fits your needs. Your dojo and your gym are often your "home away from home." You know what we mean, and if you're new to the world of combat sports and hardcore training and don't now know, you soon will. There's a feel, or even a smell to a gym that, to some, may be a turnoff, but to others may be like finding the perfect spouse. Your gym, like your dojo, has to have character and be a place where you can, and will, give everything you have in training.

You'll spend a good part of your life in a gym, so make sure it's a "good fit" for you. Some of the best gyms the authors have trained in were far from the finest in terms of modern, state of the art equipment. That's not to say that training in a modern, well-equipped gym is a bad thing. It's not. You get out of your gym what you put into it. If you're willing to bust your butt, train hard and train smart when in the gym, you'll get the most out of your experience and time there. The intent of what's presented in this part of the book is to show exercises using the equipment you will find in most gyms or equipment that you can build yourself. Not everyone has access to the latest equipment, and if you do, consider yourself fortunate and take advantage of it. However, most people make the best use of what they have and with this in mind, the exercises presented here can be performed in most gyms.

These are the exercises that we believe to be of real benefit to grapplers and fighters. Not every exercise that's been invented is shown in this book, so you may have something that works for you that you don't see here. However, there are some tried and true gym movements shown here, and there are also some others that may not be as popular or well known, but certainly will help in your overall development.

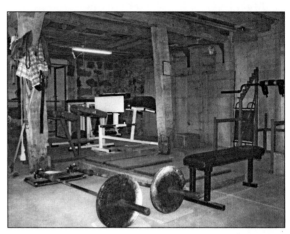

This is a hardcore gym, and while this atmosphere might not be for everyone, it certainly is the type of place that engenders serious, hard training. Located on the bottom floor of John Saylor's Barn of Truth, this gym is part of John's Shingitai Jujitsu Association training facility.

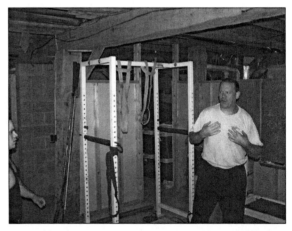

This photo shows John Saylor coaching David Fortin on using the Heavy Elastic Bands attached to the Power Rack in his weightroom at the Barn of Truth.

TECHNICAL TIP: Always use safety precautions in a weight room. Use a spotter, especially when lifting heavy weight. Take the time to learn how to perform an exercise or lift in the mechanically correct way to avoid injuries. Poor lifting form is a major reason people get injured in gyms. Train hard and train smart.

EXERCISES FOR LEGS AND HIPS

Your legs are your foundation. They must be strong; there are no two ways about it. From that strong base of your legs, your hips and core must be strong as well. Your "chain of power" extends form your legs through your body and into the power you exert when throwing, striking or grappling with an opponent. If any link in that chain is weak, then your chances of success are diminished. As author Steve Scott tells his athletes, "If your legs are weak, so is your technique." Sure, it's bad poetry, but it makes a good point.

SQUAT

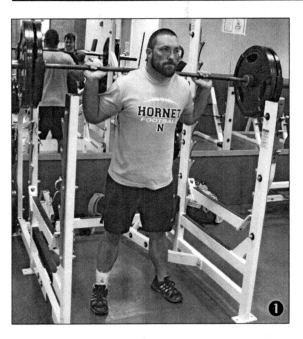

The Squat is the king of exercises because it develops real strength. The Squat develops your legs and hips and builds the foundation that is required for genuine, functional strength. To start, Jake unracks the bar and carefully steps out from it, giving himself room to perform the exercise. When Jakes unracks the bar, he takes slow, deliberate steps as he moves away from the rack. The bar rests high on Jake's shoulders, but not on his neck. Jake makes sure to hold and control the bar with his hands. Jake's head is held in an upright position and his back is straight. Jake makes sure to inhale as he unracks the bar to maintain adequate intrathoracic pressure and keep himself from bending forward. Do not bend forward or bend over at any time when performing the Squat. Jake's feet are positioned slightly wider than his hips where he has good balance. A good thing to remember is that the bar should be placed (whether the barbell is placed on your shoulders or in front of your body as in a Front Squat) in a straight line directly over your feet. If someone looked at you from the side when you're doing a Squat, the bar would be directly over your feet (not your knees). Keeping an erect, straight back will ensure this happens.

TECHNICAL TIP: Bending the spine with a heavy weight may cause back injuries, most often in the lumbar (lower back) area. A ruptured or slipped disc is painful and will put you out of commission for a long time. Use good lifting form at all times, especially when squatting.

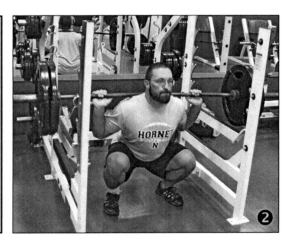

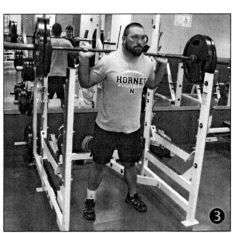

Jake squats until his upper thighs are parallel to the floor. It's a good idea to inhale while going down and exhale while coming up. Look at how Jake's head is still upright and his chest forward, with his back straight. Jake makes it a point to keep his eyes looking straight ahead. If he allowed his head to lean or drop forward, too much stress is placed on his lower back and not as much on the quadriceps, where you want the workload to be placed.

Jake finishes the Squat by standing. He makes sure to keep his back straight and erect when standing up.

OLYMPIC STYLE SQUAT

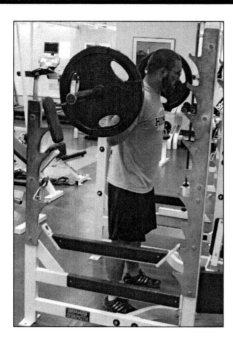

BREATHING SQUAT

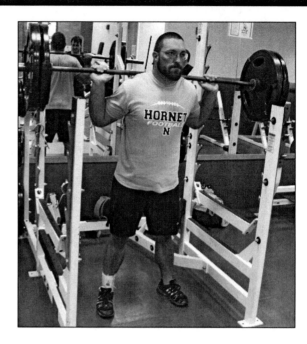

This side view of the Squat shows how Jake's back is erect and not bent over. This "Olympic Style" of doing the Squat is named such because Olympic-style weightlifters train on the Squat in this fashion. This style of Squat also uses a narrower leg base than the Power Squat used by powerlifters. Powerlifters tend to bend forward with a wider leg base, using more low back effort than used when doing an Olympic Style Squat. You won't usually squat as much weight when doing an Olympic Squat, but will reduce the risk of injuring your back when using this variation. The authors highly recommend performing Squats in this fashion as it emphasizes excellent lifting form, and the better the form in lifting, the less chance of injuries and the more benefit you get out of the exercise.

Whenever you take in 2 or more full breaths, and then perform a Squat, you are doing a Breathing Squat. There are several variations of how to perform Breathing Squats, but the basic concept is to perform the squat in the following way: 1. Take in 2 or more breaths between each repetition. 2. Perform the squat slowly and methodically; in fact, pause slightly for a second or two when you're in the bottom position. 3. Perform an Olympic Style Squat with a good, upright posture. 4. Use moderate to heavy poundage and perform 15 to 20 reps, usually only in 1 set. The purpose of a Breathing Squat is to provide additional work to your rib cage and torso increasing intrathoracic pressure as you perform the lift in a slow, methodical manner. The Breathing Squat is a tough workout. Proponents of this style of Squat have seen excellent results in their overall strength and gains in size.

QUARTER SQUAT OR HALF SQUAT

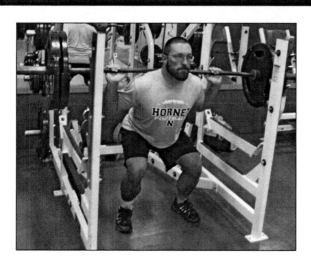

Jake squats about a fourth or half of the way down, rather than performing a full squat. You can handle more weight when doing Quarter Squats, and this form of the Squat is useful when you want to work your hips and glutes with more weight thereby developing more power and mass. Remember to use strict lifting form when using heavy weight in the Quarter or Half Squat.

FRONT SQUAT CLEAN STYLE GRIP

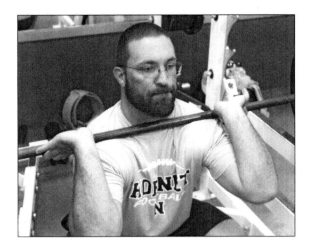

Jake rests the bar on the front of his shoulders and holds the bar in his hands as shown. This is a "Clean" style of doing the Squat with the bar resting in front of your front body rather than at your back. This style of Squat really puts a lot of the workload on your quadriceps as well as your glutes, but really keys in on your quads.

ZERCHER SQUAT

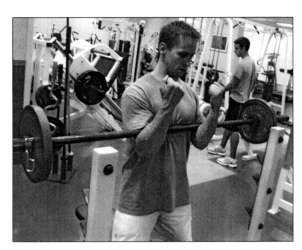

Drew uses his arms to hook up and under the barbell and rests the bar in the inside of his elbows, then takes the bar off of the rack (as shown here) and performs a Squat. This places a lot of stress on your elbows, so be careful. The Zercher Squat places the workload toward the front of Drew's body, making his quads and hips work extra hard.

FRONT SQUAT CROSS ARMS GRIP

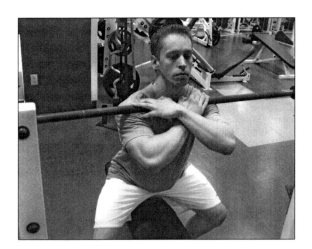

Drew places the bar on his upper chest, resting on his shoulders and upper chest as shown. He crosses his arms with his elbows forward. This balances the bar on his upper chest and shoulders and places the workload mostly on his quads, but really works his glutes as well. When you perform Front Squats, make sure your back is straight and don't bend forward. You can use can use a block of wood placed under your heels to improve your balance, but it also might make your knees move too far forward, which may place your body off-balance. Experiment with using a block of wood under your heels to see if it works for you.

TRAINING TIP: The foundation of your strength-training program should be the Squat. No other single lift or exercise can take its place. Your body is your house and if that house is built on a weak or flimsy foundation, the entire structure will be weak.

SQUAT WITH CHAINS

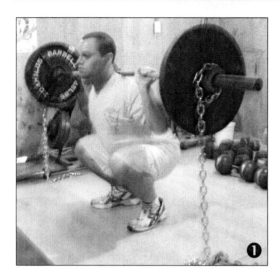

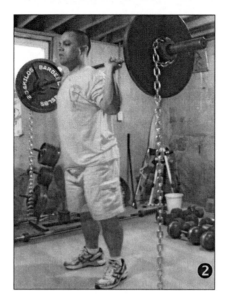

One of the major advantages of chains is that they allow you to come up out of your squat quickly, thus developing tremendous starting and accelerating strength and speed. This is the strength and speed you need for all throws and takedowns, as well as kicking techniques.

Chains provide accommodating resistance. As David squats, the weight of the chains is unloaded as they pile on the floor. As you explode upward, weight is added to the bar as the chains come off the floor. In other words, the chains accommodate your strength curve, giving you less resistance at the bottom of the squat and more as you stand erect and explode upward into your strongest position of the lift.

Switch to lifting with chains 2 to 3 weeks before a fight or tournament. Bands makes you too sore because they speed up and overload the downward (eccentric) portion of the lift beyond what naturally occurs with gravity.

SQUAT WITH BANDS

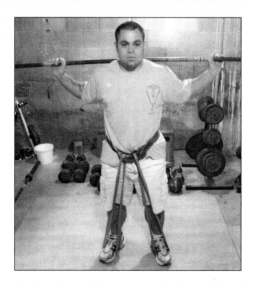

Normally, bands or chains are attached to each end of the bar and then the other end is looped to the bottom of the power rack. In this case, the bands are attached to David's belt and then an end is looped under each foot. This method will have an awkward feel at first, as well as making your legs feel wobbly, but it also works your muscles much differently, and will make you very strong and explosive.

BOX SQUAT

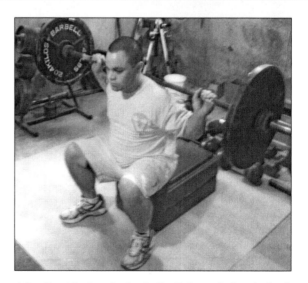

After David takes the barbell off the rack, he sits back on the box until his shins are vertical. He relaxes his hips and glutes while he keeps the rest of his muscles tight and pushes his knees out to the side. David breathes in to increase his intrathoracic pressure (which stabilizes his spine and keeps his posture erect) and explodes upward using his glutes and legs.

BOX SQUAT WITH CHAINS

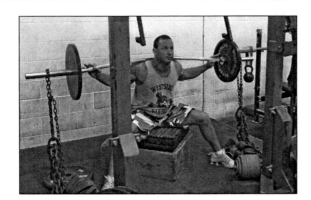

Tony Ramos adds chains on each side of the barbell, increasing his workload. Look at how Tony has looped chains around each side of the bar and draped heavier chains on them. Tony squats back onto the box until his shins are just past vertical position, then explodes off the box to an upright position.

BOX SQUAT WITH HEAVY BANDS

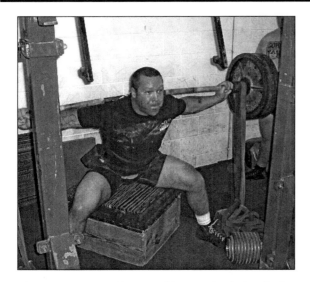

Shawn Nutter uses heavy rubber or elastic bands, increasing the resistance in his Box Squat. The bands are looped over each end of the bar and the bottom of the bands are looped over the bottom of the rack or attachment on the floor. As Shawn stands erect off the box, the bands stretch. The stretched bands pull him downward faster than gravity itself and this creates a powerful reflex and kinetic energy for the concentric (upward) portion of the lift. It's the activation of this stretch reflex that enables you to develop explosive power. Also, at the top of the squat, when the bands are fully stretched, you are handling much more resistance or workload. This allows you to get an explosive start off the box and as you get to the strongest part in the range of motion, to work through more resistance.

TRAP BAR SQUAT

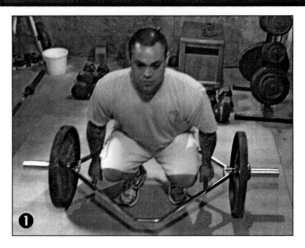

The diamond-shaped Trap (for trapezius) bar is a great addition to any gym. David shows how to use the bar in this photo. Initially, one of the primary uses of this bar was to work the trapezius, but it's also been used for years as an excellent piece of equipment to work the legs. The Trap Bar Squat enables you to perform heavy squats without placing any weight or stress on your spine. If you have any lower back injuries, or don't have access to a Squat Rack or Power Rack, the Trap Bar is ideal for working your legs. David starts by grabbing the handles and squatting inside the bar.

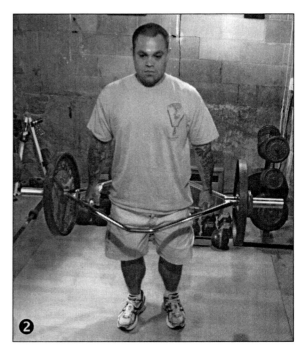

David completes the movement by standing erect. The Trap Bar works your quads a great deal. You can expect to use a bit less weight on the Trap Bar than you would in a regular squat, as this exercise keys in on your quads and gives them a tremendous workout.

TRAP BAR SQUAT ON BOX

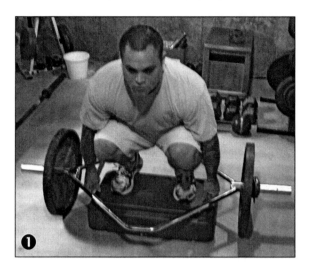

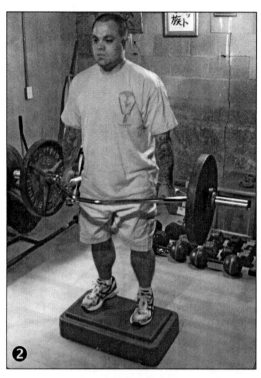

1 David adds to the workload by placing a box or riser inside the Trap Bar and stands on it.

2. David completes the Trap Bar Squat by standing upright on the box as shown.

TRAP BAR SQUAT WITH CHAINS

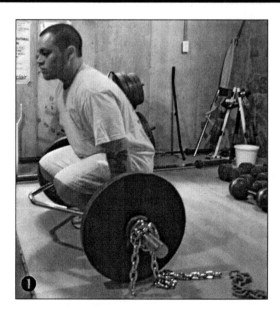

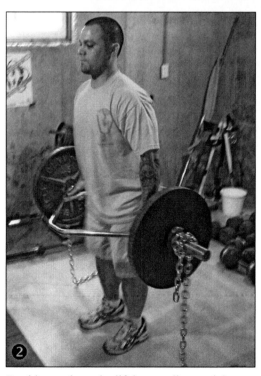

As with any squat, using chains will increase the overall effort throughout the lift by providing accommodating resistance. Look at how David's back is straight and his chest is extended forward and not hunched forward. David looks straight ahead and doesn't allow his head to droop forward.Good lifting form is essential to avoid injuries and to get the most benefit from the exercise.

David completes the lift by standing upright.

TRAP BAR CALF RAISES

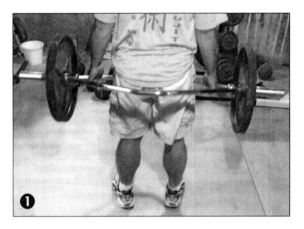 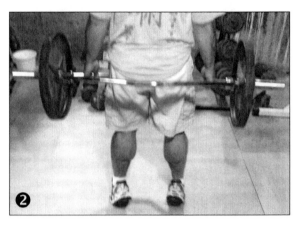

You can work your lower legs, performing calf raises with a good amount of weight using the Trap Bar. David holds the trap bar as shown.

David lifts his heels up, working his calf muscles. Notice that David holds .he Trap Bar with his arms straight and doesn't use his arms to lift the bar. You may be tempted to use your arms to lift the bar as you perform these calf raises, but don't let yourself do that. Place the entire workload your lower legs. Use enough weight to be able to perform sets of 25 reps safely.

CABLE MACHINE LEG KICKS

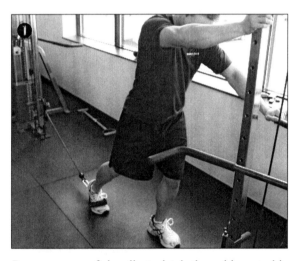 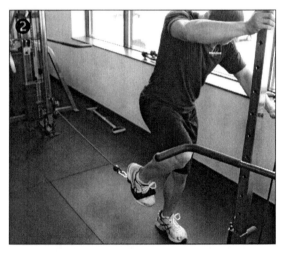

Drew uses a soft handle to latch the cable onto his right foot. Use light weight in this exercise so that you can perform it in a smooth, controlled fashion.

Drew lifts his right knee forward as he supports himself with his hands as shown. You can perform this movement slowly or in a faster, "kicking" motion. It is especially good for developing the hip flexors, which are vital to all kicking motions and Muay Thai knee strikes.

SNATCH SQUAT

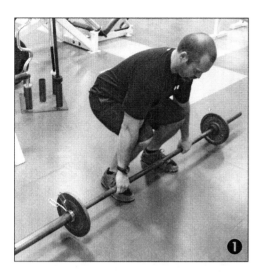

1. An enjoyable variation to doing the Squat is to perform the Snatch Squat once in a while. Chris grabs the barbell as shown. You won't use as much weight as in any of the other forms of Squat, but this is an athletic exercise that incorporates a lot of different muscle groups.

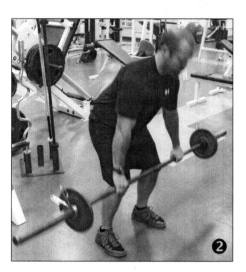

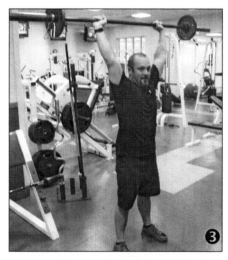

2. Chris performs a Snatch, where he swings the barbell up from the floor (with his arms straight) to over his head.

3. Chris completes the Snatch.

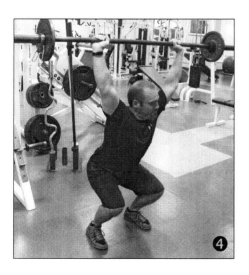

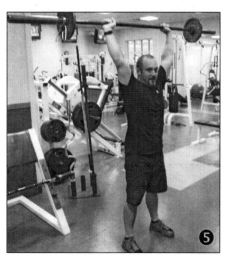

4. Chris holds the barbell overhead and performs a Squat.

5. Chris finishes the Squat and lowers the barbell back to the floor to start his next repetition. This is a good exercise to break up the monotony of training. Use weight that is heavy enough so that you can perform 3 to 5 sets of 5 reps.

BARBELL LUNGES

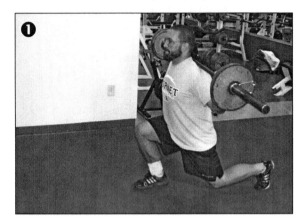

Jake places the barbell on his shoulders and starts by standing upright as if he were doing a regular Squat. He steps forward as far as possible with his right foot so that his right thigh is almost parallel to the floor. Jake's left knee almost touches (but doesn't) the floor. Jake then steps back to the starting position.

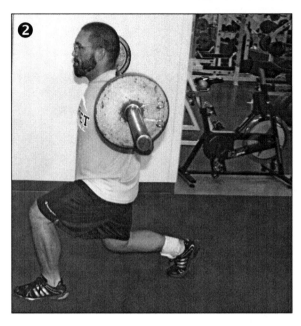

Jake then lunges forward with his left leg to complete the rep. Use light to moderate weight so that you can perform 6 to 10 reps per set. When you step forward, you place all of your weight on your leading leg. This exercise places a lot of the workload on your quads, especially down low near the knee, so if you have knee problems, use light weight and deliberate, slow lunges when performing this movement. Your glutes also receive a lot of work in this exercise, and because of this, it's a good exercise for grapplers.

A variation of this is the BARBELL LUNGE STEP.
To perform the Barbell Lunge Step, Jake simply walks forward in a lunge step so the he does 10 reps on each leg. Use light weight and make sure to keep a good, upright posture. This is an excellent exercise for grapplers who shoot in for a Double Leg Takedown and need a strong, penetration or lunge step. For strikers, this exercise is good for developing punching and kicking power from the legs, hips and core.

BARBELL SNATCH LUNGE STEPS

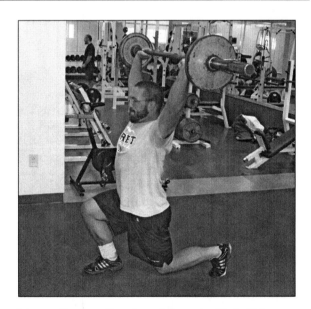

Jake performs a Snatch and does the Barbell Lunge with the barbell over his head as shown. Use light weight. This exercise adds more upper body work to the Barbell Lunge. This is not an exercise for beginners!

BELT SQUATS

The Belt Squat provides for a safe and exceptionally effective way to work your entire lower body. Using a belt takes the pressure off your spine and you are better able to safely perform full squats. One of the disadvantages of using barbell squats is the fact that the bar, loaded with heavy weight, compresses the lifter's spine. The Belt Squat completely removes stress on your spine. In fact, it serves as traction for the spine and can even correct pelvic tilt.

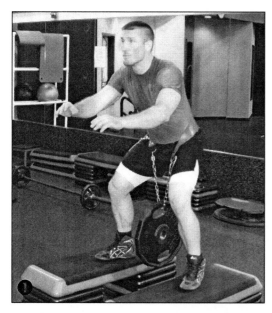

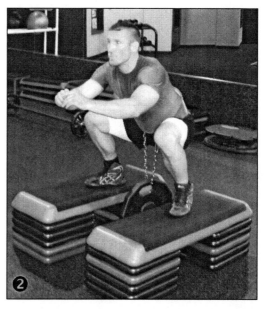

Mike is standing on a pair of boxes, cardio steps or any object that is safe and can support the weight of the lifter and the weights. The belt harness should be placed low on your hips.

Mike performs a full squat, making sure he is balanced in his stance. The two elevated boxes or steps Mike is standing on provide a place for the barbell plates to go safely.

BELT SQUATS TAKE THE PRESSURE OFF YOUR SPINE

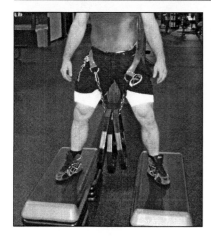

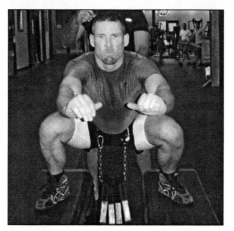

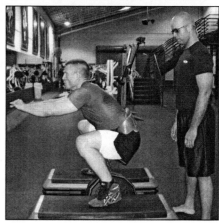

In a regular squat, even with a front grip, there is tremendous pressure on the spine. Using a belt to hold the weights, Mike will be able to perform a full squat with less chance of injury than if he would rest a barbell on his shoulders.

With the weight not pressing down on Mike's spine, he can squat lower with less chance of injury and efficiently works his quadriceps and inner thighs. Belt Squats give you a well-rounded leg workout because of the location of the weight between your legs.

For safety's sake, make sure you have a spotter. If you lose balance, your partner can quickly help you out.

LEG PRESS

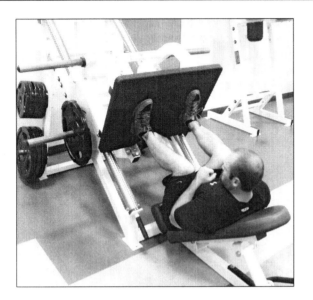

Chris is pushing with both of his legs in this photo, but you can also use this machine safely pushing with one leg. Bend your legs as far as possible and make sure your knees move to the sides of your chest and torso. Your foot placement is important, but the basic way is to place your feet about shoulder-width apart. There are several effective variations for this exercise, so use your imagination and add this machine to your leg routine.

> **TECHNICAL TIP:** Your foot placement in the Leg Press Machine determines where the workload takes place. If your feet are high on the footplate, the emphasis is mostly on the glutes and hamstrings. If your feet are low on the footplate, the primary emphasis is on your quadriceps. If your feet are wide apart with your toes slightly pointed outward, the emphasis is on your adductors (your inner thighs). If your feet are placed close together on the footplate, the workload is mostly on your quadriceps.

CALF RAISES USING LEG MACHINE

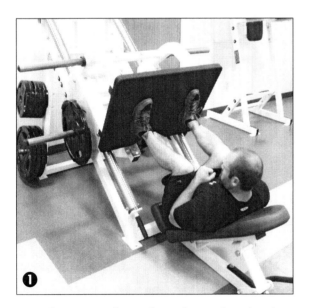

❶

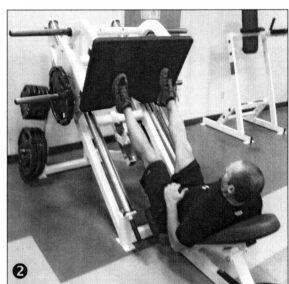

❷

A good way to work your lower legs at the calves is to do Calf Raises with the Leg Machine.

Chris pushes with both feet using the balls of his feet forcing his calf muscles to take the bulk of the work. Having a strong lower leg is important to every grappler or fighter.

LEG PRESS POP UP FOR EXPLOSIVE POWER

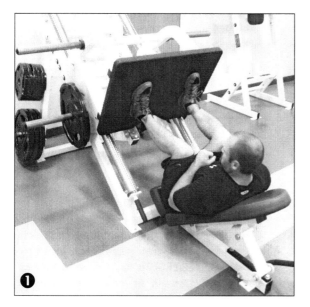

A plyometric exercise useful for grapplers and fighters is to perform Pop Ups on the Leg Machine. Use light weight, and if you have any ankle injuries, don't do this exercise.

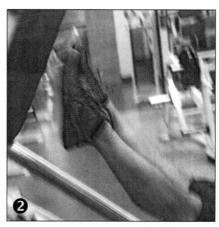

Chris has his feet shoulder-width apart on the footplate as shown.

Chris pushes or pops the footplate with the balls of his feet. Perform this exercise with light weight and in sets of 10 to 15 repetitions.

PLATE FOOT SWEEPS

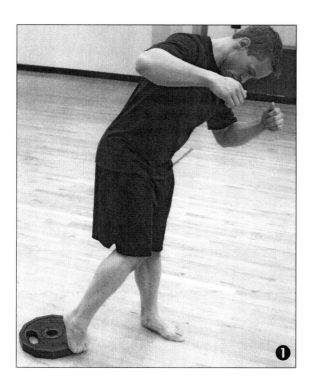

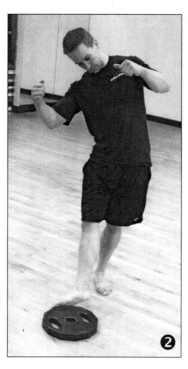

1. Drew moves a weight plate around on the floor with his foot simulating how he would use his foot and leg in a throwing technique. Drew is using his toes and the ball of his foot to reap or hook the plate, moving it around the floor.

2. Drew uses his foot in the same way he would a foot sweep or foot prop, moving the weight plate around the floor.

EXERCISES FOR THE CORE, ABDOMINALS AND LOWER BACK

The "core" is the part of the body that extends from your hips and upper leg area to the bottom of your thorax, in the front, sides and back. This is a vital link in your body's chain of power, extending from your feet and legs, to your core, then into your torso, and then through your shoulders, arms and head. The core is the middle of your body and must be strong enough to allow your lower body's strength to perform at its full potential in synergy with your upper body.

CRUNCHES ON BENCH WITH WEIGHT

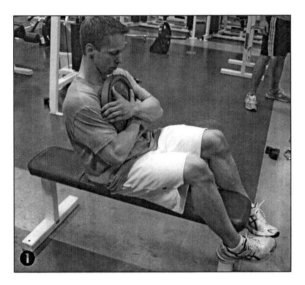

Drew holds a weight plate on his chest, but he can wear a weighted vest, hold a dumb-bell, kettlebell or heavy medicine ball when performing this exercise. Use enough weight to make the exercise harder. It's common to see guys in most every gym using a 45-pound plate when doing this exercise. Drew hooks his feet on the bench as shown, sitting upright to start.

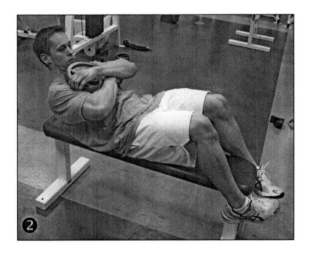

Drew lowers his body, not allowing his shoulders to touch the bench. Drew will sit back up to complete the movement. Use this exercise as a good warm-up or finisher. Perform 2 to 4 sets of 25 to 50 reps, depending on your fitness level and goals.

DANEK (RUSSIAN) TWISTS

DANEK TWISTS WITH LEGS RAISED

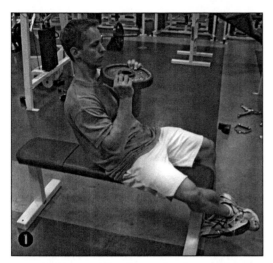

Drew holds a weight plate as he sits on a bench.

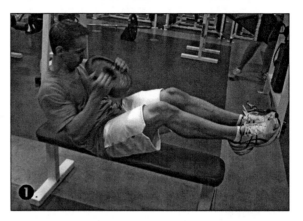

Drew makes this exercise harder by sitting on the bench on his buttocks with his legs raised and his upper body arched as shown.

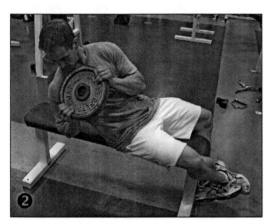

At a moderate to slow speed, Drew rotates to the right, and then to the left, holding the plate on his chest. This is an excellent core exercise, working all angles of the middle part of your body.

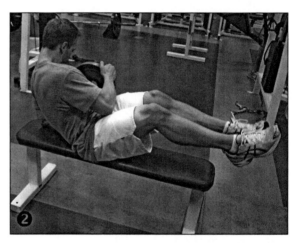

Drew rotates to his left, holding the plate close to his body.

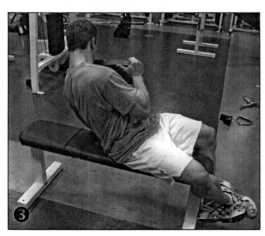

Perform this exercise using 2 to 4 sets of 24 to 50 reps, depending on your fitness level and specific goals.

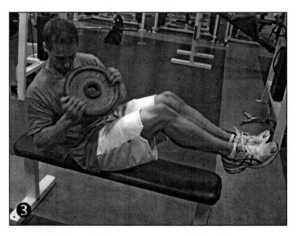

Drew rotates to his right to complete the exercise. This is a great core exercise and should be used as an integral part of your workout.

HANGING LEG RAISES TO CURL UP

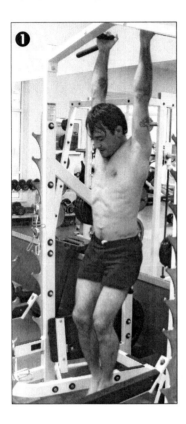

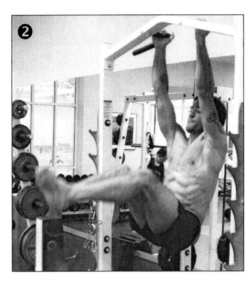

1. Using the weight of your body to develop strength is effective. Nikolay holds onto a bar or set of handles, allowing his lower body to hang.

2. With minimal (or no) swinging, Nikolay raises his legs.

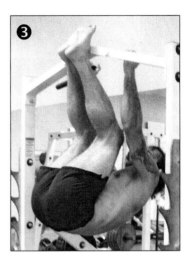

3. Nikolay raises his legs, touching the upright. He will lower his legs, completing the repetition. This is an excellent finisher to a workout. Perform one set of as many reps as possible. This is a tremendous core exercise that also works your legs and hips, stressing your abs, hip flexors, quads and obliques.

LEG RAISES

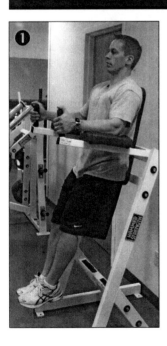

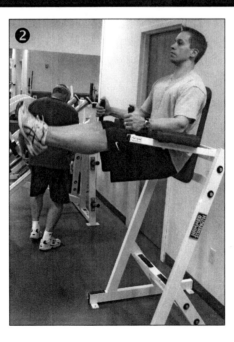

1. The Leg Raise unit is common to many gyms. Drew points his toes and keeps his back and legs as straight as possible when performing this exercise.

2. Drew lifts (and does not swing) his legs up, keeping his toes pointed. This is an excellent core and lower body exercise, working your hip flexors, six-pack and obliques. To complete the movement, Drew lowers his legs gradually, making sure not to allow them to drop or swing back. Perform one set of as many reps as possible as a great finisher to your workout or add this exercise in as a part of your training circuit.

BACK RAISES (HYPEREXTENSIONS)

The Hyper unit is seen in most gyms and is often one of the loneliest pieces of equipment on the floor. A lot of "old-timers" still call this piece of equipment the Roman Chair. This exercise is commonly called "Hyperextensions" but to actually hyperextend the back could cause injury, so we call them Back Raises.

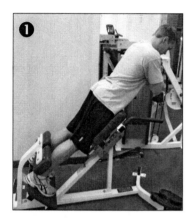 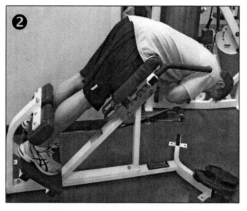 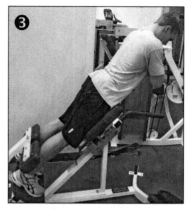

Drew starts the exercise by crossing his hands at his chest and making sure his back is straight. Drew can make this exercise harder by holding a barbell behind his neck or wearing a weight vest.

Drew lowers his upper body gradually and with control. This exercise places a lot of work on your glutes (rear end) and hamstrings (biceps femoris), as well as your spinal erectors and lower back. If you use a barbell behind your neck, use weight you can safely handle and perform 3 to 5 sets of 5 repetitions.

Drew completes the exercise by straightening his body. He can make the exercise a bit harder by holding his body rigid for a few seconds before bending forward to start his next repetition.

BACK RAISES (HYPEREXTENSIONS)

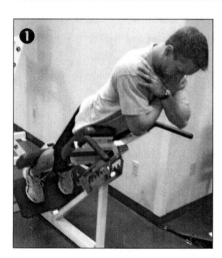 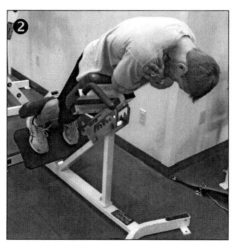 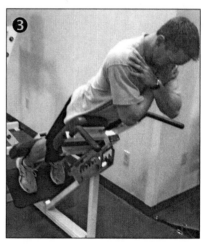

This is a great variation of the Hyperextension that adds extra work to your abdominals. Drew starts off with his body upright.

As Drew bends forward, he also curls his body and draws his shoulders forward as shown. Drew can hold this position for a few seconds to make it harder.

Drew straightens his body to complete the exercise.

SIDE RAISES

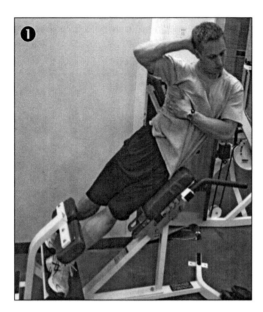

Performing this exercise keys in on your obliques and rectus abdominus on the side. Drew is bending, and also works the opposite side by contracting in an isometric way to keep his body from going below horizontal.

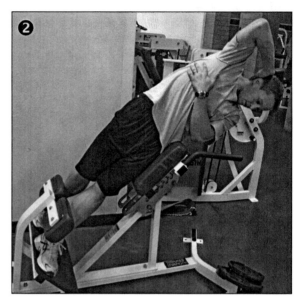

Drew keeps places his left hand on his right ribcage to keep his left arm from lowering too far and giving him the opportunity to bounce. This hand placement keeps Drew's movement strict, making the exercise more effective.

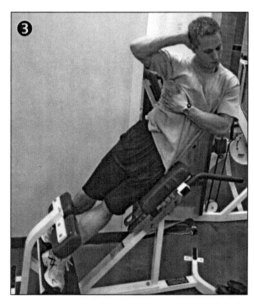

Drew finishes the movement by arching or curling to his right, keeping stress on his entire upper body with emphasis on his obliques and six-pack.

BACK RAISE TWISTS

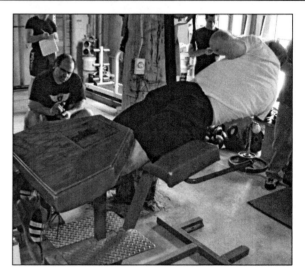

Danny Goss performs the Hyperextension and as his body straightens, he rotates to his left and then to his right on the next rep, gradually and with control. This is an excellent lower back, core and glute/hamstring exercise. To make it more difficult Danny can wear a weighted vest or hold a weight plate.

EXERCISES FOR THE LOWER BACK, GLUTES, HAMSTRINGS AND HIPS

What is often called the "glutes" are actually the muscles extending from the hip to the upper leg, called the Gluteus Maximus and Gluteus Medius, and then the muscles that form the entire back of your upper leg. The "hamstrings" are the muscles that comprise the back of your legs. While it looks good to have big, bulging Quadriceps in the front of your legs, the development of your glutes and hams is essential to success in fighting.

REVERSE HYPER MACHINE

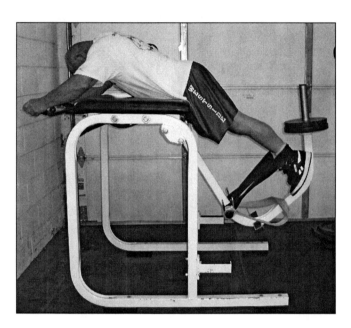

Louie Simmons is training on his invention, the Reverse Hyper Machine. The Reverse Hyper Machine is being used in more gyms and is great for increasing strength in the lower back, glutes and hamstrings and for rehab or restoration. If you don't have access to this piece of equipment, you can do the exercise by leaning over a strong, high table, attaching the weights to your feet and performing the exercise just as with the machine. To see how to perform this exercise, you can visit Louie's web site at www.westside-barbell.com or search for Louie Simmons or the Reverse Hyper Machine on the Internet. The part where your legs swing under you is very beneficial to your spine and discs, since this motion elongates the spine and even allows fluid to re-enter the discs. This isn't true of most other conventional weight lifting exercises in which the spine is compressed. This is why Reverse Hypers are so important for rehab of injuries and for developing a strong, healthy back. For more information on the Reverse Hyper, contact Louie Simmons at Westside Barbell, 3884 Larchmere Drive, Grove City, Ohio 43123 or call (614) 801-2060.

45 DEGREE ANGLE REVERSE HYPER MACHINE

Jerry Obradovic is working out on the 45 Degree Reverse Hyper Machine. The 45-degree angle of this Reverse Hyper unit really focuses in on the glutes and hamstrings.

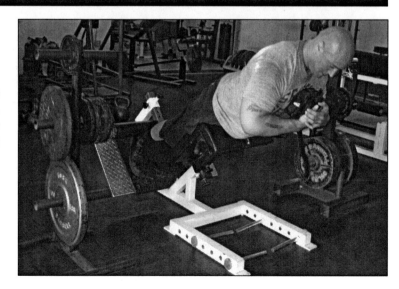

DEADLIFT

If you perform the Deadlift right, it's a tremendous total body exercise. People who don't use it right or who don't use it at all have given this exercise a bad reputation. The Deadlift works virtually every muscle in your body and builds tremendous functional strength.

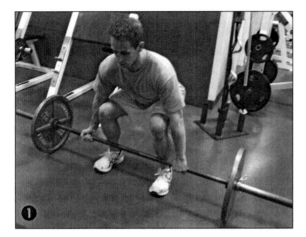

Drew starts the lift by grabbing the bar slightly wider than shoulder width as shown. One hand grips the bar palm forward and the other hand is palm backward as shown. Look at how Drew's shins are touching the barbell.

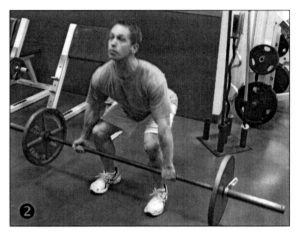

Drew sticks out his chest and takes in a deep breath as he lifts the barbell. Doing this allows his rib cage to stiffen and keeps his torso from bending or arching forward. Drew also makes it a point to keep his lower back straight and slightly arched. Doing all of this prevents poor lifting form and prevents injuries when doing the Deadlift.

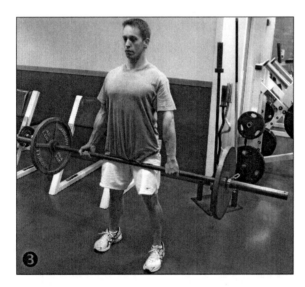

Drew completes the deadlift by standing erect, pulling the bar up along his legs. Drew will hold this position for a couple of seconds, and then lower the weight to the floor to complete the repetition.

PALMS IN GRIP

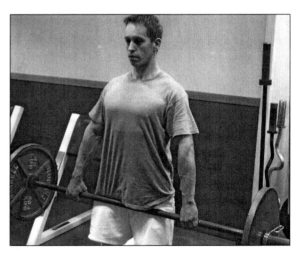

Drew is performing the Deadlift with the Palms In grip rather than the normal way of grabbing the bar in the Deadlift with one palm forward and the other palm facing backward when grabbing the bar.

DEADLIFT (SUMO STYLE)

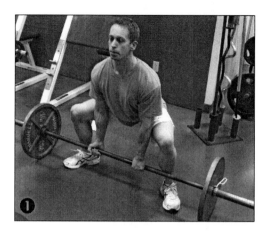

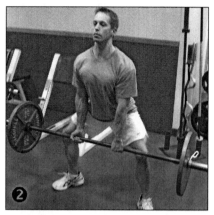

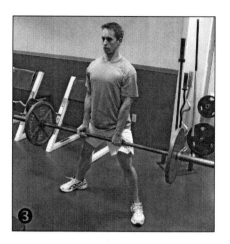

Drew squats at the bar as shown, with his legs wide. Look at how Drew's arms are between his legs and not on the outside of his legs as in a regular Deadlift. Drew makes sure to stick his chest out and arch his lower back as he did in the regular Deadlift.

Drew lifts the barbell, making sure his chest is extended forward with his lower back straight as he lifts. Excellent lifting technique is essential for the Sumo Style Deadlift to avoid injuring the hips and inner thighs as well as the lower back.

The big difference between the Sumo Style Deadlift and the regular Deadlift is that the Sumo Style focuses on the quadriceps and adductors (inner thighs) with less emphasis on your lower back. It also places a lot of stress on your traps as you pull the bar upward.

STIFF LEGGED DEADLIFT

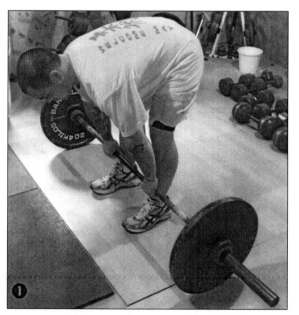

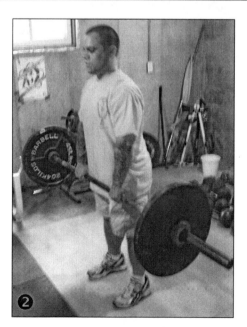

This exercise really works your entire lower back, hamstrings and glutes. You can also use a pair of dumbbells when doing this exercise.

David places his shins against the bar, bends over at the waist and grabs the bar with his hands about shoulder width. David makes sure to have his head up and not droop forward, keeping his back as straight and possible. David knees are locked and straight.

David straightens up, holding the bar at arms' length. He inhales as he comes up and exhales as he lowers the bar to the floor.

STIFF LEGGED DEADLIFT (SUMO STYLE)

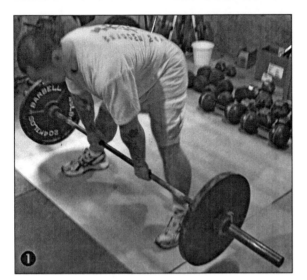

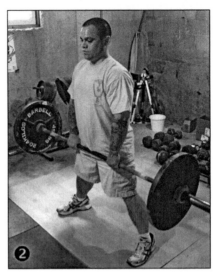

Use weight that allows you to perform 3 to 5 sets of 10 repetitions.

A variation of this exercise is to perform it Sumo Style. Doing it this way places more work on your inner thighs and quadriceps.

David makes sure to use good lifting technique and doesn't jerk the weight up to complete the lift.

DEADLIFT USING IMPLEMENTS WITH HANDLES

If you have access to any type of lifting bar, you can perform this Deadlift. It works just about every muscle in your body and develops excellent strength in the hips, lower back and trapezius area. Your glutes and leg structure also get a great workout. Doing Deadlifts like this is a good way to break the monotony in training.

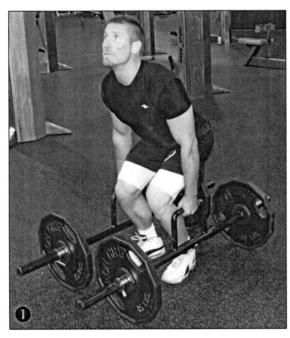

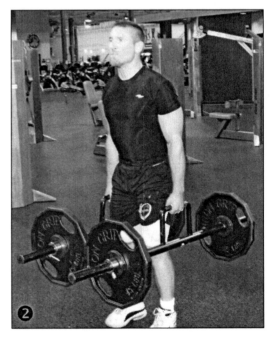

The workload is placed on the side of Mike's body rather than in front of it, giving him a different angle and ability to lift a bit more weight.

Mike completes the lift by standing erect. As with every Deadlift, use good lifting form to get the most out of the exercise and to avoid injuries.

JEFFERSON LIFT (ALSO CALLED KENNEDY LIFT)

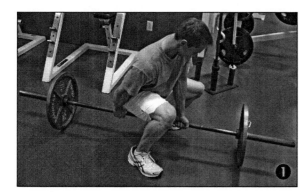

Drew straddles the barbell with his feet wider than his hips and squats down and holds the front of the bar with his left hand (palm down) and the rear of the bar behind him with his right hand (palm up). Drew's thighs are parallel to the floor and his back is straight.

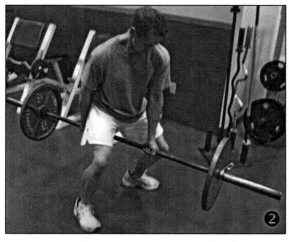

Drew squats up and rises with the bar at arms' length. Inhale as you lift and exhale on the way down.

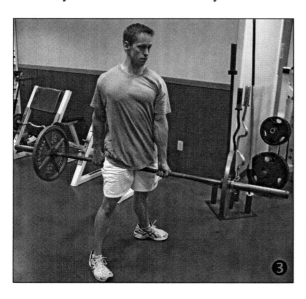

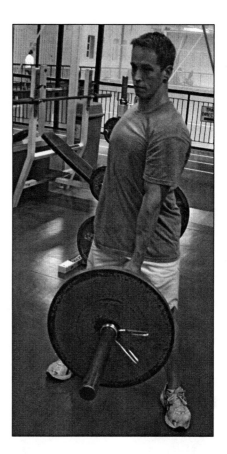

This front view of the Jefferson Lift shows how the body is turned to accommodate the movement in the lift. This is a good exercise for the adductors in the inner thighs, your quadriceps and almost all the muscles in your hip area. It also works your lower back, so make sure you perform it carefully and use good lifting form. The twisting action in the lower back can be harmful if you don't use proper lifting technique or if you jerk the weigh to get it off the floor.

Drew stands up, keeping his head up and body erect as he completes the lift. Drew makes it a point to keep the bar at arms' length with his elbows locked.

GOOD MORNINGS

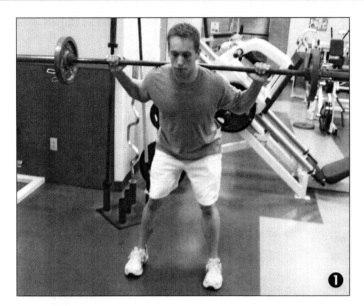

This exercise strengthens the lower back, glutes and hamstrings, all of which will help you lift and throw an opponent. Drew has his feet slightly wider than shoulder width and with his knees slightly bent. Drew makes it a point to inhale as he starts the exercise. This keeps his chest forward and his spine erect.

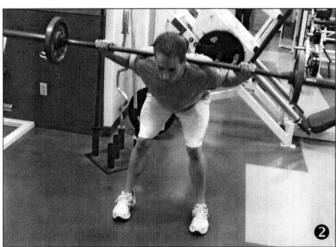

Drew bends forward at the waist until his body is at about a 90-degree angle. You can perform this exercise with straight legs rather than having them bent, but our preference is to bend the knees. Bending the knees poses less risk of injuring your lower back when performing this movement.

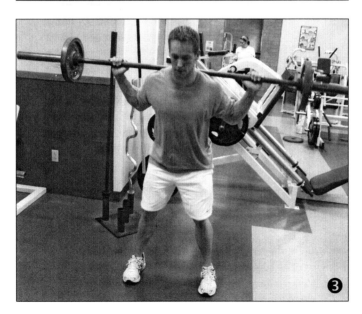

Drew returns to the starting position and will repeat the exercise to complete the set. After a warm up of 10 reps with light weight, perform 3 to 5 reps per set doing 3 to 5 sets. Good Mornings pose a very real risk of injury to the lower back, so it's important to use moderate weight rather than heavy weight when performing this movement. Don't jerk or bounce the weight to complete the lift.

BAR PLACEMENT ON SHOULDERS FOR THE GOOD MORNING

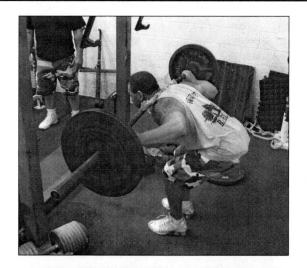

Tony Ramos doing some Good Mornings as Louie Simmons offers some coaching. Make sure the bar is placed on your upper back and traps and not resting on your neck. Resting the bar on your neck is dangerous and can cause injuries.

GOOD MORNINGS USING A WEIGHT PLATE

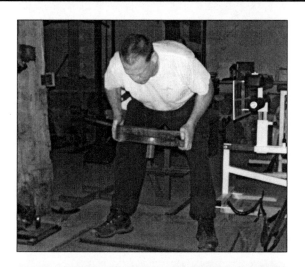

John Saylor holds two 45-pound plates in his hands rather than using a barbell across his back. This places less strain on your lower back, and especially your spine when performing this exercise. Actually, you can use any heavy object such as a large stone, anvil, bag filled with any material or anything that will give you a good workout.

BACK PRESS

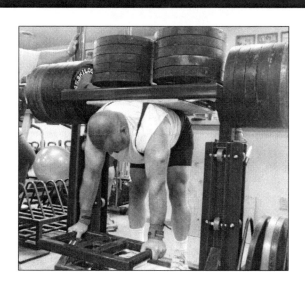

Dr. Al Myers shows how to perform the Back Press. While definitely not for everyone, this exercise develops extreme strength in the low back, core, hips and legs. Very few gyms have the Back Lift machine, but if yours has this piece of equipment, you can use it once in a while in the place of Good Mornings. Massive poundages are lifted in this and Al's personal best is 2,915 pounds.

EXERCISES USING THE GYM GRAPPLER

The "Grappler" was developed by Louie Simmons and has a variety of uses. Shown here are some of the exercises that you can do using this piece of equipment. If you don't have a Grappler, you can wedge one end of an Olympic bar in a corner and make your own. However, the safety of having a Grappler with one end bolted to the floor is certainly recommended over wedging a bar in the corner.

GYM GRAPPLER PRESS

Avoid swinging the Grappler or jerking it when pressing it. Perform 3 to 5 sets of about 5 repetitions. Use weight that allows you to use good lifting form. The upper back, especially the latissimus dorsi, rhomboids, traps, and even the side and back heads of the deltoids are worked in this exercise.

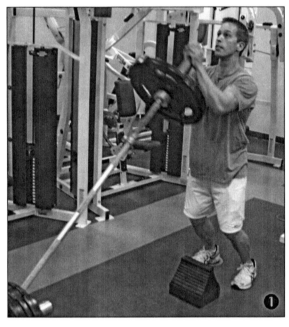

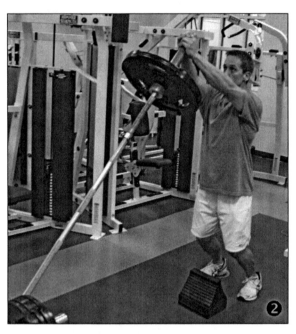

Drew grabs the end of the barbell and performs an Overhead Press with it.

Drew completes the exercise by pressing the Grappler to arms' length.

GYM GRAPPLER 1 ARM PRESS

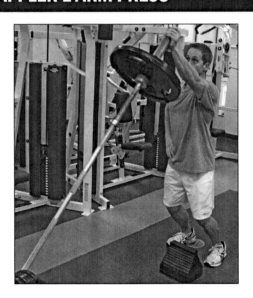

Drew performs an Overhead Press with 1 arm. Alternate arms and perform 10 reps with one hand, then switch to the other hand and perform 10 reps to complete the set.

GYM GRAPPLER ROTATIONS

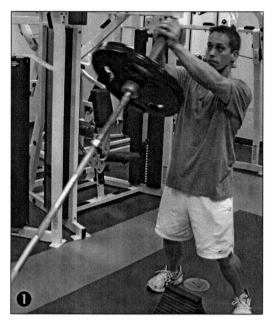

Drew grabs the Grappler at the end of the bar with his arms slightly bent.

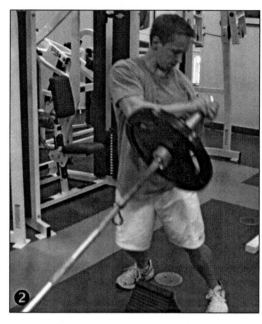

Drew rotates as far as possible to his left, moving the bar to his left hip or side.

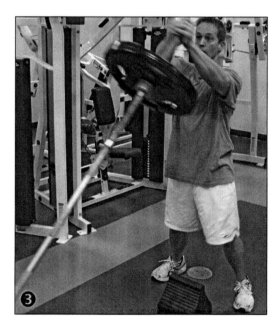

Drew rotates back to the starting position.

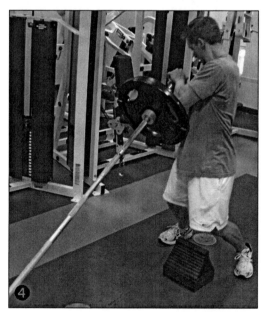

Drew rotates to his right as far as possible to complete the exercise. Use enough weight so that you can rotate or twist safely and perform 10 repetitions. Perform 3 to 5 sets depending on your goals and fitness level. This is a great finisher to any workout in the gym.

GYM GRAPPLER SIDE TO SIDE

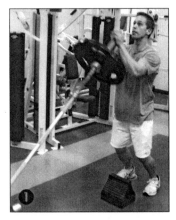 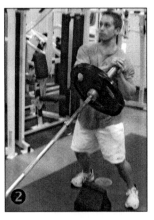 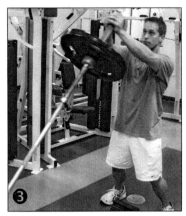 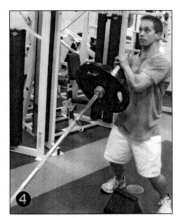

This exercise is similar to the Grappler Rotations, but Drew doesn't rotate. Start with the bar in front of your body

Drew moves the bar to his left, going as low as possible with it and still maintaining good control.

Drew moves the bar back to the starting position.

Drew completes the exercise by moving the bar to his right.

This exercise works your arms, shoulders, upper chest and upper back really well. Using the Grappler also forces you to have good, stable lower body position, which is a secondary benefit of using this piece of equipment.

GYM GRAPPLER 1-ARM BENT OVER ROWING

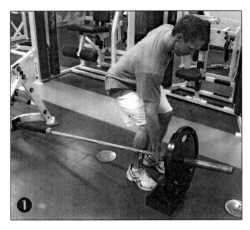 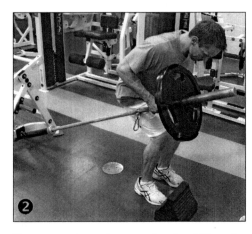

Drew uses the Grappler to perform a 1-Arm Bent Over Row.

Drew completes the exercise by lifting the bar to his chest, making sure not to jerk it as he lifts it. Use weight that you can safely perform 10 reps.

TECHNICAL TIP: Use your imagination when training with the Grappler. There are many different exercises that are effective for combat sports using this piece of equipment. Working this thing simulates a human body in many ways, so make it a point to get one and use it. You can find the Grappler at www.westside-barbell.com.

PRESSES, PULLS, CLEANS AND SNATCHES FOR UPPER BODY STRENGTH

The lifts presented here really develop strength in your upper body. Remember that your physical abilities dictate how well your technical skills are performed. For example, the most basic defense against a choke is to have a strong, muscular neck!

HIGH PULLS

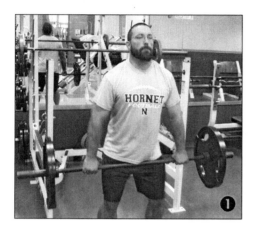 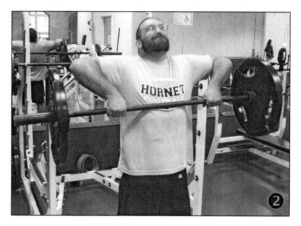

Jake holds the bar at arms' length, touching the front of his hips. Jake's head is erect and he is looking forward to insure his back is erect and his shoulders are square. Jake's grip on the bar is a bit wider than the width of his shoulders.

Jake pulls (not jerks) the barbell upward as high as possible with his elbows out wide, making sure to keep the barbell close to his body. This is a great exercise for your trapezius, shoulders, entire upper back and upper arms.

BENT OVER BARBELL ROWING

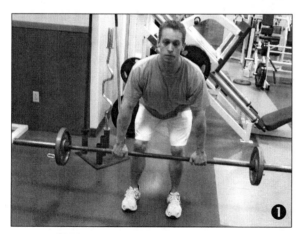 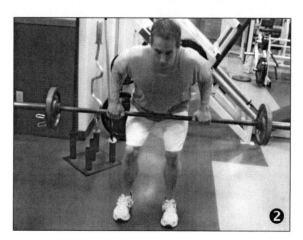

Drew bends over, making sure his knees are slightly bent to avoid injuring his back. He holds the barbell at shoulder width.

Drew pulls the barbell to his torso or chest, touching the bar to his torso or chest with each repetition. This exercise is good for your entire back, but especially for your latissimus dorsi and upper back structure.

UPRIGHT BARBELL ROWING

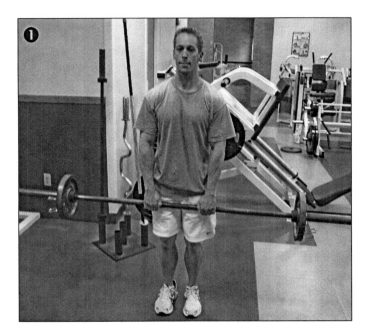

An exercise that is similar to High Pulls is the Upright Row. Drew holds the bar at a width a bit narrower than his shoulders and stands upright with his head forward, keeping his back erect and shoulders square.

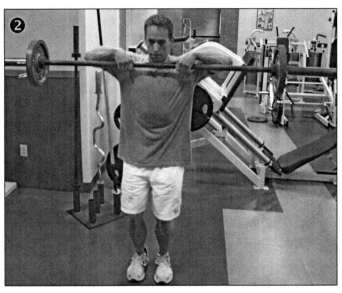

Drew pulls (not jerks or swings) the barbell up to his chin with his elbow out wide. Notice that you will have a slight bend in your wrists as shown here. That's a natural movement and won't hurt your wrists. This exercise is ideal for development in your traps, shoulders and upper back.

TECHNICAL TIP: When loading plates on a bar, load them with the flat side out. Seasoned lifters have, for years, loaded plates onto bars with the flat side out. This is a custom that is a holdover from the sport of Powerlifting. Some of the new plates made today don't have a flat side, so this "rule" doesn't apply in that case. It's really a silly thing, but we've seen old-timers get highly upset at a new guy in a gym that made the mistake of loading a barbell plate on a bar the wrong way. Does it make the weight any heavier or make the exercise more efficient? No. It simply is an old ritual used in countless weightrooms all over the world. However, if you want to load the bar with the flat side in, feel free to do it, but please not in our gyms!

POWER CLEANS

This exercise is a popular one, although the authors don't always recommend it. It is a good overall strength developer, especially for your upper body, but you have a potential of injury if you use bad form or too much weight. Use moderate weight and perform 3 to 5 sets of 5 to 10 reps per set depending on your goals and fitness level.

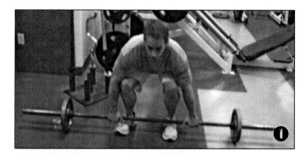

Drew starts the exercise by squatting and grabbing the bar just a bit wider than the width of his shoulders. Drew's head is up and he is looking ahead to keep his back straight, with his chest extended forward.

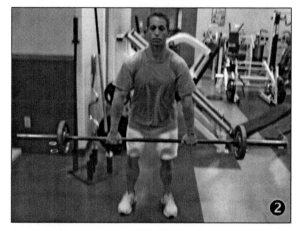

Drew pulls the bar up the line of his body.

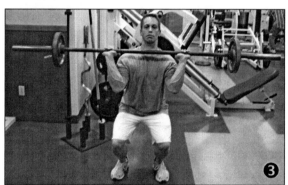

Drew cleans the barbell by swinging it upward and onto the front of his shoulders high on his chest. His elbows are forward. As he pulls the barbell up, Drew dips under the barbell by doing a partial squat.

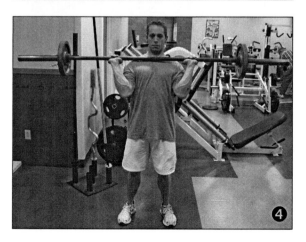

To complete the lift, Drew stands erect with the barbell resting on his upper chest. Drew will lower the weight to the floor and start over to begin his next repetition.

HANG CLEANS

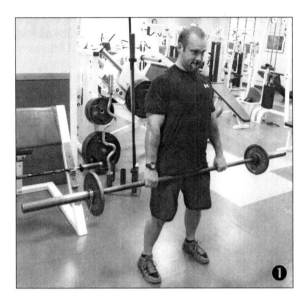

A common variation of the Power Clean is the Hang Clean. It's called the "Hang" Clean because Chris is holding the barbell at arms' length as shown, thus "hanging" in front if him.

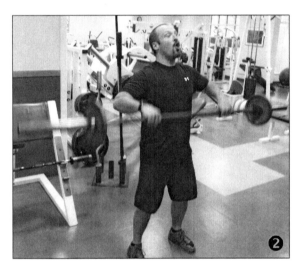

Chris cleans the barbell upward as shown. Another variation of the Hang Clean is that Chris doesn't squat or dip under the barbell as he cleans it.

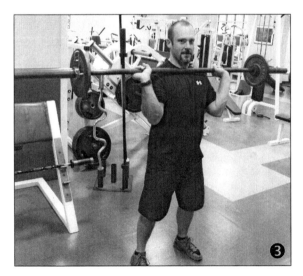

Chris completes the lift by resting the barbell on his upper chest.

OVERHEAD BARBELL PRESS

Pressing a barbell over your head is a fantastic way of developing your strength. Before the Bench Press became popular in the 1960s, the Overhead (or Military) Press was the primary exercise used to develop the upper body. The Overhead Press develops just about every muscle in your upper body and requires a strong lower body (legs and hips) to handle the workload. We recommend this exercise as a serious, tried and true exercise to increase the strength in your upper body. Perform 3 to 5 sets of this exercise, using 5 to 10 reps per set, depending on your goals and strength level.

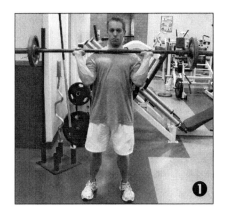

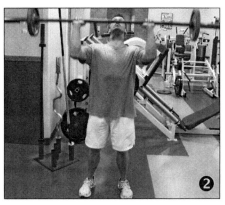

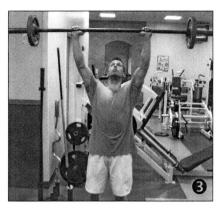

Drew starts the exercise by either cleaning the barbell or taking it from a rack.

Drew's hands are about a shoulder width apart. He presses the barbell upward, making sure not to jerk, swing or bounce as he lifts the barbell.

Drew presses the barbell overhead to arms' length. He will lower the weight to his chest and perform another repetition.

SEATED BARBELL PRESS

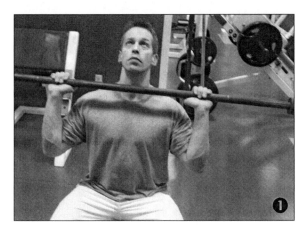

A good variation of the Overhead Press is to perform it when seated on a bench. Drew holds the barbell at his upper chest.

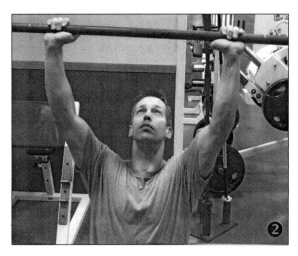

Drew presses the barbell overhead. Performing this exercise when seated forces you to use only your upper body, making it more difficult to do. Use less weight than when doing this exercise standing.

PUSH PRESS

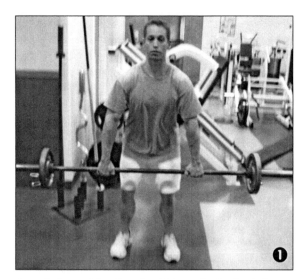

A variation of the Overhead Press is the Push Press. Drew cleans the barbell to his chest as he would the Overhead Press.

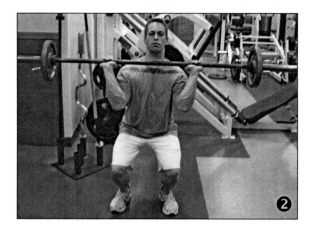

As Drew cleans the barbell, he dips under it slightly, making sure not to squat down too far (just bend his knees). As Drew presses the bar upward, he "pushes" it upward by using his legs to help in the lifting action.

2 MAN OVERHEAD PRESS

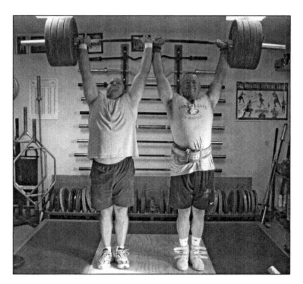

Here's a lift that relies on some real strength and team-work! World All-Round Weightlifting Team Champions Chad Ullom and Al Myers perform a heavy 2-Man Overhead Press with an extra-long bar. As a grappler or fighter, you may not do this type of lifting on a regular basis, but there's nothing wrong in trying some different types of lifting and having some fun in the gym from time to time. For information on All-Round Weightlifting, visit their web site at www.USAWA.com.

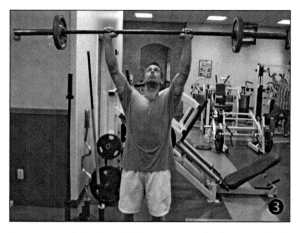

Drew completes the lift by pressing the bar overhead in one "pushing" motion. The Push Press is a good variation of the Overhead Press and is sometimes called the "Cheat Press" because of the use of the legs when performing the lift.

SNATCH

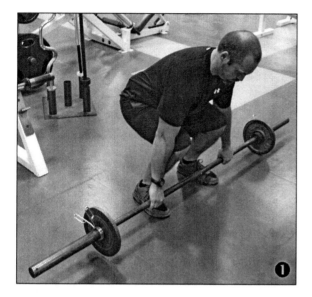

The Snatch is one of the 2 Olympic-style lifts and is a good all-round lift requiring strength, coordination and speed. Chris uses a wide grip to hold the barbell as he squats down, making sure his back is erect.

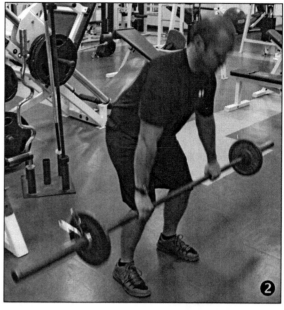

In a quick, explosive movement, Chris lifts the barbell off the floor.

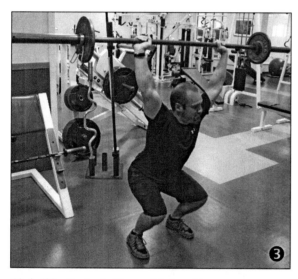

Chris lifts the barbell over his head in one movement as he dips or slightly squats under the bar as shown. Look at how Chris has his arms straight as he holds the bar overhead.

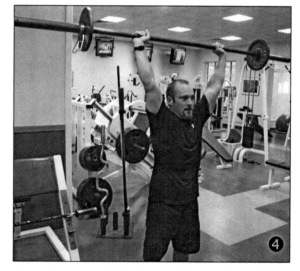

Chris finishes the lift by standing upright with the bar extended over his head. Chris will lower the bar to the floor and repeat the exercise. For fighters and grapplers, the authors recommend that you perform this exercise once in a while to break the monotony of training. A routine of 3 to 5 sets of 5 to 10 reps per set will give you a good workout. Use moderate weight so that you maintain good lifting technique to avoid injuries.

PRESSES USING THE BENCH

You can use a bench for more than simply the Bench Press. A bench is a handy tool and can be used in a variety of ways. Presented here are just a few exercises you can do using a bench.

SEATED SNATCH

The Seated Snatch really isolates your upper body, forcing it to do most of the work. In a standard Snatch, the legs get a workout as well, and this variation keys in on your upper back and shoulder strength. The goal when performing a Snatch, especially when doing it off the bench, is to keep your back erect, chest forward, head upright and keep your elbows as straight as possible. You want to swing the barbell up and over your head in one explosive movement.

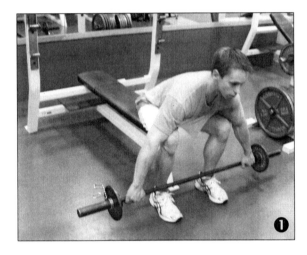

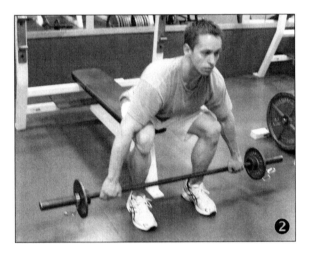

1. Drew is seated on the end of a bench and grabs the bar very wide as shown.

2. Drew lifts the barbell off the floor as he straightens his body.

3. In one explosive movement, Drew lifts the bar overhead. He will lower the bar to the floor with control and start his next repetition.

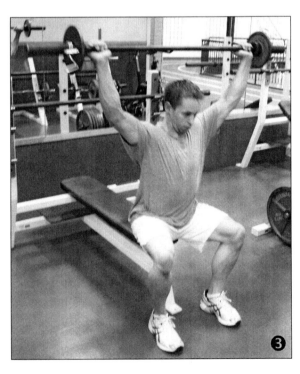

FLAT BENCH PRESS

The Bench Press is a standard lift in all gyms, but fighters and grapplers should use it with discretion. This lift is a good upper body developer, but if you spend too much time doing it, you take time away from other lifts or exercises that are more beneficial for grapplers and fighters. Big man-boobs aren't that important for athletes in combat sports. However, in an overall strength program, using the Flat Bench Press, as well as the Decline and Incline Bench Presses, can be beneficial to you.

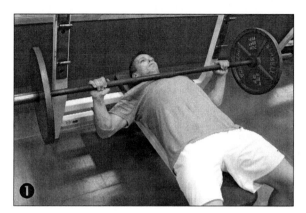

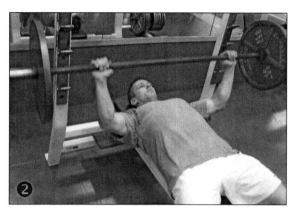

Drew grabs the bar using a medium-width grip. He lowers the bar to his chest so that it touches his chest.

When pressing the bar, Drew makes sure not to arch his back up and keeps his back flat on the bench.

Depending on your goals, level of strength and personal preferences, perform 3 to 5 sets of 5 to 10 reps. As with other lifts such as the Overhead Press, Squat, Snatch, Deadlift and others, you will use a variety of lifting routines when performing this standard lift. The Bench Press works your chest, shoulders, upper back and triceps. A lot of people spend a lot of time lying on a bench, looking up at the ceiling and pressing a bar off of their chests. As said before, use this lift once in a while. The authors favor using the Overhead Press as the primary upper body strength development lift, and recommend using the Bench Press once a week at most.

NARROW GRIP BENCH PRESS

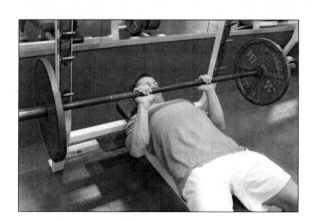

This variation of the Bench Press is to grab the bar slightly wider than your chest as Drew is doing here. You won't lift as much weight, but this is an excellent exercise for your triceps and inner pecs.

INCLINE BENCH PRESS

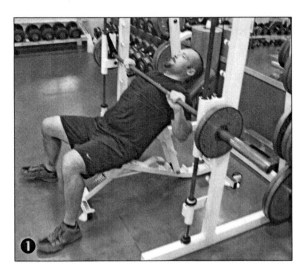

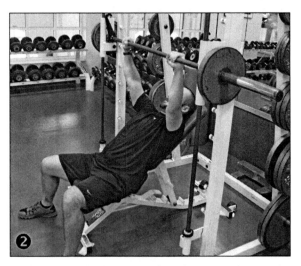

Performing a Bench Press from this position works your upper chest and front deltoids. Chris uses a medium-width grip on the bar as he lowers the bar off the rack, touching his chest.

Chris presses the bar upward as shown. He lowers the bar to his chest with control to complete the lift. Use 3 to 5 sets of 5 to 10 reps to get a good workout.

SMITH MACHINE INCLINE BENCH POP-UPS

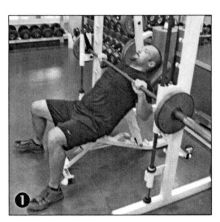

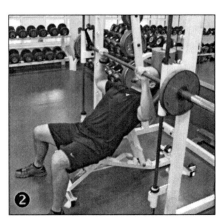

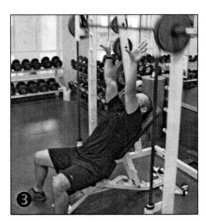

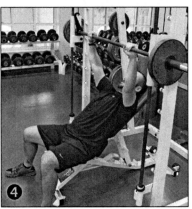

1. The Smith Machine is fairly common in most gyms today. It affords you a good degree of safety in lifting and keeps the bar in a straight track. Chris holds the bar with a medium-width grip and uses light weight to perform this exercise. **CAUTION:** Only perform this exercise when using a Smith Machine!

2. Chris starts to press the bar.

3. As he presses the bar, Chris "pops" it out of his hands and throws it upward as high as possible.

4. Chris catches the bar, lowers it to his chest and starts his next repetition. This is a good exercise to develop "push-off" power. Remember, use light weight!

DIPS, PULL UPS, CHIN UPS, PUSH UPS AND USING THE BAR OR PLATES

Using the weight or your own body to develop strength is highly recommended! Most gyms have dip racks, pull up bars and other pieces of equipment where you can perform exercises using your body weight. You are encouraged to add more weight to these exercises by using a weighted vest, weight belt that holds weight plates, kettlebells or dumb-bells or even wearing wrap-around ankle weights making the movement more difficult.

DIPS

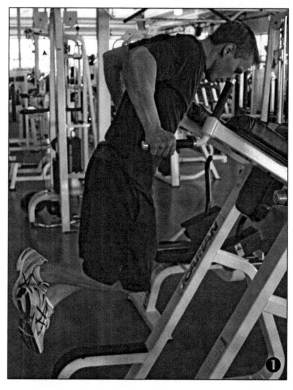

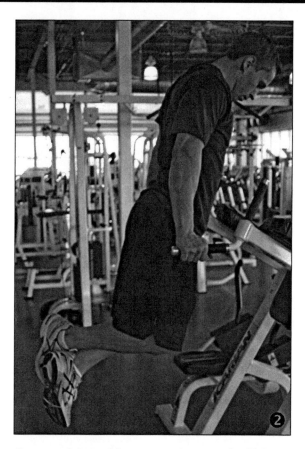

One of the best exercises anyone, whether they're a fighter or not, can ever do in the gym is the Dip. This exercise develops your entire upper body, but it really focuses on the structure of your shoulders, pectorals and upper back. Also, there are few better triceps exercises than the Dip. Drew assumes the position as shown here, making sure to keep his body upright and hooking his feet to avoid swinging.

Drew straightens his arms as shown and will lower himself to complete the rep. A good routine to follow when performing Dips is to perform 3 to 5 sets, doing as many strict reps as possible per set.

TECHNICAL TIP: Dips are a great "test" of strength. Every so often, test yourself to see how many strict Dips you can do without stopping. Really gut them out. You can also get some of the guys your train with to have a "Dip Contest" for bragging rights in your gym.

WEIGHTED DIPS

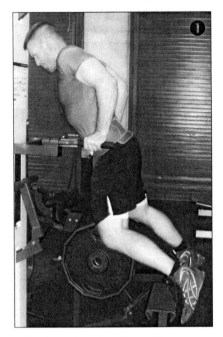 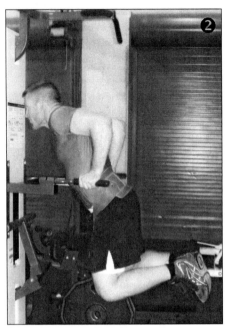 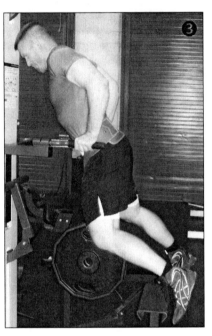

Mike is performing dips while wearing a hip belt with weight plates.

Mike cranks outs the dips, making sure his legs are bent to emphasize the work for his upper body.

Mike can also wear a weighted vest or use strap-on ankle weights to add more resistance to this exercise.

BENCH DIPS

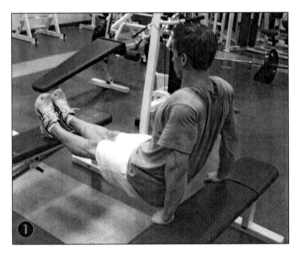 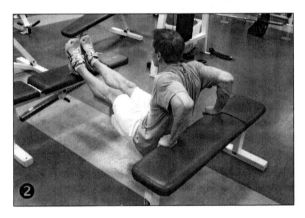

An excellent variation when doing Dips is to perform them as shown here. Drew rests his feet on a bench with his legs straight as he places his hands on another bench, supporting his body.

Drew lowers his body as far down as possible and then presses up, straightening his arms to come to the starting position. Bench Dips really isolate your triceps, and give your upper back, shoulders and chest a tough workout as well. Use this variation once in a while when performing your Dip routine. Also, if you don't have access to a Dip bar, this is a great way to perform Dips.

NARROW GRIP BENCH DIPS

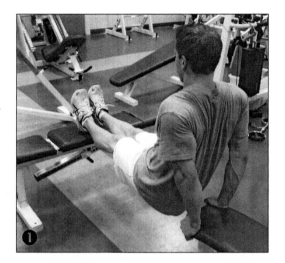 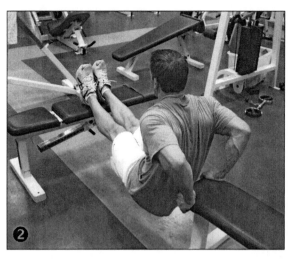

Drew really focuses in on his triceps in this variation of the Bench Dip. Look at how narrow his hands are grabbing the bench.

Drew makes sure to not allow his elbows to go out wide when dipping down. Try to keep your elbows back and not flair out to the side so that your triceps get the full benefit of this exercise.

BENCH DIPS WITH PARTNER HOLDING FEET (LOW POSITION)

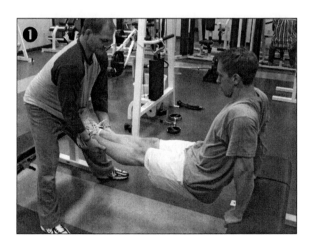 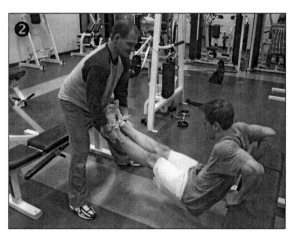

In this Bench Dip variation, Bryan holds Drew's feet as shown.

Bryan makes sure not to allow Drew to sag, so he stands back far enough to make Drew keep his legs straight when performing this exercise.

BENCH DIPS WITH PARTNER HOLDING FEET (HIGH POSITION)

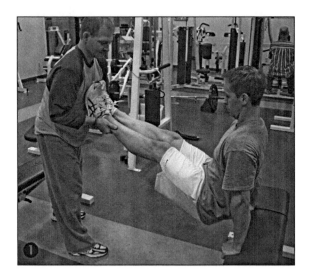

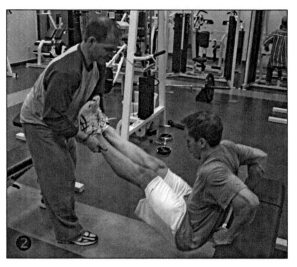

To make this exercise harder, Bryan holds both of Drew's feet high at Bryan's chest. This variation puts a lot of stress on Drew's upper body when he performs the dipping movement.

Bryan makes sure to keep Drew's legs straight and not allow him to sag as he does the dipping movement.

DIP BAR PUSH UPS

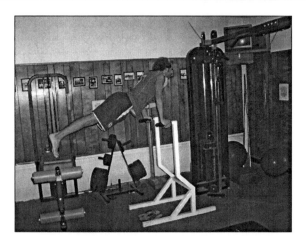

Josh Henges performs push-ups on a dip rack with his feet resting on a box sitting on a piece of gym equipment. Doing push-ups this way will give you a deep, full range of movement and work your entire upper body.

TECHNICAL TIP: Be creative in using the equipment you have in your gym or weightroom. Be safe, and don't do anything foolish, but use your imagination. Just because someone named a piece of equipment "Dip Bars" doesn't mean the only thing you can do on it are dips. Anything can be used as a tool, implement or object to increase your strength or fitness level.

COMPOUND EXERCISE USING PUSH UP, BURPEE AND PULL UP

Performing a series of exercises is an excellent way of pushing yourself in your training. You can combine any number of exercises together based on your needs, interest and level of fitness.

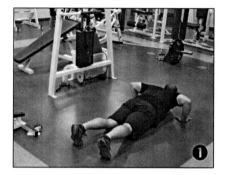

Chris starts his routine by performing a Push Up.

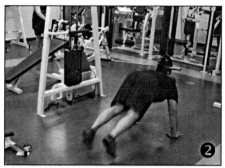

After completing his Push Up, Chris immediately performs a Burpee (Squat Thrust).

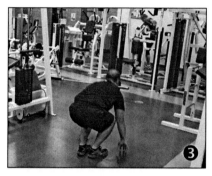

As soon as Chris completes his Burpee, he jumps up.

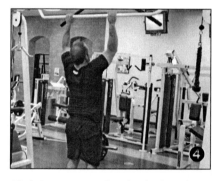

Chris jumps up and grabs the bar above him.

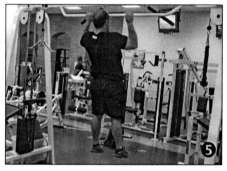

Chris performs a Pull Up.

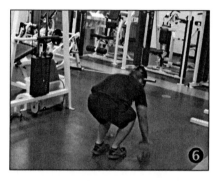

Chris lets go of the bar and drops to the floor. He will immediately perform another Burpee.

As soon as you shoot your legs out to complete the Burpee, finish with a Push Up. Chris will perform this series of exercises doing as many as possible in a specified time, or doing a specified number of times he performs this circuit. **Wearing a weight vest will add resistance to this exercise and make it harder.**

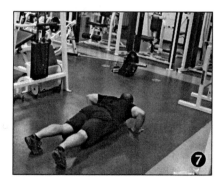

PULL UPS WITH PALMS FACING AWAY

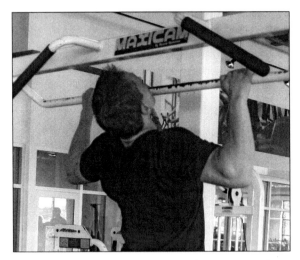

Pull Ups are one of the best exercises you can do to develop serious and functional strength in the upper back, shoulders, upper chest and arms. Along with Dip, this exercise is one of the best strength developers ever invented. Performing this exercise with your palms facing forward is an excellent workout. Perform 5 sets, doing as many reps as possible per set. Wear a weighted vest or a hip belt with weights to make this exercise harder.

ONE ARM PULL UPS

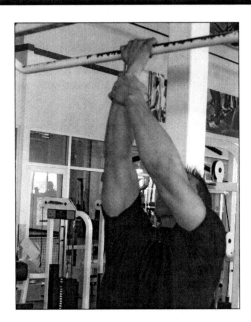

Drew isolates one side of his body when doing 1-Arm Pull Ups. He uses his left hand to grab his right forearm and wrist when performing this exercise to keep his shoulders square and avoid swinging.

PULL UPS WITH PALMS FACING YOU

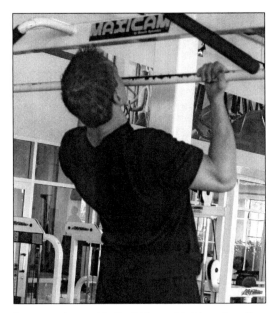

Drew performs his Pull Ups with his palms facing him as shown here. This places the emphasis on his biceps with additional work for the latissimus dorsi.

HANG FOR TIME

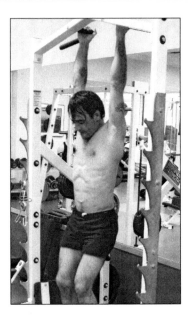

Jump up and grab the bar or handles and allow your body weight to relax. Hang as long as possible. This exercise is tougher than you might think. This is a tough grip exercise and works your arms, shoulders, back and entire body. This can be used as a finisher after a hard workout.

PULL UP FROM A HANG

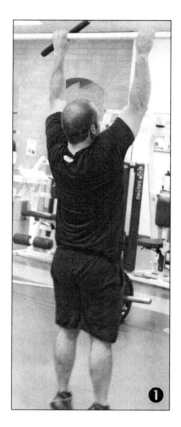
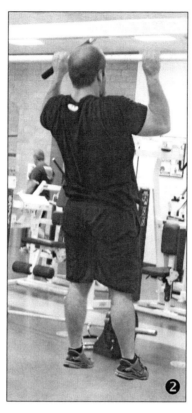

1. Chris will jump up and hold onto the pull up bar and hang there for a count of 10. He then performs as many pull-ups as he can do. Perform 5 sets of this exercise.

2. By hanging for a count of 10, and then performing your pull-ups, you add far more work to this exercise.

BARBELL PUSH UP

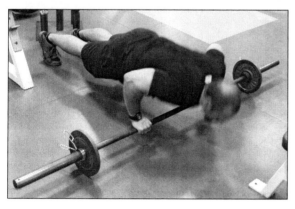

Chris holds a barbell while doing Push Ups. Chris can vary this exercise by rolling the barbell out in front of him or back toward his lower body to make it more difficult. This is a good variation of the Push Up and can be used to break the monotony in your training.

PLATE HOLD LEAN BACK

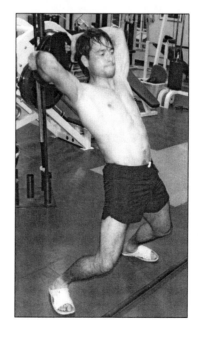

You can hold a weight plate over your head and lean back with a slight arch in your body as Nikolay is doing in this photo. Hold the plate for a specified period of time, doing several sets depending on your interest and fitness level.

FRONT PRESS USING EMPTY BAR (AND BANDS FOR MORE RESISTANCE)

A good exercise for explosive power in punching or pushing an opponent away form you is this Front Press. You can use just the bar or attach an elastic band on the bar and loop it around your shoulders and back to make it more difficult.

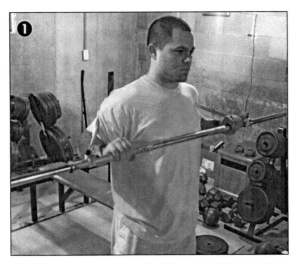

David uses an empty bar, in this case a 25-pound bar, to perform this exercise. He grabs the bar a little wider than his pectorals and holds it to his chest as shown.

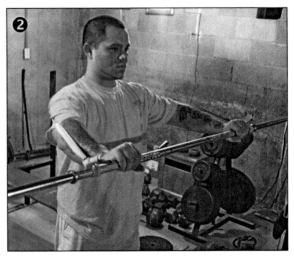

David pushes the bar directly to his front so that his arms are fully extended. Using the elastic band makes this movement more difficult.

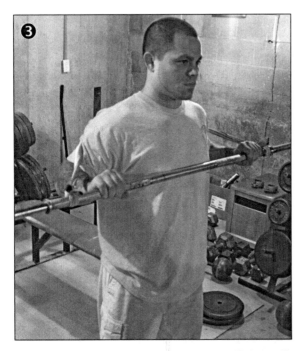

David returns the bar to his chest and will immediately perform another rep. This is a great warm-up as well as a finisher to any workout. Perform this exercise quickly, doing as many reps as possible in a specified time limit.

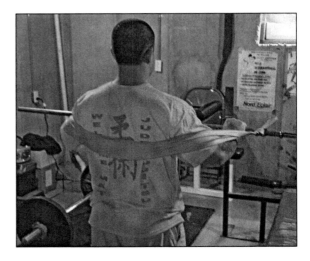

David has looped the elastic band around his shoulders and chest as shown here to add resistance to this exercise.

WEIGHT PLATE STEERING WHEEL

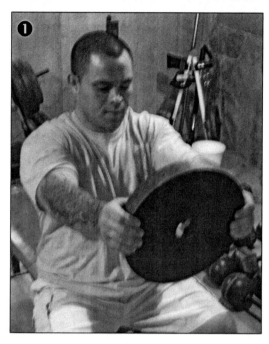

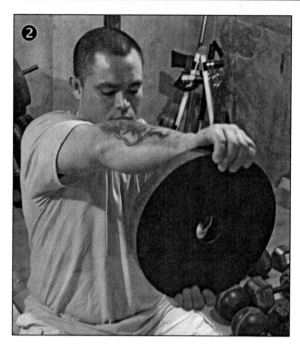

This is a good forearm exercise with benefits for your shoulders and upper back. David holds a weight plate out in front of him with his arms extended.

David turns the plate in the same way he would a steering wheel. He will turn the plate back and forth doing as many reps as he wishes. This is a good finisher for any workout to develop your forearms and grip.

HORIZONTAL PULL UPS ON BENCH OR POWER RACK USING BAR

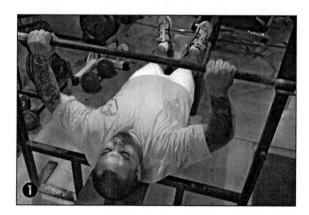

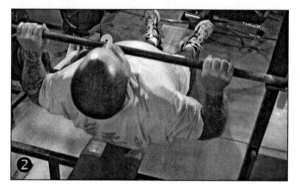

Pull yourself up you until your chest touches the bar. Keep your body rigid as you can throughout the movement. Repeat this exercise for as many reps as you can for several sets. Vary your grip from workout to work out and try varying the angle of your body by raising your feet, or by lowering them to the floor. Another variation is to secure a band over your chest and each end to the bottom of the rack. The added resistance of the band will make you very strong.

This develops the pulling muscles of your arms, rear delts and upper back. This is a good exercise to perform after doing Push Ups or Bench Presses so that you work opposing muscle groups. Grab a horizontal bar and place your feet out in front of you so that you are in a prone position.

AROUND THE WORLD USING WEIGHT PLATE

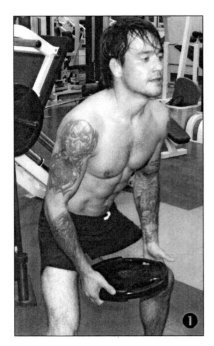 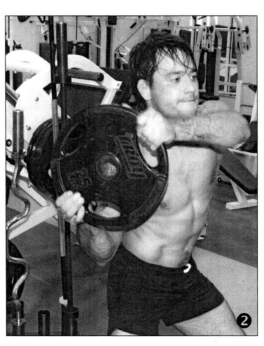 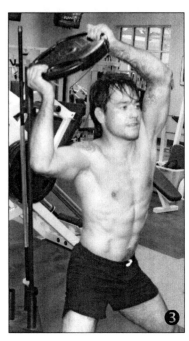

Nikolay holds a weight plate with both hands in front of him as shown here.

Nikolay moves the plate to his right, over his right shoulder.

Nikolay moves the plate over his head.

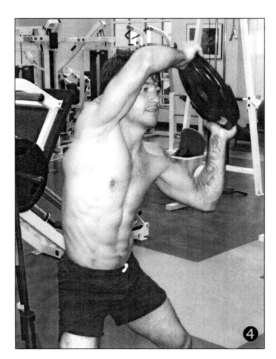 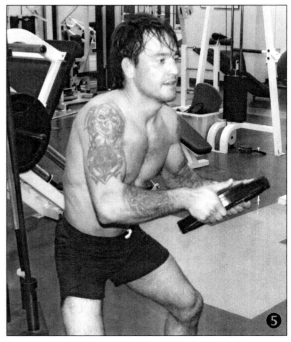

Nikolay then moves the weight over his left shoulder.

Nikolay moves the plate over his left shoulder, returning it to the starting position. He will rotate the plate in the other direction to balance his workout. Perform several sets of this movement as a great warm-up before a workout.

CABLE MACHINE EXERCISES

One of the best pieces of equipment in any gym is the Cable Crossover Machine. You can use this machine for many exercises and get a fantastic workout. Working with the cable machine offers a safe, controlled way of performing every gym movement and gives you excellent resistance. Almost every movement you can do with a barbell or dumb-bell can be replicated on a cable machine. Presented here are some exercises recommend for fighters and grapplers.

CABLE CROSSOVERS (CRUNCH STYLE)

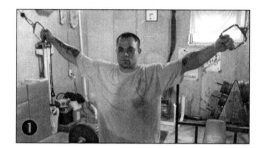

David grabs a handle with each hand as shown, making sure to extend his arms fully.

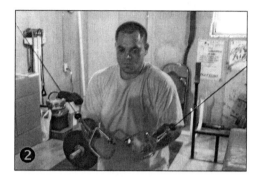

David pulls each cable in to his front midline, emphasizing an inward squeeze towards the stomach. Perform 3 to 5 sets of 10 reps using enough weight to make your work hard for the entire routine.

CABLE CROSSOVERS TO FRONT WITH STRAIGHT ARMS

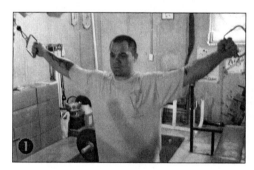

David grabs each handle with each of his arms, making sure they are fully extended.

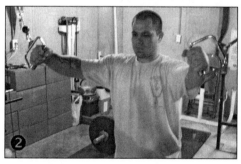

David keeps his arms fairly rigid and pulls the handles to his front.

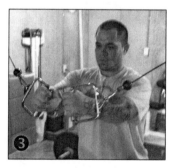

David brings the handles together as shown. This is a good variation of this exercise and places a lot of the workload on your front deltoids, entire length of your pectorals, upper back and entire arm structure.

BENT OVER CABLE CROSSOVERS

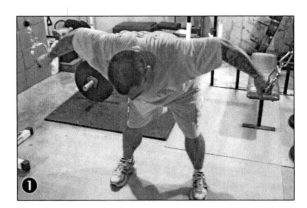

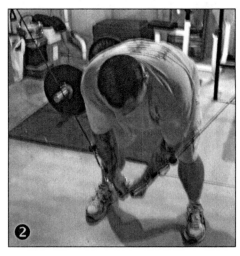

This is an excellent pectoral developer, and you can work your chest hard by varying how far you bend over as you perform the movement. David bends over at the waist as he holds the handles in each hand with his arms extended.

David pulls the handles inward so that they meet together in front of him. This is a really good movement to work your chest, shoulders and upper back.

SIDE CABLE PULL-DOWNS

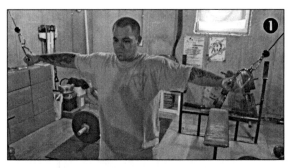

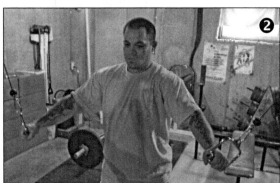

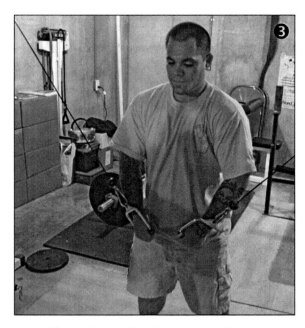

3. David pulls the handles downward so that they meet in front of him. Perform 3 to 5 sets of 10 reps.

1. This exercise isolates your side deltoids and has an additional benefit for your upper back. David holds the handles out to his side with his palms down as shown.

2. David pulls the handles downward keeping his arms rigid as he does.

STRAIGHT ARM CABLE PUSHDOWNS

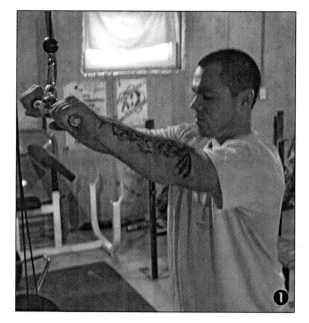

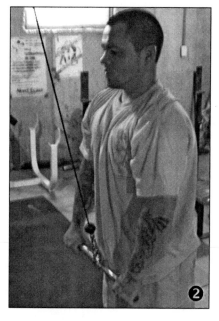

This is a good exercise for grapplers and fighters who like to use the Cable Crossover Machine. It works the lats and high into the triceps. This type of exercise helps develop strength for punching and pulling an opponent when grappling.

David stands facing the machine and takes a shoulder-width grip on the bar, keeping his arms straight. David makes sure not to move his back and keeps his abdominals contracted.

Davis pushes the bar downward until it touches the front of his body at the hips.

CABLE PALMS UP PULLDOWNS

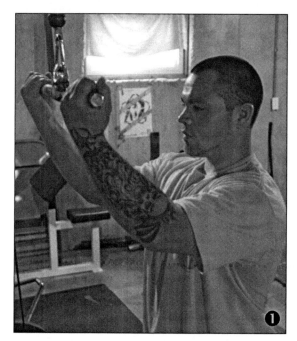

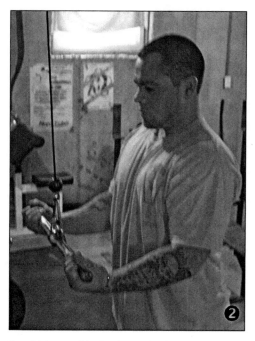

A good variation of the Straight Arm Pushdowns is to perform this Straight Arm Pull Down.

It works the same muscle groups, but places more emphasis on your triceps. David grabs the bar with his palms up and arms fairly rigid.

David keeps his back motionless as he pulls the bar downward until it meets the front of his hips. Perform 3 to 5 sets of 10 reps.

CABLE LAT PULLDOWNS (TO UPPER CHEST)

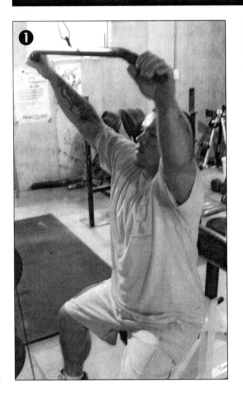
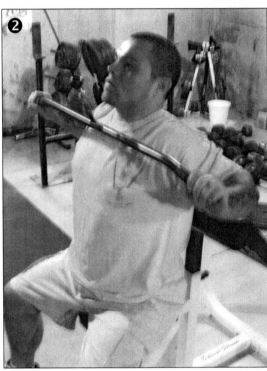

1. There are several ways to perform the Lat Pulldown, but this one emphasizes the muscles that you often use in grappling. Davis takes a wide grip on the bar as shown.

2. David pulls the bar to his upper chest as shown, making sure to flair his elbows back as far as possible as he pulls.

CABLE CHEST PULLS (SEATED)

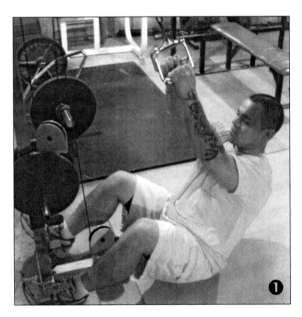
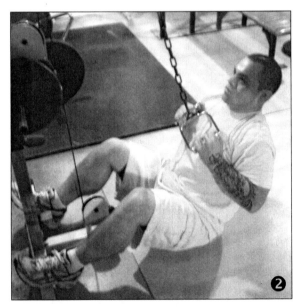

David sits on the floor as shown, with the handles above him in a higher position.

David pulls the handles to his chest making sure his elbows are pulled back far. Pull, don't jerk the weight and use a fairly heavy weight. This is excellent for your upper back, shoulders, arms and chest.

CABLE CROSSOVER CURLS

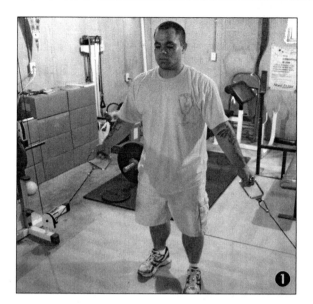

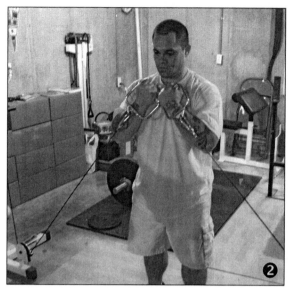

This movement is a good biceps developer, but it also works your entire upper body. David holds the handles down low as shown.

David curls the handles to his chest as shown, making sure to not jerk or swing the weight. This is an excellent exercise for grapplers because it strengthens all the muscles you use when you pull an opponent.

CABLE CROSSOVER CURLS (1 ARM)

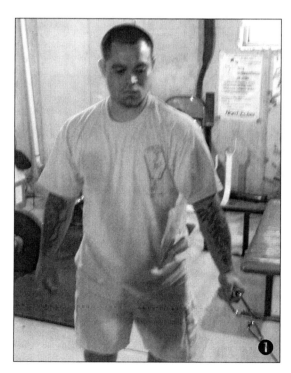

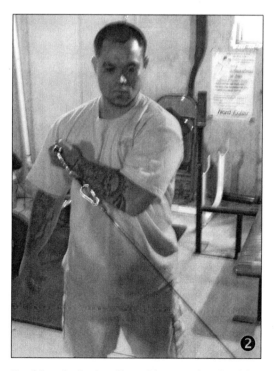

This is a good biceps exercise, but also works the entire side you pull with. David holds the handle as shown.

David curls the handle to his opposite shoulder. Do not jerk or swing the handle; emphasize a smooth curling motion. This exercise works the biceps (and entire arm), as well as the shoulder, upper back and pectoral.

CABLE PREACHER BENCH CURLS

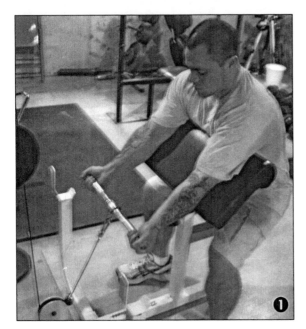

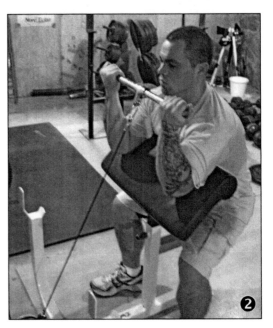

The Preacher Bench is a great tool that forces you to perform curls in a stricter fashion and doing the Preacher's Bench Curls with the cable machine offers more safety in training than using a barbell for novice as well as advanced lifters. David grabs the bar with both hands.

Davis curls the bar in a smooth controlled motion, making sure not to jerk the bar. Preacher Curls give you a serious biceps workout, so make it a point to perform this exercise as often as possible.

CABLE PREACHER BENCH CURLS (1 ARM)

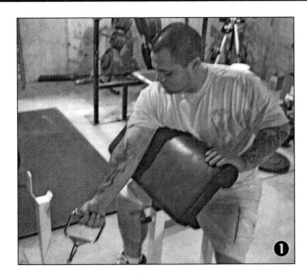

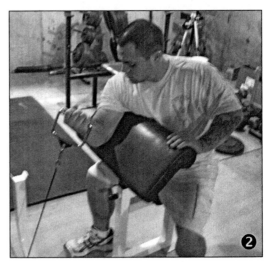

The 1-arm version of the Preacher Bench Curl isolates your arm as shown. Make sure to use a moderate weight and don't yank or jerk the handle.

David curls the handle with control to get the full benefit of the movement. You can perform this movement with a dumb-bell as well if you prefer not to use a cable machine.

CABLE SKULL CRUSHERS

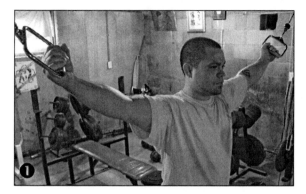

David holds the cable out wide to each side with his arms extended and palms up.

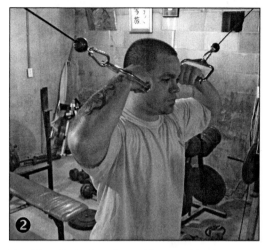

David curls the handles to his ears. This is a good biceps workout.

CABLE UCHIKOMI

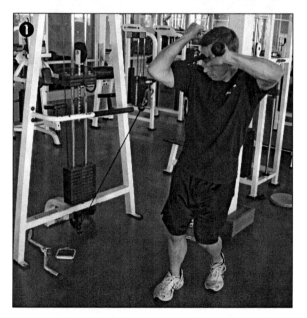

Drew performs Uchikomi drills on the cable machine by using a rope. You can use a towel, judo belt or anything to hold onto while doing Uchikomi.

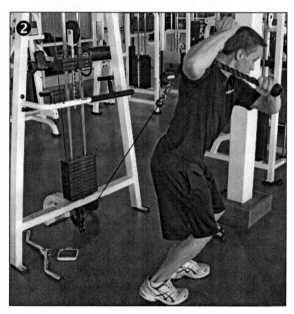

Drew turns, and as he does, he performs the same movement he would if he were throwing an opponent.

EXERCISES FOR THE ARMS

While doing "curls for the girls" will indeed, give you large strong arms, the more important reason to have strong arms is that we use our arms to control our opponent, strike our opponent, grab our opponent, and generally use our arms as an extension of our bodies. You use your arms to grab, hold, hit and manipulate your opponent, as well as use them in many other ways when fighting or grappling. Arm strength is extremely important.

TRICEPS BARBELL CURL

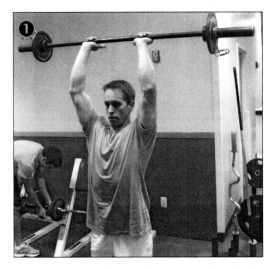

The Triceps Curl or Triceps Extension is the fundamental exercise to develop your triceps. Tri means "three" and ceps means, "head." The triceps is the largest muscle group in your upper arm and does a tremendous amount of work.

MANHANDLE YOUR OPPONENT WITH ARM STRENGTH

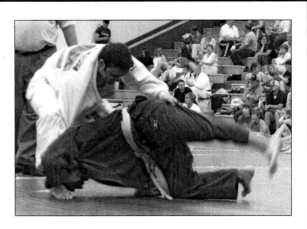

Arm strength is mandatory for success in any fighting sport. You grab, pull, push and manipulate your opponent with your arms and hands. Pulling an opponent over onto his back takes tremendous arm strength. Derrick Darling pulls his opponent over onto his back to start a hold-down.

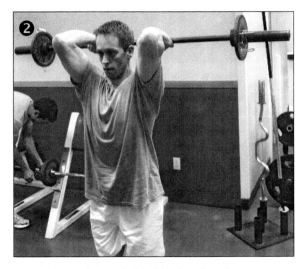

Drew lowers the bar behind his head as shown.

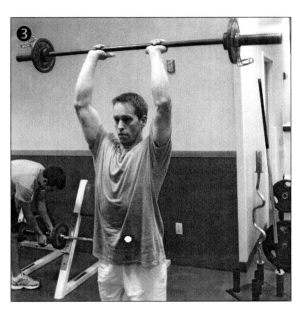

Drew curls the barbell back to its original position overhead.

TECHNICAL TIP: When doing Triceps Curls, point your elbows directly forward and don't allow them to flair out wide. Keeping your elbows forward works your triceps harder.

TRICEPS CURL WITH E-Z CURL BAR

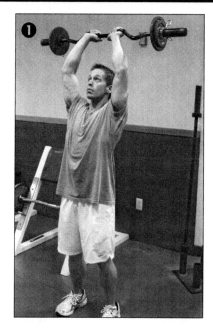
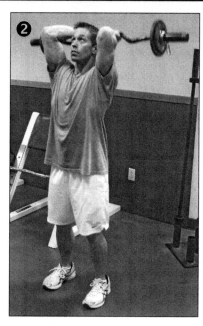
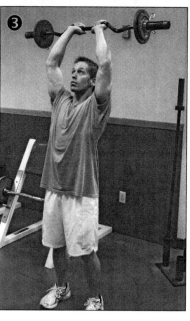

Drew's grip is a bit narrower on this variation of the Triceps Curl. Doing this changes the angle of how his triceps are worked. Drew holds the bar overhead.

Drew lowers the bar slowly behind his head.

Drew curls the bar back to its original position overhead.

SEATED TRICEPS CURL WITH E-Z CURL BAR

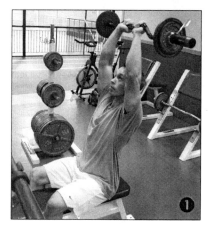
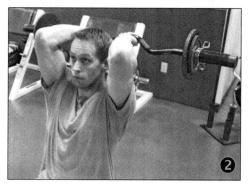
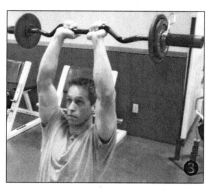

Seated Triceps Curls do not allow you to use your lower body and reduce the chance that you will cheat or swing the weight as you lift it. We recommend this form of this Triceps Curl to really isolate your triceps and gain serious strength. Drew has the bar extended overhead with his palms forward as shown.

Drew lowers the bar behind his head as shown, making sure to slowly lower the bar and not allow it to drop.

Drew curls the bar back to its original position overhead.

> **TECHNICAL TIP:** You can also use a short straight bar or even a long Olympic bar when doing the Seated Triceps Curl.

TRICEPS PRESS ON BENCH USING E-Z CURL BAR

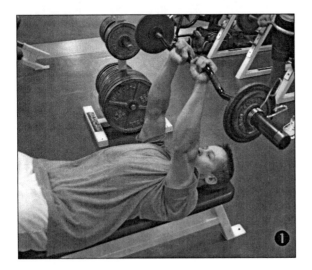

Drew holds the bar above his head as shown while lying on the bench.

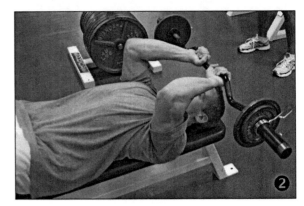

Drew bends his elbows as shown, lowering the bar slowly to his forehead.

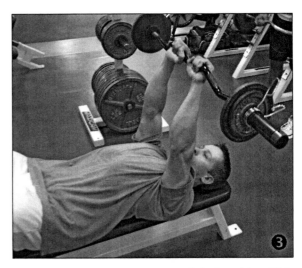

Drew presses the bar back to its original position. This way of performing the Triceps Curl forces you to do strict controlled and measured movement that develops real strength. Use moderate weight on this movement and don't jerk the weight.

WRIST ROLLER

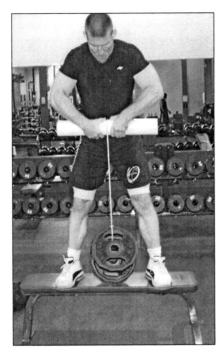

This exercise is terrific for forearm and grip development. Mike is using a PVC pipe that is about 2 to 3 inches in diameter. Drill a hole through the PVC and run a strong nylon rope through it. Attach some weight plates on the end of the rope. Mike rolls the weight up, then back down, repeating for as many reps as possible. Don't be surprised if you feel a hellacious burn in your forearms and hands.

BARBELL CURL

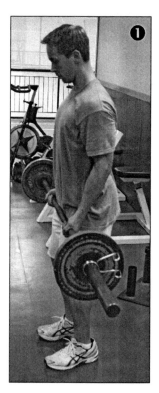
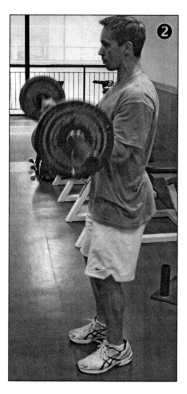
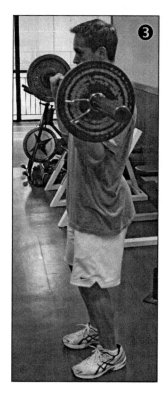

The biceps are important for grappling and fighting. Sure, big arms look good, but strong arms are what you want to have. Doing Barbell Curls with an Olympic bar is an excellent overall arm developer. The straight Olympic bar, rather than an E-Z curl bar, is preferred because it provides the angle necessary to develop the muscles in the entire forearm and elbow joint as well as the biceps.

Drew makes sure not to swing the barbell or "cheat" when he performs this lift. Also, don't "hump" the weight with your hips to help move the barbell. Use enough weight so that you can perform a strict curl movement and also provide enough resistance so that you can perform 6 to 10 repetitions. A good workout is to perform a Pyramid where you do 10 reps at a moderate weight, then 8 reps with a little more weight, then onto 5 reps with more weight, then 4 reps with even more weight, and then 2 reps with heavy weight. It might look like this: Set 1: 10 reps at 110 pounds; Set 2: 8 reps at 125 pounds; Set 3: 6 reps at 140 pounds; Set 4: 4 reps at 150 pounds; Set 5: 2 reps at 160 pounds.

Drew curls the barbell to his chin, making sure not to swing or hoist the weight. Good, strict curls help you develop real strength, but also help you avoid injuries.

TECHNICAL TIP: Never underestimate the importance of arm strength for any combat sport. Your arms enable you to "reach out and touch someone." You hold, hook and hit with your arms. The stronger your arms are, the better chance you have of winning a fight.

TREADMILL AND GYM RUNNING

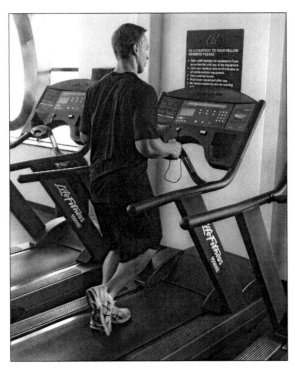

To wrap up this part of the book presenting exercises you can do in the gym, it's important to remember to work on your cardio in the gym. If the weather's bad, or yuo simply prefer to train on your cardio in the gym, don't forget to get your time in on the treadmill or other cardio machines.

ELLIPTICAL MACHINE

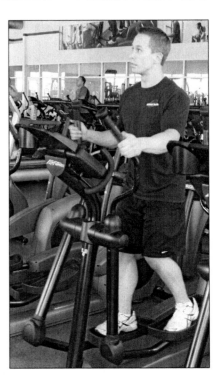

A great addition to any cardio workout is to work on the Elliptical Machine. If you've developed shin splints or other injuries from running, the gliding movement of this machine is excellent for your cardio development. This machine really gives you a strenuous workout and if you haven't tried it yet, be sure to jump on one and work up a sweat!

STATIONARY BIKE

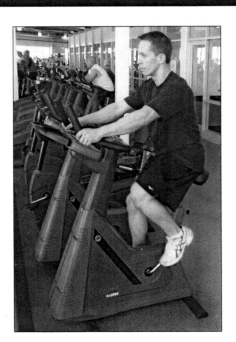

Training on a Stationary Bike is a great workout and used by a lot of athletes as a warm-up before a lifting workout. If you have knee or ankle injuries but still need to work on your cardio, working out on a bike in the gym will give you a good workout. Often not as tough of a cardio workout as the Treadmill or Elliptical Machines, the Stationary Bike is still a good addition to every fighter or grappler's training program.

SECTION 2: PART 4:
TRAINING WITH DUMB-BELLS AND KETTLEBELLS

● ● ● "If you want to get strong, get in the gym. When you get there, work your ass off." Wayne Gardner

Training with a weight that you can hold in one hand provides a lot of versatility in your overall workout program. Every piece of equipment in the gym has a valid purpose and dumb-bells and kettlebells are two of the handiest implements you will find. You can lift them with both arms working together, each arm doing a different movement or just about any way you wish. You can swing them, throw them, carry them, lift two of them or just lift one of them. Some athletes use dumb-bells and kettlebells as an addition to their overall training while others prefer to focus their training program almost entirely around the use of dumb-bells and kettlebells.

If you have an injury and a barbell limits your movement when trying to perform an exercise, kettlebells or dumb-bells provide more variable training enabling you to work around the injury and focus in on a body part. Many of the circuits in Section 1 emphasize the use of dumb-bells or kettlebells. Both authors have used dumb-bells and kettlebells extensively during their individual careers as athletes and as coaches. Use your imagination when training with these implements, but always remember to use good lifting form. This part of the book presents some dumb-bell and kettlebell exercises that you will find useful for any combat sport, or for strength and fitness training in general.

DUMB-BELL JUDO SWINGS

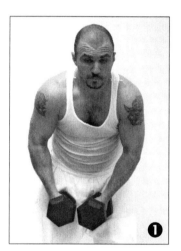
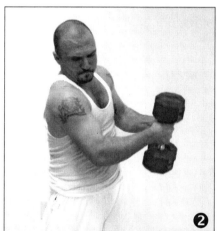
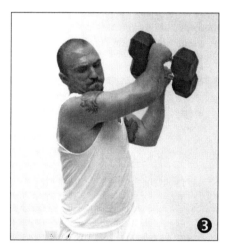
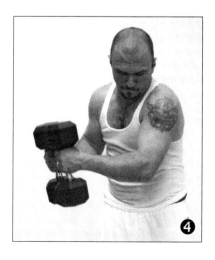
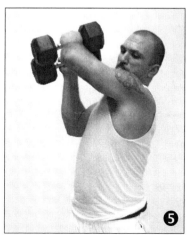

1. Hold a dumb-bell in each hand and in front of the body as shown.

2. Swing the dumb-bells in unison as you rotate to the left.

3. Swings the dumb-bells above the left shoulder.

4. Swing the dumb-bells to the starting position and then swing them in unison to the right.

5. Finish the movement by swinging the dumb-bells over the right shoulder. Repeat this movement for 10 reps.

DUMB-BELL PULLOVERS

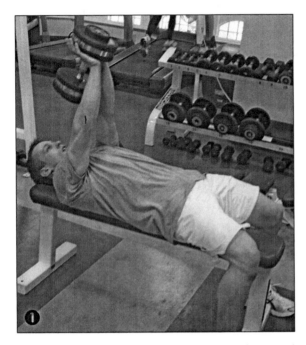

This is a great exercise for triceps and total pectoral development, shoulders and the upper back. Drew lies flat on a bench and holds the dumb-bell above him.

TRAINING TIP: When doing Dumb-Bell Pullovers, inhale deeply as you perform the pullover and exhale as you bring it back to your front. This deep breathing expands your ribcage and helps in the overall development of the area. Breathing in this way also tightens your core muscles, enhancing your core strength as well.

STRONG BODY ROTATION FOR BIG THROWS

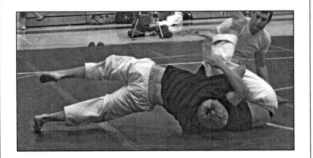

Dumb-Bell Judo Swings, among other exercises, develop the dynamic and functional muscles needed to throw opponents with control and force.

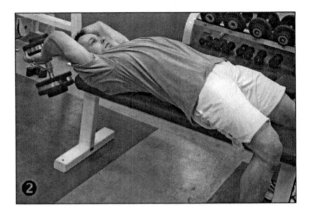

Drew performs the pullover as shown and lowers the dumb-bell as far down as possible getting a full and complete stretch in his chest and back as he does. Drew keeps his back flat on the bench and makes sure not to arch.

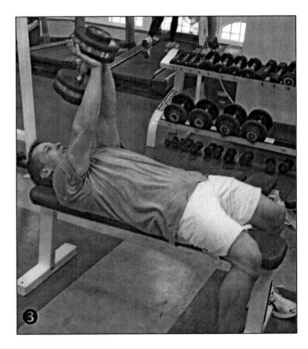

Drew completes the exercise by pulling the dumb-bell over his head to the starting position. This exercise is excellent for enlarging and stretching the rib cage. Make sure to inhale as you lower the dumb-bell and exhale as you bring the dumb-bell back to the starting position.

DUMB-BELL PULLOVERS ACROSS BENCH

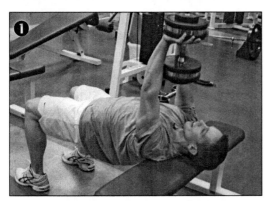

This popular variation of the Dumb-Bell Pullover has Drew lying across the bench. Drew starts the exercise by holding the dumb-bell above him.

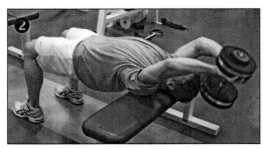

Drew lowers the dumb-bell over his head.

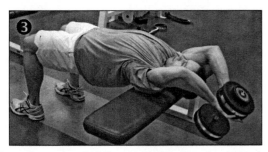

Drew gets a good, full stretch, allowing the dumb-bell to go as low as possible with full arm extension.

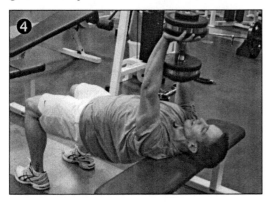

Drew returns the dumb-bell to the starting position above him. Like the other variations, this is excellent for triceps and pectoral strength and really works your upper back and shoulders. Perform 3 to 5 sets of 8 to 15 reps per set.

DUMB-BELL AROUND THE WORLD

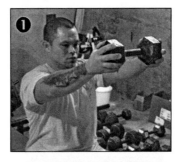

David holds each end of a dumb-bell as shown. He holds the dumb-bell out in front of him with his arms extended.

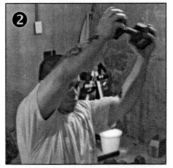

David moves the dumb-bell to his left, keeping his arms extended as he does.

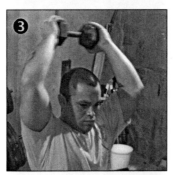

David continues to move the dumb-bells in a circle around his head.

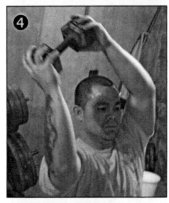

David continues to rotate the dumb-bell. This is a good exercise for the deltoids as well as the upper back. You can also get some benefit to your core and even into your lats.

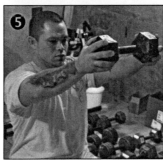

David completes the movement and returns to the starting position. Use moderate weight and make sure not to swing the weight or move it around too fast.

KETTLEBELL ROLLBACKS

This is an excellent total body exercise and useful for every grappler, no matter what his specialty is. This is an unusual exercise not seen in many gyms but very useful for grapplers and fighters. Performing this exercise toughens the entire body, as well as strengthening the core and lower back muscles so important for fighting. Perform about 10 repetitions as a finisher after a workout using a weight that you can control, but as heavy as possible. Don't hold your breath when performing this exercise; inhale at the start and exhale at the finish.

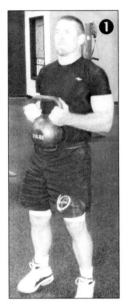 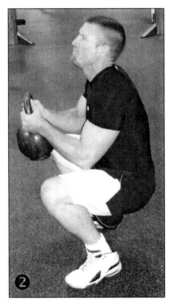

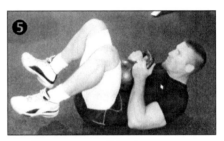

5. Mike starts to roll back.

1. Mike holds the kettlebell at his front as shown.

2. Mike holds the kettlebell in close to his body as he squats low.

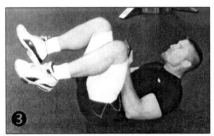

3. Mike tucks the kettlebell in to this body as he rolls back as shown. Mike makes sure to stay round and not flatten out.

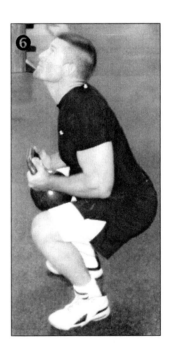 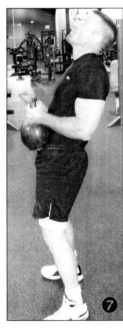

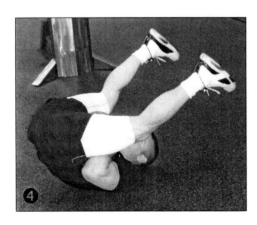

4. Mike rolls back onto his shoulders with his feet extended over his head.

6. Mike rolls back up and into a squat position.

7. Mike rolls back and up and back to a standing position.

KETTLEBELL 1-ARM ROWING TRIPOD

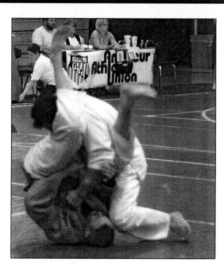

Mike holds a kettlebell in each hand. He assumes a wide stance as he leans forward. Mike performs a set of 10 reps with his right hand, and then performs a set with his left hand. You can also alternate back and forth, doing one rep with your left arm, then one with your right, and so on until you complete the desired number of reps. A good variation is to move forward as you alternate pulls from one arm to the other. After completing the pull simply place the kettlebell in front of you and immediately execute a pull with the other arm. Continue like this for a designated distance or until you've completed the desired number of reps.

STAYING ROUND IMPROVES YOUR MOBILITY

**STAYING ROUND IMPROVES YOUR MOBILITY
IN GROUNDFIGHTING**
A functionally strong body in the rounded position can switch from one technique to another in groundfighting. This spinning armlock from the guard is the result of a strong core, hips and legs.

KETTLEBELL CRAB WALK

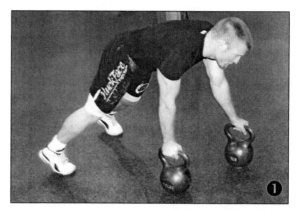

Mike holds a pair of kettlebells as he assumes the position shown here. Make sure your feet are spread wide.

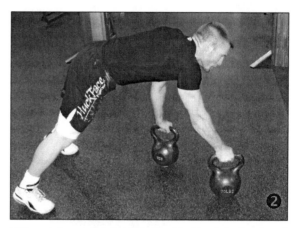

Mike picks up the kettlebell with his right hand and "walks" it forward, stepping with his feet as well.

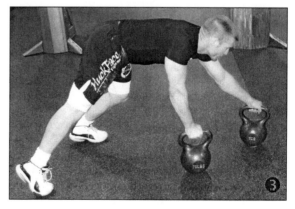

Mike picks up the kettlebell with his left hand and "walks" it forward. Mike continues to do this for about 10 repetitions in one direction, and then walks back about 10 repetitions to finish the set.

KETTLEBELL PASS THROUGH LEGS

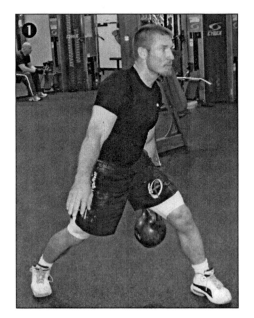

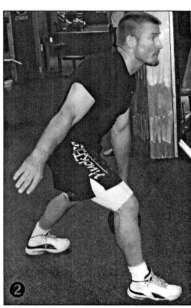

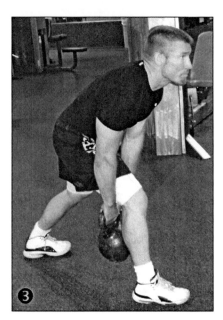

Mike assumes a wide stance with his left leg forward He holds a moderately heavy kettlebell in his right hand.

Keeping his knees flexed, Mike moves the kettlebell in his right hand through his legs and grabs it with his left hand.

Mike holds the kettlebell with his left hand as shown.

TECHNICAL TIP: When performing this exercise, bend your knees. As Mike is showing here, a slight bend forward at the waist is okay, but don't bend forward too far or you will strain your lower back.

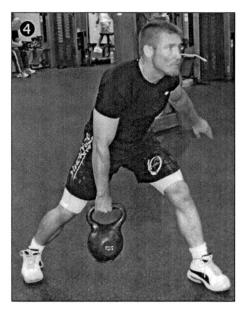

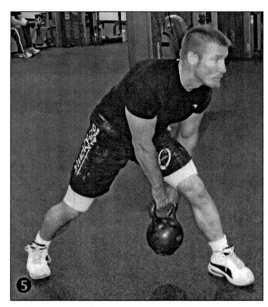

Mike moves the kettlebell through his legs with his left hand.

Mike completes the repetitions by grabbing the kettlebell with his right hand. He will perform 10 passes through his legs to complete the set.

FARMER'S WALK WITH HEAVY DUMB-BELLS

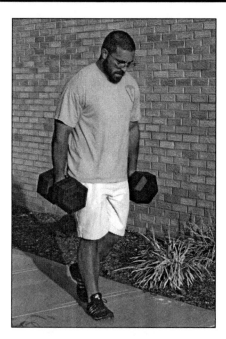

The Farmer's Walk is one of the best total body exercises you can perform. Jake holds a pair of heavy dumb-bells in each hand and starts walking. Jake walks as far as possible before dropping or setting the dumb-bells down. He rests briefly, picks the dumb-bells up again and continues to walk. When starting this exercise, use light to moderate weight, but you will quickly find that you will be able to use heavy weight. The Farmer's Walk works your trapezius and exhausts your legs. It's also fantastic for developing a strong grip.

FARMER'S WALK W/ CARRY IMPLEMENTS

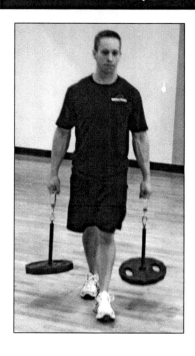

You can use any implement you wish when performing the Farmer's Walk. Drew is using a pair of loading pins and handles in this photo.

FARMER'S WALK WITH KETTLEBELLS

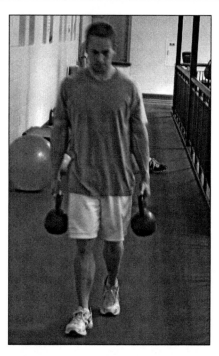

Drew holds a pair of kettlebells instead of a pair of dumb-bells in this variation of the Farmer's Walk.

1-ARM CURL WITH IMPLEMENT WALK

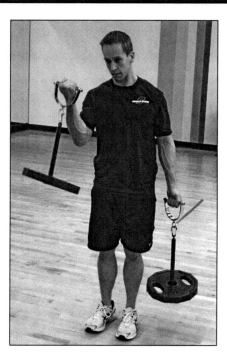

As a variation to the Farmer's Walk, Drew performs curls as he walks to make the exercise harder. He can also walk for a specific number of steps or period of time and then stop to perform a set of 10 curls on each arm as a variation.

CONDITIONING FOR COMBAT SPORTS

1-ARM BENT OVER ROWING

This is one of the best exercises any grappler can use to develop real, functional strength. It is excellent for the lats and rear deltoid. It also works your trapezius, rhomboids, triceps and biceps. You will be amazed at how thick your arms get. This is a good exercise to do immediately after performing the Overhead Press or Bench Press. Perform 3 to 5 sets of 5 to 10 reps per set depending on the weight of the dumb-bell.

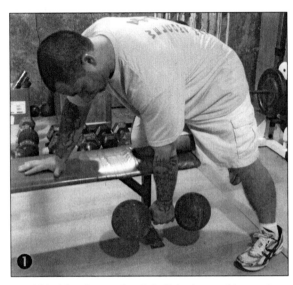 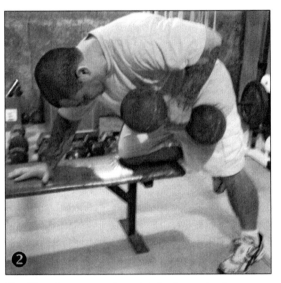

David holds a heavy dumb-bell (or he could use a kettlebell) in his left hand as shown. David rests his right hand and right knee on the bench with his left foot stable on the floor.

David makes sure to keep his body as steady as possible as he pulls the dumb-bell as high as possible to his chest. It's important not to jerk or swing the dumb-bell as he lifts it. David inhales as he lifts the dumb-bell and exhales as he lowers it.

1-ARM BENT OVER ROWING WITH PALM DOWN

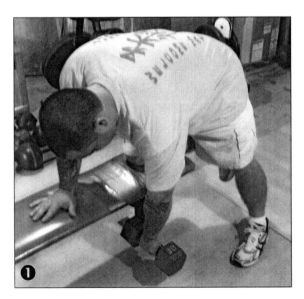 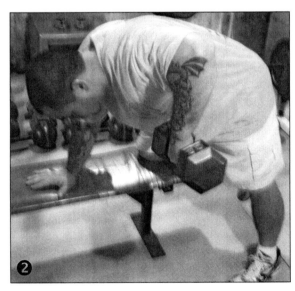

This is a good variation of the Bent-Over Rowing with David holding the dumb-bell palm-in as shown.

David pulls the dumb-bell up to his chest. This variation emphasizes latissimus development in the upper back.

DUMB-BELLS & KETTLEBELLS

DUMB-BELL SHOULDER SHRUGS

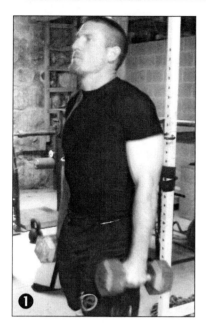

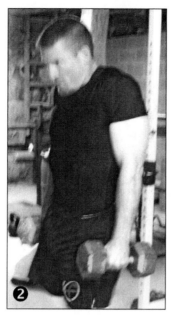

One of the best trapezius exercises you can use is the Dumb-Bell (or Kettlebell) Shoulder Shrug. Mike makes sure not to use his arms to lift the dumb-bell at any time, keeping his arms straight. He holds a dumb-bell in each hand with his head upright and looking forward.

Mike shrugs his shoulders up as high as possible and rolls them forward.

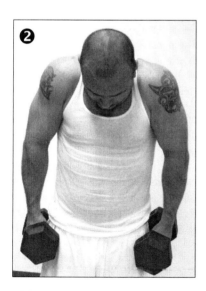

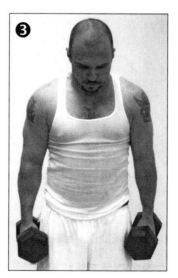

This front view shows how the shoulders roll forward as you dip your head.

He completes the movement by finishing his shoulder shrug and moving his head up. Use heavy weight, performing 3 to 5 sets of 6 to 10 reps.

BACK AND ARM STRENGTH

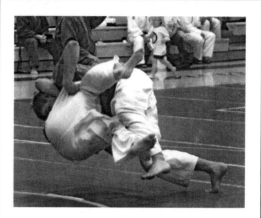

BACK AND ARM STRENGTH HELP WHEN SHOOTING IN

This double leg during a freestyle judo match is the result of not only good technical training, but also good training in the weight room. Upper back and arm strength from towing movements in the gym create a good, strong base to develop your technical skills.

A STRONG NECK CAN PROTECT YOU

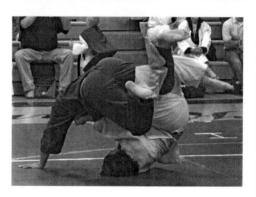

Sometimes, a strong neck can keep you from getting injured. This athlete was thrown hard on his head and shoulders and got up to continue the match. A strong trapezius, along with the many other muscles in the upper body and neck can help you avoid an injury.

BOTH ARM DUMB-BELL BENT OVER ROWING

This variation of Bent-Over Dumb-Bell Rowing is an old exercise, but has stood the test of time. Instead of doing the 1-Arm Bent-Over Row, you can do this from time to time to break the monotony of training.

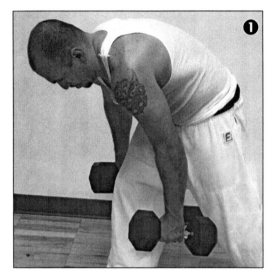

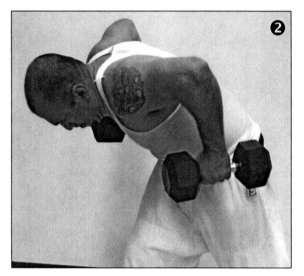

Mike holds a pair of dumb-bells in each hand as he bends over at the waist.

Mike pulls each dumb-bell to his chest as shown.

BENT-OVER DUMB-BELL SIDE RAISES

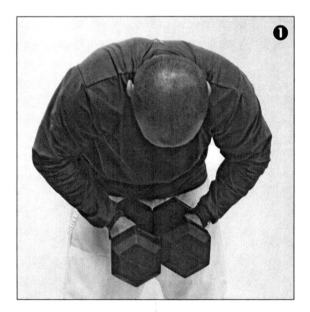

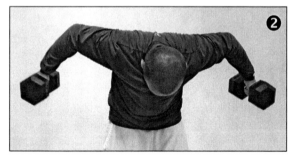

Mike raises each dumb-bell out wide to the side as shown making sure to flair his elbows up high as he does. This is a good exercise for the entire pectoral area, as well as the rear delts and arms. Perform 3 to 5 sets of 10 reps.

Mike bends over at the waist as he holds a pair of moderately heavy dumb-bells in each hand. Mike holds the dumb-bells in close to his body with his arms bent.

DUMB-BELL CLEANS

This is a good shoulder exercise. You can use moderate to heavy weight when performing it. Use 3 to 5 sets of 5 to 10 reps per set, depending on the weight of the dumb-bells.

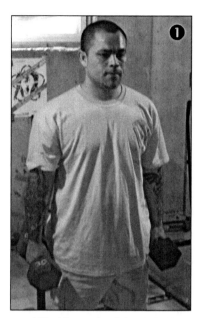

David holds a pair of dumb-bells in each hand as shown.

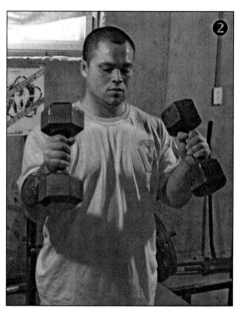

David swings or "cleans" the dumb-bells up.

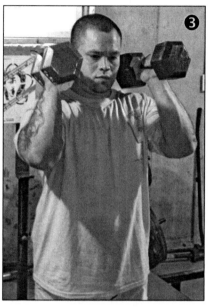

David completes the dumb-bell clean as he brings the dumb-bells to about the level of his ears.

DUMB-BELL PRESS

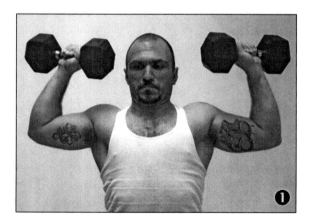

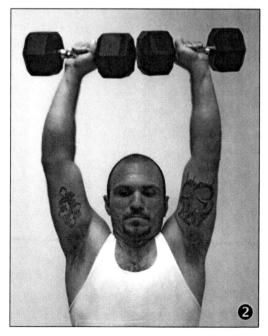

1. Mike holds a pair of dumb-bells as shown. You can do this standing or while seated.

2. Mike presses the dumb-bells overhead. Use moderate weight with a routine of 3 to 5 sets of 10 reps per set. Make sure to keep your back erect and press the dumb-bells rather than jerking or swinging them overhead. Dumb-Bell Presses are an excellent shoulder exercise, working all three heads of your deltoid.

DUMB-BELL 1-ARM ALTERNATING PRESS

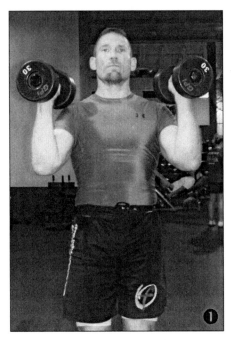

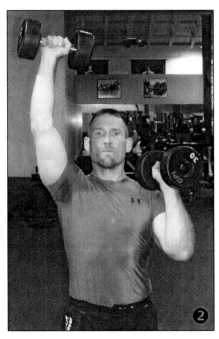

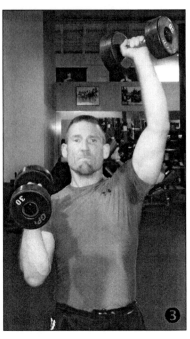

Mike holds a pair of dumb-bells at his shoulders. He can perform this standing or seated. This exercise works all three heads of the deltoid as well as the upper pectoral near the clavicle.

Mike alternately presses the dumb-bell overhead with his right arm, rotating his wrist so that his palm faces forward.

Mike lowers the dumb-bell with his right hand and presses the dumb-bell in his left hand overhead.

DUMB-BELL ARM TWIST

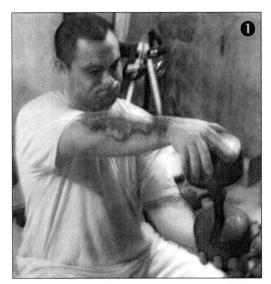

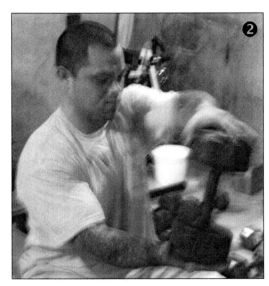

David holds a dumb-bell on each end with both hands, making sure his arms are extended forward. He rotates the dumb-bell end over end.

David rotates the dumb-bell end over end for 10 to 25 reps using a light to moderately heavy dumb-bell. The heavier the dumb-bell you use, the fewer the reps you perform.

KETTLEBELL PRESS

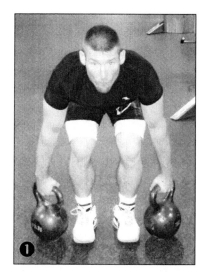 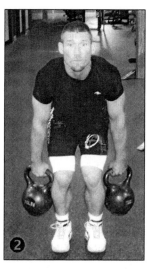 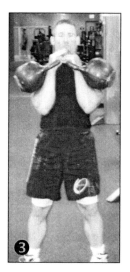 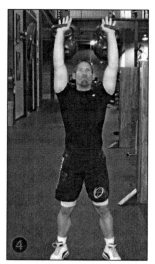

Mike squats and bends forward as he holds a pair of kettlebells in each hand as shown. His head is looking forward and his back is straight.

Mike starts to clean the kettlebells.

Mike cleans the kettlebells to his shoulders. He holds them with each implement on the outside of each wrist with his elbows close in.

Mike presses the kettlebells overhead. This is a good variation of the Barbell or Dumb-Bell Press and works the same muscle groups. Use it to break up the monotony of training.

1-ARM KETTLEBELL PRESS

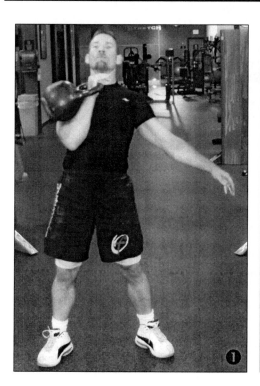 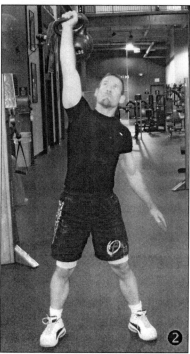

1. Anytime you press a kettlebell or dumb-bell overhead with 1 arm, it forces your body to stabilize the lifting movement in a way that replicates the dynamic action and movement in a fight or grappling match. Mike cleans the kettlebell with 1 arm.

2. Mike presses the kettlebell over his head. Many athletes find that pressing a kettlebell overhead is more difficult to do than pressing a dumb-bell. Use anywhere from a light to heavy kettlebell, depending on your goals and fitness level.

1-ARM KETTLEBELL TRIPOD PRESS

This is a dynamic, functional movement and is a total body exercise. Use light weight initially to learn how to perform this exercise safely and correctly. Then progress on to moderate to heavy weight. Do 1 set of 10 on each arm, and perform 3 to 5 sets.

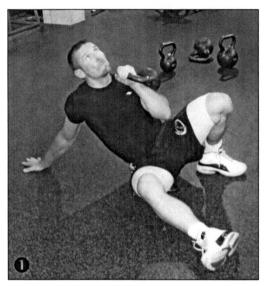

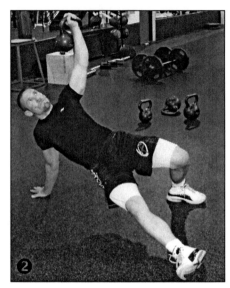

Mike assumes a sit-through or tripod position on the floor, making sure his right arm is posted out wide for stability. Mike shoulders the kettlebell.

Mike presses the kettlebell over his head and toward the ceiling as he uses his right arm and left leg to push his body upward.

1-ARM DUMB-BELL SNATCH

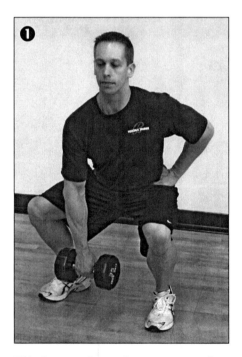

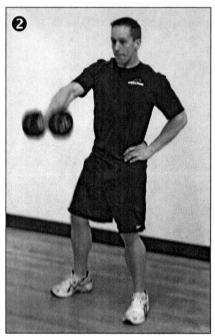

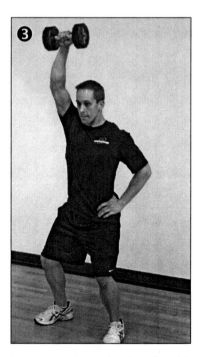

This is a good exercise to use once in a while and is a good test of plyometric strength. Drew holds the dumb-bell with his right hand as shown as he squats low.

Drew swings (or snatches) the dumb-bell upward, keeping his right arm extended. Drew springs upward with his body. You can use heavy weight as a test of explosive strength for single reps.

Drew completes the Snatch with the dumb-bell over his head. When performing this exercise, alternate the lift from right to left hand to avoid overtraining each arm.

DUMB-BELL CROSS-BODY TO SHOULDER RAISES

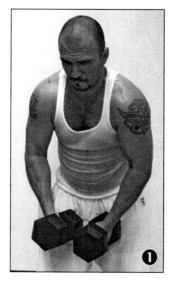

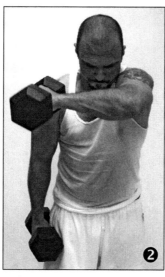

1. Mike holds a pair of moderately heavy dumb-bells at his front. This is a functional exercise that works the front and side deltoids along with the pectorals. It also gives your trapezius muscles a lot of work.

2. Mike raises the dumb-bell and rotates his left arm, bringing the dumb-bell to his right shoulder. He lowers the weight to the starting position and repeats with his right arm. Use weight where you can perform good, strict repetitions and don't swing or jerk the dumb-bells as you lift them. Perform 3 to 5 sets of 10 reps, depending on the amount of weight used. You can also use this as a good warm-up before a heavy Bench Press or Overhead Press workout.

DUMB-BELL LATERAL RAISES

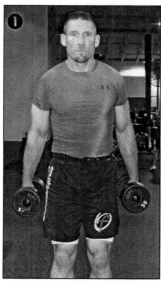

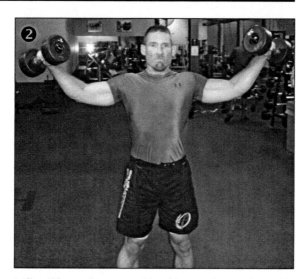

Mike holds a dumb-bell in each hand while standing in a straight, upright posture with his head up and looking forward. A common mistake is to shrug your shoulders forward when doing this exercise.

Mike lifts each arm to his sides, trying to keep his arms as straight as possible. Don't swing or jerk the weights. This focuses in on the side deltoids, but gives all 3 heads of the deltoid a good workout. This exercise also works the trapezius really hard. Perform 3 to 5 sets, doing anywhere from 10 to 25 reps per set, depending on the amount of weight used.

STRENGTH TO SKILL

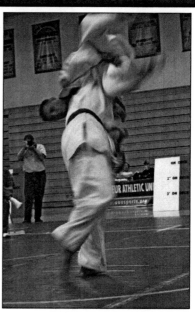

STRENGTH IS A PRE-REQUISITE OF SKILL

It takes functional strength to perform the techniques of any combat sport against a skilled, resisting, fit opponent. This Kata Guruma (Shoulder Wheel or Fireman's Carry) at the AAU Grand Nationals by Scott Brink shows how functional strength translates to results on the mat.

DUMB-BELL LATERAL HOLD FOR TIME

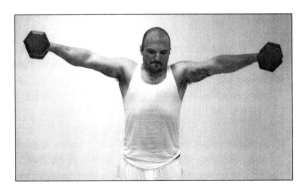

Mike holds the dumb-bells out laterally for a specified time or count. Mike can vary this exercise by holding the dumb-bells and raising his arms above horizontal for a 10-count and then lowering slightly below horizontal, holding for another 10-count. Make sure to use light weight.

DUMB-BELL FRONT RAISE HOLDING SIDES

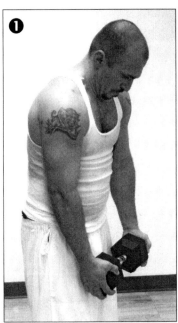

1. Mike performs a variation of the Front Dumb-Bell Raise by holding each side of a dumb-bell as shown. A heavier dumb-bell can be used for this variation since you are using both hands.

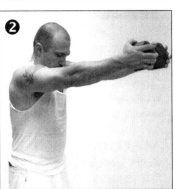

2. Mike raises the dumb-bell to shoulder height as shown. Depending on the weight used, perform 3 to 5 sets of anywhere from 10 or more reps per set. To make this exercise harder, Mike can stand with his back pressed against a wall, forcing him to stand upright and not allow him to swing or jerk the dumb-bell as he lifts it. Mike can also perform this exercise using a barbell or kettlebell.

DUMB-BELL 1 ARM FRONT RAISES

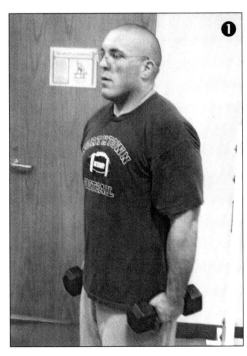

Jake stands upright holding a dumb-bell in each hand at his sides. This exercise is good for working the front deltoids, and it indirectly works all the muscles in the scapula and upper back, including the trapezius and gives the entire arm a good workout as well.

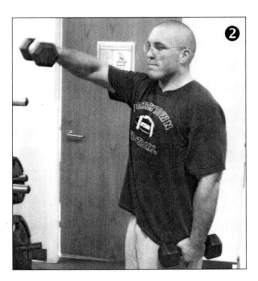

Jake raises his right arm upward to about shoulder height with control, making sure not to swing or jerk the dumb-bell. He lowers the dumb-bell and then repeats the movement with his left arm. Use light weight, performing 3 to 5 sets of 10 to 50 reps per set.

DUMB-BELL ROTATOR CUFF FRONT PRESS

When author Steve Scott tore both of his rotator cuffs a number of years ago, he learned the value of this exercise (and the other rotator cuff exercises) first-hand! These movements provide a great warm-up and they are effective at developing functional strength. Important: Use light weight (5 pounds or less) when performing rotator cuff exercises. Heavy weight could cause injuries. Perform about 3 sets of 10 to 25 reps per set using very light weight.

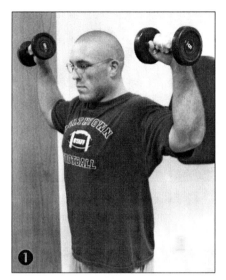

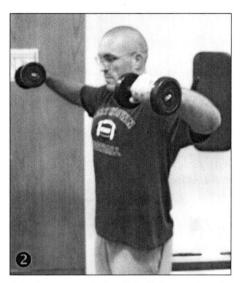

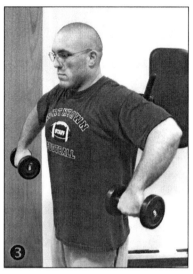

Jake holds a pair of dumb-bells to his sides. Notice that his palms are facing forward.

Jake lowers each dumb-bell forward, making sure to keep his elbows motionless.

Jake lowers the dumb-bells forward and down, with his posture straight and his chest lightly arched forward. Jake will raise the dumb-bells to complete the exercise.

DUMB-BELL INCLINE BENCH ROTATOR CUFF PRESS

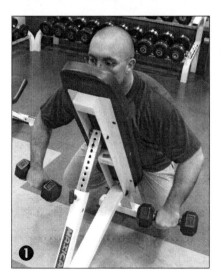

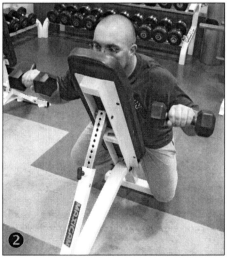

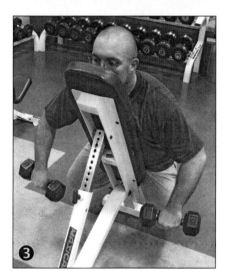

This works the entire shoulder area more intensely. Jake holds light dumb-bells in each hand as he lies face forward on the incline bench. Jake starts the exercise with the dumb-bells in the low position with his palms facing backward.

Jake raises each dumb-bell upward and forward as shown, making sure not to swing or jerk the weight or move his body on the bench. Jake raises the dumb-bells to shoulder height.

Jake finishes the exercise by lowering the weight to the starting position. As with any Rotator Cuff Press, use light weight and strict form, and perform 3 sets of anywhere from 10 to 25 reps per set.

CONDITIONING FOR COMBAT SPORTS

DUMB-BELL INCLINE BENCH 1-ARM ROTATOR CUFF PRESS

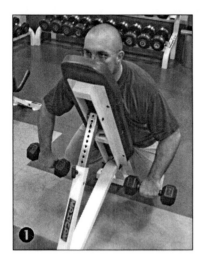 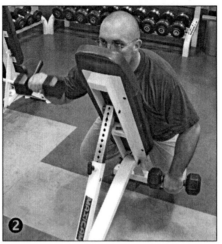 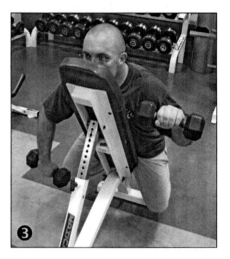

This is the 1-arm variation of the Front Rotator Cuff Press on the incline bench. Jake starts the exercise holding both dumb-bells at his side with the palms down.

Jake raises his right arm, making sure his elbow is as motionless as possible. Jake raises the dumb-bell in his right hand to shoulder height.

As Jake lowers his right arm, he repeats the movement with his left arm. Use light weight and perform 3 sets of 10 to 25 reps per set.

INCLINE BENCH SEATED ROTATOR CUFF PRESS

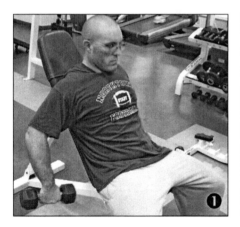 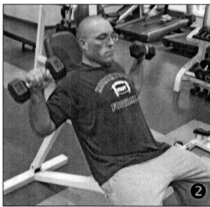 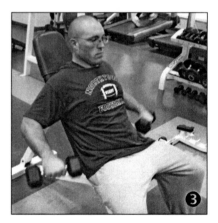

Jake is positioned on an incline bench as shown. He holds a pair of light dumb-bells in each hand with the palms facing backward. Look at how Jake flairs his arms out to the side with his elbows bent.

Jake moves each hand holding a dumb-bell forward and upward, making sure to keep his elbows as motionless as possible. Don't swing or jerk the dumb-bells when lifting them. Jake lifts the dumb-bells to shoulder height.

Jake lowers the dumb-bells back to the starting position to complete the exercise. As with the other rotator cuff exercises, perform 3 sets of 10 to 15 reps using light weight.

TECHNICAL TIP: Rotator cuff surgery and the therapy that follows aren't pleasant. If you train a great deal on heavy bench presses, you are vulnerable to rotator cuff injuries. Rotator cuff injuries are also common in many sports including combat sports. Use these rotator cuff exercises as an effective warm-up before each lifting session to help prevent rotator cuff strains or tears. The exercises shown here are often used as part of the overall therapy for rotator cuff injuries and have great prevention value as well. When performing therapy or rehab for any injury, follow the advice of your doctor and physical therapist.

DUMB-BELL ROTATOR CUFF FRONT CURLS

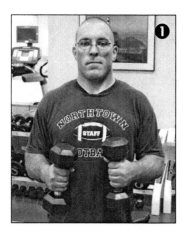 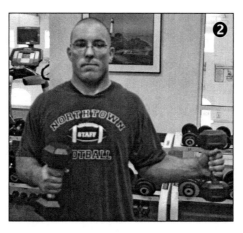 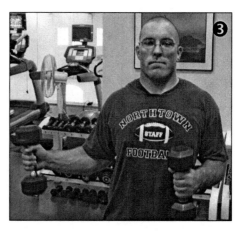

Jake holds a pair of dumb-bells in front of his body with palms facing in as shown.

Without moving his left elbow, Jake moves his left arm to his left side while holding the dumb-bell with his palm now facing forward. Jake returns his left hand to the starting position to finish the exercise on his left side.

Jake repeats the movement with his right hand. Use light weight and don't swing or jerk the dumb-bell. Perform this exercise slowly. Do 3 sets of 10 to 25 reps per set.

DUMB-BELL THROWING (TAI OTOSHI-BODY DROP) DRILL

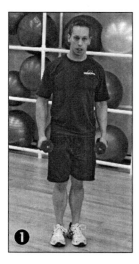 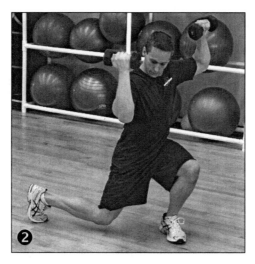 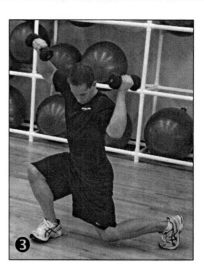

This is a good drill for improving your throwing skill using a pair of dumb-bells or kettlebells. Drew stands with a pair of light to moderately heavy dumb-bells in each hand.

Drew shoots his right leg back toward his right rear side as he turns his body to his left. Look at how Drew positions his right foot on the floor and bend his right knee, almost touching the floor with it. As he does this, Drew lifts the dumb-bells upward as shown.

Drew quickly switches to the other side, replicating his initial movement. Perform this drill for a high rep count, doing anywhere from 25 to 100 reps per set.

KETTLEBELL 1-LEG BALANCE

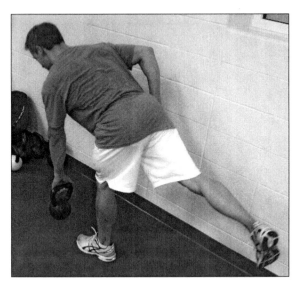

Drew holds a kettlebell in his left hand as he balances on his left leg. leans forward, keeping his back straight, and lifts his right leg, keeping it as straight as possible. Drew lowers the kettlebell to the floor and then straightens back up to complete a repetition. You can perform 10 reps on each side. This is a good total body exercise, and is excellent for balance development and can be used after a good cardio workout.

TAI OTOSHI (BODY DROP) IN ACTION

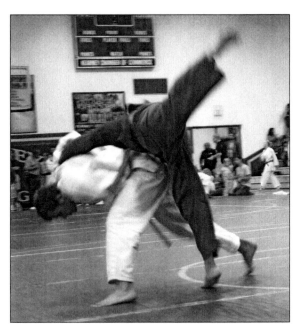

The explosive and powerful action needed to throw a resisting opponent comes from directed and specific training based on having a solid foundation of speed and strength.

KETTLEBELL HOLD ON STABILITY DISC

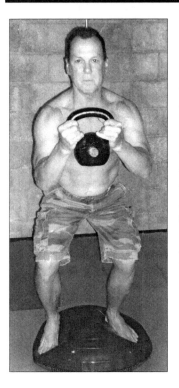

Dan holds a kettlebell while balancing himself on a soft Stability Disc. You can perform squats from this position, hold the weight for time or even practice front kicks or leg lifts. This is a good exercise for all the small stabilizer muscles in your entire body. Use a much weight as you feel safe in using.

KETTLEBELL BOTH HANDS ON STABILITY DISCS

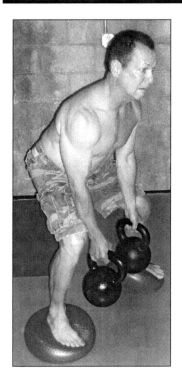

Small Stability Discs are commercially available and can be used for excellent balance, core and stabilizer training. Dan is holding a pair of kettlebells while balanced on a pair of Stability Discs. He can perform Overhead Presses, Curls or any number of exercises while standing on these discs.

KETTLEBELL STEP UPS

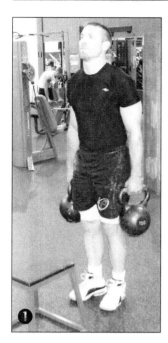

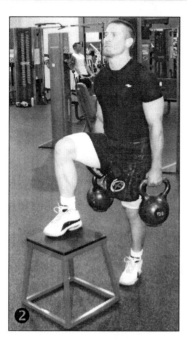

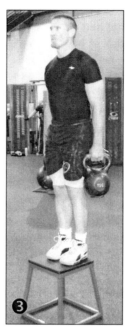

When he starts his second rep, Mike will step up with his left leg, alternating legs each time he steps up and steps down. Perform 3 to 5 sets of 10 reps per set for a good overall leg work-out. This is also a good exercise for your traps, shoulders and upper back.

TECHNICAL TIP: Walk; don't run, when carrying heavy weights or implements whether it's up stairs or on flat ground. Take it one step at a time and don't hurry. Serious ankle, knee or back injuries can take place if you're not careful when carrying heavy objects.

① Mike holds a heavy pair of kettlebells as he stands in front of a low step or box.

② Mike steps up onto the box with his right leg as shown.

③ Mike steps up onto the box and will step down to start another rep.

KETTLEBELL STAIR CLIMB

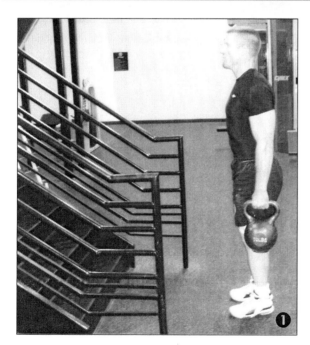

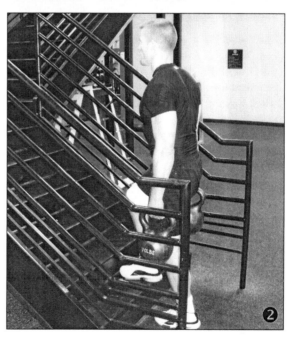

① Mike holds a heavy pair of kettlebells at the bottom of the stairs. He can hold a pair of dumb-bells or carry a heavy barrel (or any heavy implement).

Mike starts his climb, holding the heavy kettlebells. Using a pair of heavy kettlebells or dumb-bells when climbing the stairs gives your legs, traps and hands a seriously hard workout. Keep an erect posture when performing this exercise, both on the way up and the way down. Walk, don't run, when doing this exercise.

KETTLEBELL THROW

You can search the Internet and actually purchase throwing implements used in the Highland Games or Strongman Contests or look at how this movement is performed in these sports. Use light to moderate weight. When tossing the weight for height, a 56-pound implement is used in the Highland Games and when throwing for distance, either a 28-pound or 56-pound implement is used. World Highland Games Champion Sean Betz has thrown the 28-pound weight for over 94 feet on a regular basis and tossed the 56-pound weight over 18 feet.

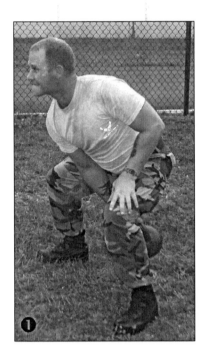

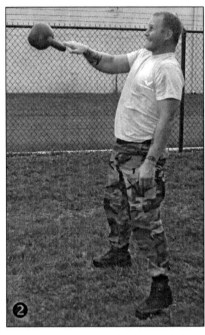

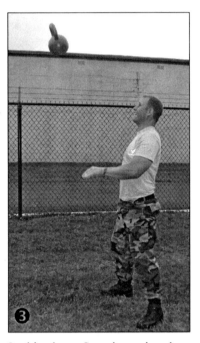

Sean assumes a wide stance with bent knees as shown, and swings the kettlebell through his legs. Sean can use 1 hand or both hands when holding the kettlebell. Basically, Sean wants to either throw the weight as far forward as he can, or toss the weight as high as possible over his head. Either way, it's a great exercise to develop explosive strength.

Sean swings the kettlebell through his legs once or twice to build momentum and releases the implement on the upswing.

In this photo, Sean is tossing the kettlebell for height.

LIFTING PIN 2-HAND SUMO SQUAT ON BOXES

Using a lifting pin to perform squats allows you to work your legs hard without placing any serious stress on your spine, much in the same way you do when using a lifting belt. The only limit is how much you can hold with your hands and arms when performing this exercise. Perform 3 to 5 sets of 5 to 10 reps per squat depending on the amount of weight you use. This exercise is a good one for both the legs and hips, but also for your upper body as well. It combines the benefits of a Squat and a Deadlift.

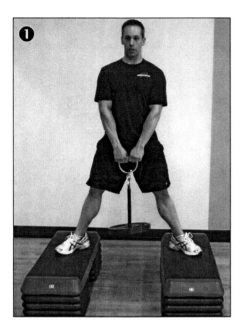 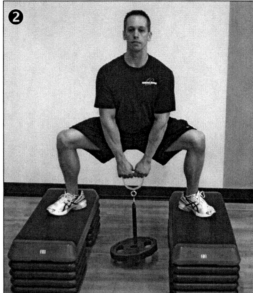

1. Drew stands on a pair of boxes or steps with a wide Sumo stance and holds a lifting pin with as much weight as he wishes.

2. Drew performs a Sumo Squat while holding the lifting pin.

LIFTING PIN 1-HAND SUMO SQUAT ON BOXES

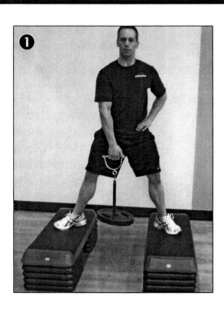 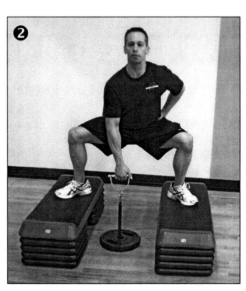

1. Drew stands on a pair of boxes or steps using a wide stance as he holds a weighted lifting pin with 1 hand.

2. Drew performs a wide or Sumo Squat while holding the lifting pin. Perform an equal number of squats while holding the lifting pin with each hand. Perform 3 to 5 sets of 6 to 10 reps using moderate to moderately heavy weight.

KETTLEBELL ON FOOT LEG LIFT

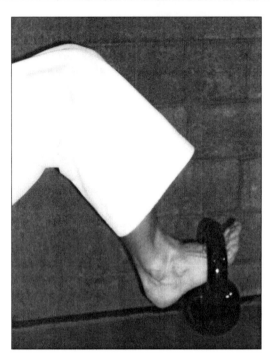

You can place your foot through the handle of a kettlebell and lift it as shown here. Dan is practicing a slow, controlled kicking movement with his leg while holding the kettlebell on his foot. Before there were specialized machines to work the legs, athletes used kettlebells and weighted shoes to develop the lower body.

DUMB-BELL CURL WALK

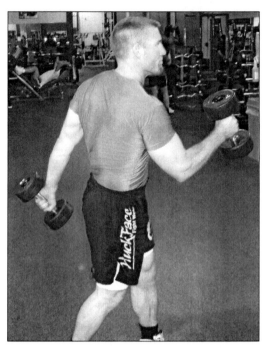

Another way to walk while working the arms is to stroll around and swing or curl a pair of dumb-bells or kettle-bells. Mike is walking and curling a set of dumb-bells, making sure to keep a good, erect posture when walking and controlling the dumb-bells as he curls them. This is a good all-around body exercise, forcing your stabilizers in the back, hips, and shoulders to control the weight as you move. This is a good exercise to use a finisher to any gym workout or workout in the dojo or wrestling room.

HAND POSITION FOR TRICEPS EXTENSTIONS

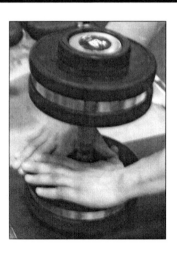

DUMB-BELL HAND POSITION FOR TRICEPS EXTENSTIONS
Look at how Drew places his hands and grabs the dumb-bell. This grip is the standard way of holding a dumb-bell when performing most overhead lifts.

HAND POSITION FOR ELBOWS IN CLOSE

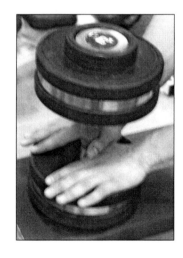

DUMB-BELL HAND PO-SITION FOR ELBOWS IN CLOSE WHEN DO-ING TRICEPS EXTEN-SIONS
Holding the dumb-bell with this hand position forces you to keep your elbows in really close and focuses the effort of the lifting movement directly on your triceps.

SEATED DUMB-BELL TRICEPS EXTENSIONS

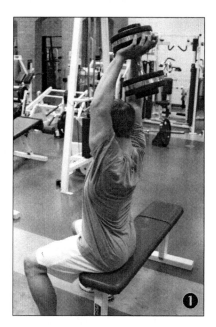 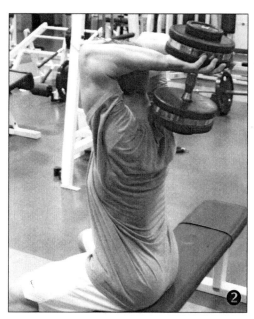 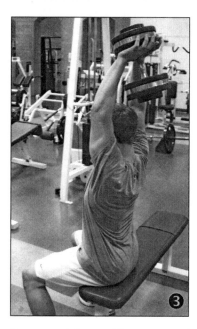

Drew sits on a bench, holding a dumb-bell overhead in the position shown here. Make sure to keep a straight back and look directly forward, not allowing your head to droop or look down. This erect posture is necessary tp get the most out of this lift.

Drew lowers the dumb-bell behind his head as shown, making sure his elbows are pointed directly forward. If your elbows flair out to the sides, then you place less stress on your triceps and make this exercise almost entirely a shoulder exercise and not a triceps movement. Drew lowers the weight with control and doesn't allow it to bounce or jerk.

Drew straightens his arms and brings the dumb-bell back to the starting position to finish the repetition.

While this exercise is primarily an excellent strengthener for your triceps, it also works your shoulders and upper back hard. You can perform 3 to 5 sets of 6 to 15 reps per set, depending on the amount of weight you use. The big rule is to keep a good, straight back and look forward and maintain good lifting form to get the most out of this triceps exercise and avoid injury.

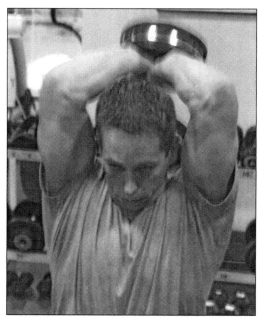

Drew keeps his elbows pointing directly forward in this photo.

DOUBLE DUMB-BELL TRICEPS EXTENSIONS

Here's a good way of working your triceps and shoulders hard. Mike holds a dumb-bell in each hand and performs a Triceps Extension. Holding a dumb-bell in each hand forces you to concentrate harder and makes each arm work independent of each other, but still move the dumb-bells in unison. Make sure not to use too much weight. Good, strict form is really necessary to get the most out of this exercise and to avoid injuries.

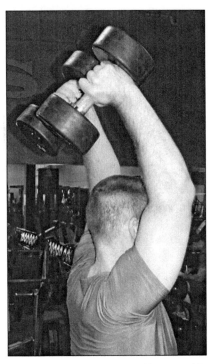

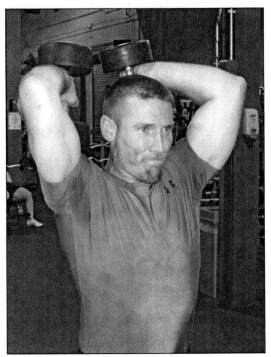

Mike holds the dumb-bells over his head as shown.

Mike lowers the dumb-bells behind his head making sure his elbows are pointed forward and not to the side. A routine of 3 to 5 sets of 8 to 10 reps per set using moderate weight is a good workout.

DUMB-BELL KICKBACKS

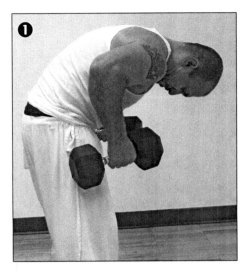

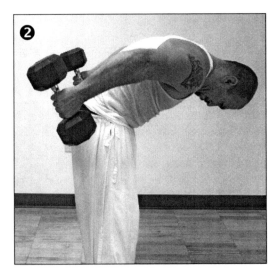

Mike holds a pair of dumb-bells as he bends forward. He holds the dumb-bells in close to his body as shown.

Mike extends his arms backward as shown making sure to not jerk or swing the weights. This is a good strength builder for the triceps.

DUMB-BELL CURLS

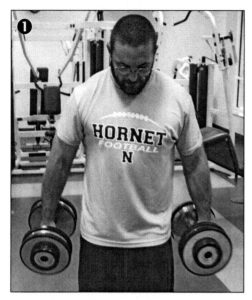

Jake holds a dumb-bell in each hand with his palms facing his hips as shown.

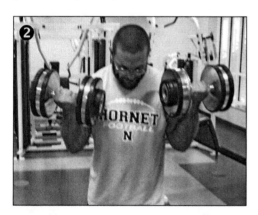

Jake curls the dumb-bells to his shoulders as shown here, making sure to not swing or jerk the weights. Use weight that allows you to perform strict exercises with good form. Perform 3 to 5 sets of 6 to 10 reps.

ALTERNATING DUMB-BELL CURLS

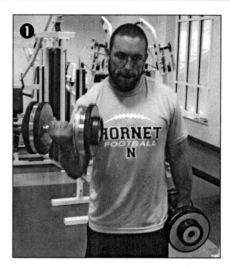

Rather than curling both dumb-bells at the same time, Jake alternates curling the weights and curls the dumb-bell with his right arm.

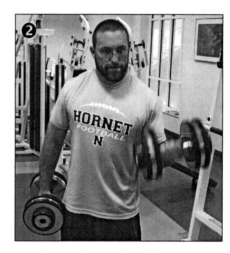

As he lowers the dumb-bell in his right arm, Jake curls the dumb-bell in his left hand. Use weight that allows you to perform good, strict form and do 3 to 5 sets of 6 to 10 reps.

TRICEPS EXTENSIONS HOLDING EACH END OF DUMB-BELL

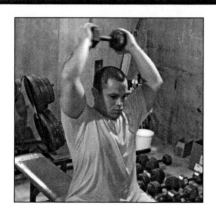

David holds each side of a dumb-bell as he performs triceps extensions. You can do this standing or seated. This is a good exercise to give some variety to your triceps training.

DUMB-BELL UPPERCUT CURLS WITH BODY TWIST

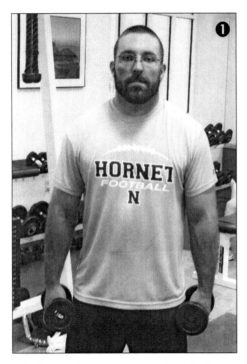

Jake holds a light to moderately light dumb-bell in each hand as shown.

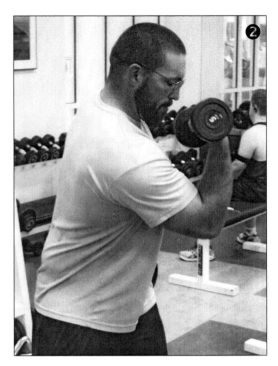

Jake returns to the starting position and holds the dumb-bells at his side as shown.

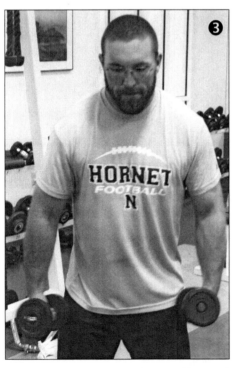

Jake rotates to his left as he curls the dumb-bell in his right hand.

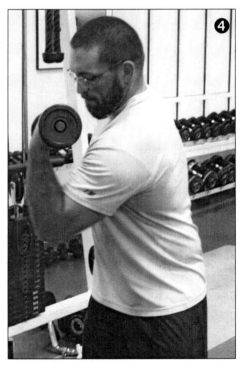

Jake rotates to his right as he curls the dumb-bell in his left hand. Use weight that allows you to perform strict, controlled movements. This is a good exercise for working on the muscles that affect punching power, including the upper back, shoulders and entire arm structure.

HAMMER CURLS

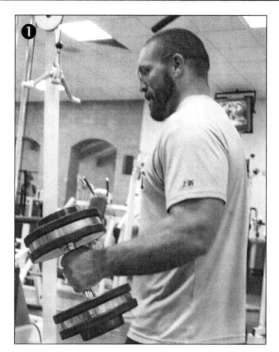

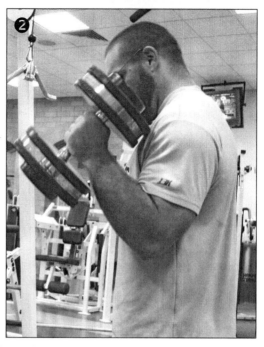

A tried and true forearm builder is the Hammer Curl. Jake holds a dumb-bell in his left hand with his palm in as shown here.

Jake curls the dumb-bell to his shoulder. This is a good exercise to use once in a while to offer some variety to your arm development, in place of Dumb-Bell Curls.

BOTH HAND DUMB-BELL CURLS

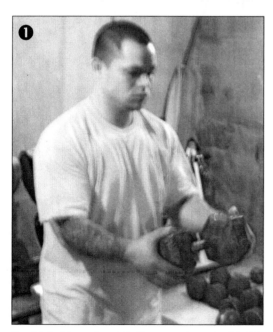

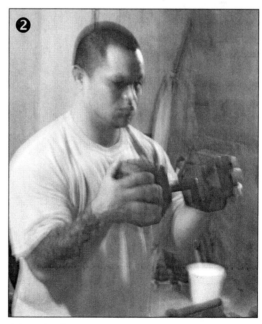

David holds a dumb-bell on each end with his hands as shown to start this exercise. This exercise is a good biceps builder and you can use a heavy dumb-bell when performing it.

David curls the dumb-bell with both hands. You can perform this standing or seated. Another variation when doing this exercise is to kneel on both knees as you perform it. If you do this, make sure to keep your back straight and don't swing the dumb-bell as you curl it.

SEATED CONCENTRATION CURLS

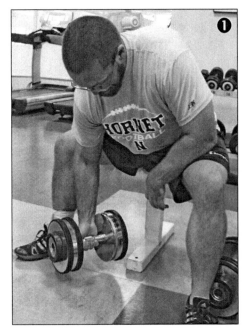
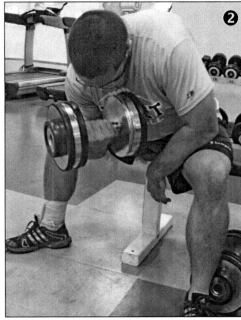

1. Jake sits on a bench or chair with his legs wide. He holds a dumb-bell in his right hand as shown to start the exercise. Jake rests his right elbow on his right upper thigh to brace his right arm.

2. Jake curls the dumb-bell with his right arm, making sure to avoid swinging or jerking the dumb-bell. Use as much weight as you wish, as this is a real strength developer for your biceps. Perform 3 to 5 sets of 5 to 10 reps, depending on how much weight you use.

HANGING DUMB-BELL CURLS

1. Jake positions himself on an incline bench with his chest on the bench. Jake holds a pair of dumb-bells in his hands as shown. Use weight that allows you to perform strict curls with good form and make sure to not swing or jerk the dumb-bells as you lift them.

2. Jake curls the dumb-bells as shown. He can also perform alternating dumb-bell curls if he wishes. Perform 3 to 5 sets of 10 reps.

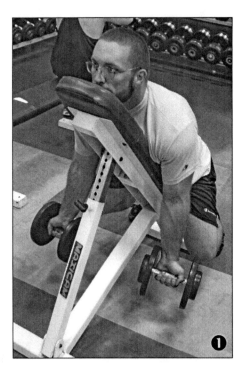
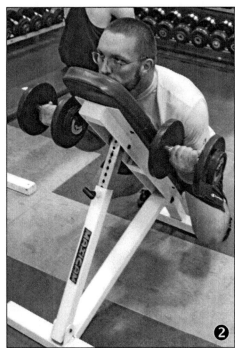

TECHNICAL TIP: This is a great exercise for strength development in your upper arms. Strong arms are vital in every combat sport, so use this exercise often.

FLAT CROSS-BODY DUMB-BELL CURLS

This is an excellent exercise that directly works the muscles you need to keep an opponent from straightening your arm in a Cross-Body Armlock. Don't jerk or swing the weight and be sure to use a light dumb-bell. If the weight is too heavy, you could inure your shoulder. Perform 3 to 5 sets of 10 to 25 reps.

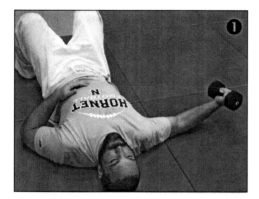 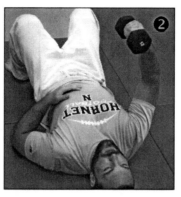 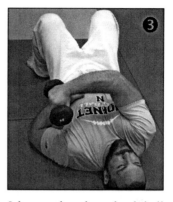

Jake lies on the mat or floor and holds a light dumb-bell in his right hand straight out to his right side.

Jake curls the dumb-bell upward in his right hand.

Jake curls the dumb-bell across his chest in a controlled and slow movement.

DUMB-BELL ALTERNATING PUNCH

This is a good exercise to develop punching power and has been used for years with good reason; it works. Perform this exercise in timed rounds. Start out with three 20-second rounds, working to three 30-second rounds, then on to three 45-second rounds and then on to three 1-minute rounds. After that, work up to performing three 3-minute rounds. Make sure to use light dumb-bells so you can maintain good punching form. Don't move your body around when doing this exercise; emphasize the punching form with your feet planted in one place on the floor.

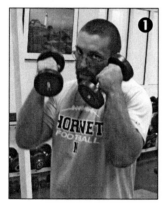 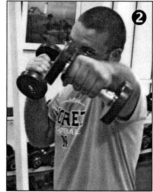 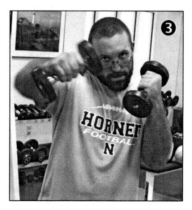 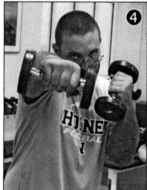

Jake holds a pair of light dumb-bells in his hands as shown.

Jake jabs with his left hand as shown, making sure to use good punching form.

Jake starts his straight right-hand punch as he brings his left hand back to his left jaw line.

Jake shoots out a straight right hand punch using good striking form.

DUMB-BELL HOOK AND SHOULDER ROLLOVER

This is a good exercise to develop the muscles that affect your left hook and shoulder as you roll with a punch. It's an old boxing exercise that significantly strengthens your entire upper body movement when using a left hook.

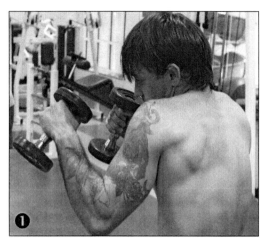

Nikolay holds a pair of light dumb-bells in his hands as shown.

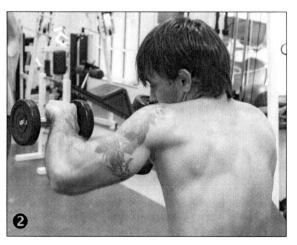

Nikolay throws out a left hook using good punching form.

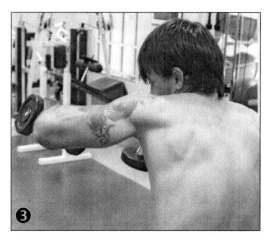

As Nikolay finishes his left hook, he makes sure to roll his left hand downward and roll his left elbow slightly upward. This movement really strengthens the left shoulder and back, which are vital for the left hook to have the power necessary to knock out opponents.

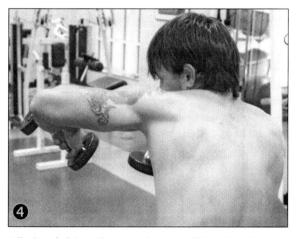

Nikolay finishes the exercise by rolling his left hand downward as shown. Perform this exercise with slow to moderate speed and use a light dumb-bell. If you want, switch the dumb-bell to your right hand and repeat it on your right side.

TECHNICAL TIP: Shadow boxing using light dumb-bells is a great way to develop power in your punching. You can use any shadow boxing routine you wish using dumb-bells to add to the workload. Just remember to not use dumb-bells that are too heavy, which will prevent you from using good punching form.

DUMB-BELL PUNCHING WITH TOTAL BODY MOVEMENT

This differs from the Dumb-Bell Alternating Punching because it involves the entire body, using the dumb-bells to strengthen your overall body movement when fighting. It's ideal for all fighters in striking sports, but is also excellent for grapplers in judo, sambo, wrestling or sport jujitsu where you must have strong gripping or pummeling power.

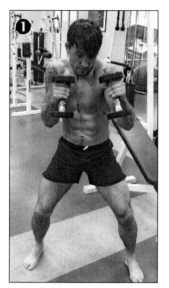

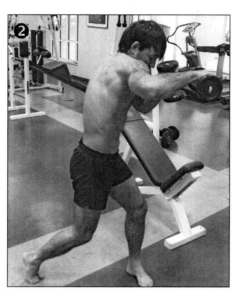

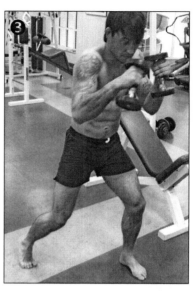

Nikolay starts the exercise holding a pair of dumb-bells as shown.

Nikolay throws out a straight right hand punch, using good form and involving his entire body.

Nikolay brings the dumb-bell back and sets himself to continue the exercise.

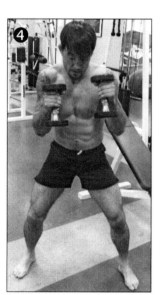

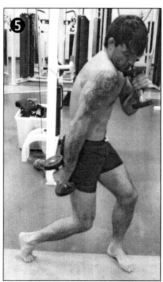

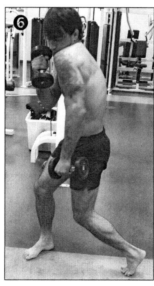

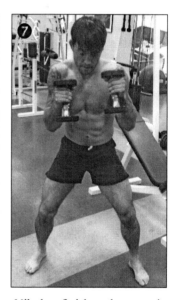

Nikolay is back to his starting position.

Nikolay rolls his right shoulder, lowering the dumb-bell as he does. Look at how he uses good form to simulate the movement used in a real boxing match or MMA fight. This also works the muscles used in grip fighting or pummeling in judo or wrestling.

Nikolay immediately rolls the right shoulder, making sure to use smooth, coordinated movement. The movement of the hips, lower body and feet are all part of this exercise, so make sure to use realistic and good form when performing it.

Nikolay finishes the exercise by assuming his initial fighting stance.

KETTLEBELL CATCH

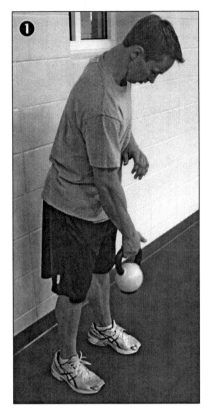

❶ ❷ ❸

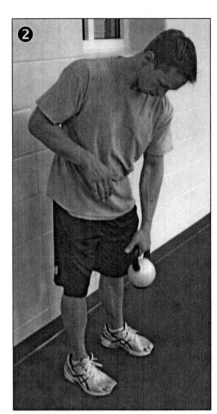

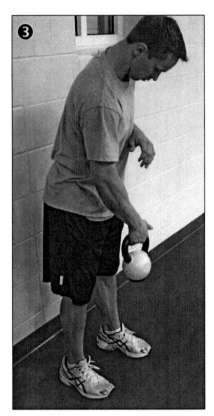

This is a good grip exercise, but it can also be a good exercise for your trapezius. Drew holds a kettlebell in his right hand to start the exercise.

Drew lets go of the kettlebell with his right hand and immediately catches it with his left hand.

Drew continues the exercise by letting go of the kettlebell with his left hand and immediately catching it with his right hand. Drew will perform as many catches as possible without stopping or dropping the implement.

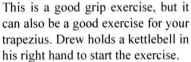

When you can perform at least 100 catches without dropping the kettlebell, move up in weight to a heavier kettlebell. This is a great finisher to any workout in the gym or after a hard practice on the mat.

KETTLEBELL PUNCHING

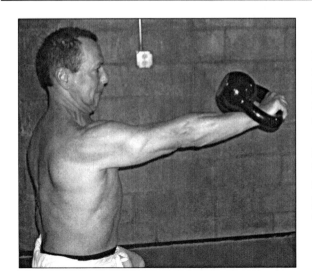

Dan holds a light kettlebell as he performs a front straight punch. Look at how the body of the kettlebell is resting on his wrist to prevent it from swinging as he punches. Perform 5 to 10 sets of anywhere from 10 to 100 reps per set depending on the weight of the kettlebell and your goals. As with all the other exercises that emphasize punching power, use good form and don't use too much weight.

SECTION TWO: PART 5:
"IT'S SO OLD-FASHIONED, IT'S COOL" TRAINING

● ● ● "You can't be normal and do this. Normal people get normal results. To achieve abnormal results, you have to be abnormal." Louie Simmons

This part of Section 2 is certainly not "normal". While the exercises presented on the following pages might be considered unusual and in some cases, a throwback to another era, the functional and scientific basis for why they work is definitely up to date. Before the introduction of the various different weights, machines and exercise equipment many people today may take for granted, the "old timers" used just about anything they could get their hands on to develop their strength and overall fitness. Lifting, pulling, pushing or swinging anything that might improve your strength and conditioning has been used for years by a lot of athletes in a variety of sports, and your imagination is your only limitation.

There are many tools to use, and many different ways to use them, that haven't been included on these pages but what we have included are exercises that we're familiar with and have used in our own training, as well as training many athletes and what we have seen used by others with success. As you progress in your training, you may collect stones, barrels, tires, or just about anything that you can use to improve your strength and fitness. It might have been the champion stonelifter and author, Steve Jeck, who once said, "Stones are nature's barbells." This pretty much sums up what this part of the book is about. To illustrate this point, this photo shows John Saylor's lifting barrel sitting alongside the other pieces of equipment in his gym during a workout with Eric Millsap.

The best way to improve your body is to challenge yourself all the time. Change your routine on a regular basis. Both your body and mind need the stimulation of doing different exercises and a varying workload. Your body adapts to a physical activity and the variety offered in this type of old-fashioned training doesn't allow your body to slip into its "comfort zone". Do exercises in the water, on sand or uneven surfaces to make your training more difficult. You can get a workout anywhere and at anytime you put your mind to it. Whatever you do, don't fall into the trap that you can only get a good workout in a gym with expensive equipment. Getting calluses on your hands is a good thing.

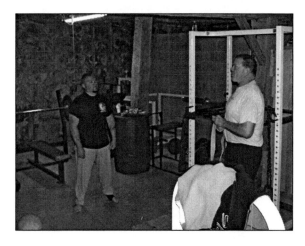

Every culture on the planet has its own unique history of strongmen as well as its own unique history of fighting and some of these traditions are reflected on the following pages in this part of the book. Some exercise and training techniques and tools come from Scotland, while other comes from Okinawa, Russia, ancient Greece or have their origins in America. Many methods of developing strength are common to many different cultures and countries.

Interestingly, some people refer to using chains, ropes, stones and other objects as "dinosaur training," "hardcore training" or "caveman training," but call it what you want, adding this type of "old-fashioned" training to your exercise program will certainly be a great benefit to you. Both authors have been long-time proponents of this approach to training in their personal lives. We both have hard-core gyms in the basements of our homes filled with various objects, rocks, ropes, chains and other tools of our trade. It's amazing what you can use to develop your strength and conditioning. Almost anything can be used as a tool to develop your strength and improve your fitness. We don't have this stuff in our gyms to impress people or be different, we have it there to use.

Several years ago, a young athlete admiringly described his coach as being "so old-fashioned, he's cool". That's an accurate description of this type of training.

STRETCH BANDS, CABLES & STRAPS

GROUND AND POUND

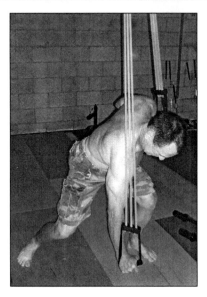

Dr. Dan Rinchuse has hooked his set of stretch bands to a ceiling beam, crossbar or any secure overhead fixture. Dan is punching downward while standing, but can be on knees as well as a variation. This exercise works the back, shoulders and every muscle group used in punching. It is also a great exercise for developing the same muscle groups for doing throws.

STRETCH BANDS ON THE POWER RACK

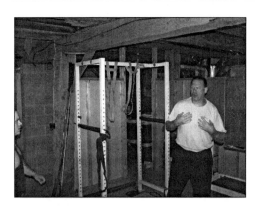

John Saylor is coaching a group of athletes in his Barn of Truth weightroom and you can see the heavy rubber bands John has tied onto his power rack. Rubber or stretch bands are versatile tools and can be taken with you if you travel and want to keep up with your training. Stretch bands come in a variety of strength levels and are usually inexpensive to buy.

STRETCH BAND DIPS

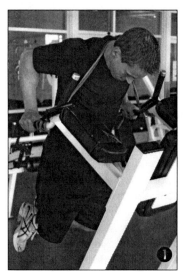 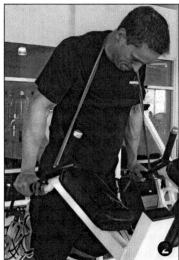

Rubber and elastic bands are commercially available in a variety of resistance levels. Drew is using some bands to add to the workload when doing Dips. Dips provide for an excellent upper body workout, blasting your triceps, shoulders, upper back and pectorals.

Drew looped the bands over his shoulders and is holding them in each hand while holding the dip bar. Use a light or heavy band, depending on your goals and level of fitness. Perform 3 to 5 sets, doing as many dips as possible per set for a tremendous workout. Dips should be a staple of every fighter or grappler's training.

HEAVY BAND DIPS

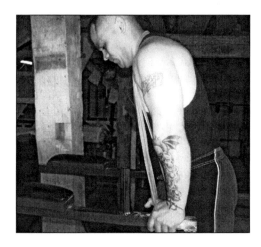

When using thicker, heavier bands, don't do as many repetitions per set. A good heavy band workout is performing a specified number of sets (for instance, let's say 3 sets) and David does as many repetitions as possible per set. David sets a time limit of 30 seconds rest between sets. He might do 12 reps on the first set of heavy band dips, 8 reps on his second set and do 5 on his last set.

BENT OVER DIPS WITH HEAVY BAND

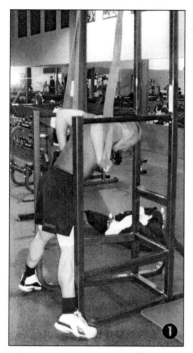 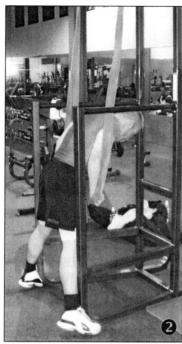

Mike is bending forward and using each hand to push down on the heavy bands that are attached above his head on the rack. Mike has his elbows pointing up and hand pointing down and is looking down to make sure he's bent over far enough.

Mike pushes down with both hands (either at the same time or alternating hands). It's a good idea to use a band heavy enough to give you a lot of resistance. Perform 3 to 5 sets, doing as many reps per set as possible.

BODY PLANK USING HEAVY BANDS

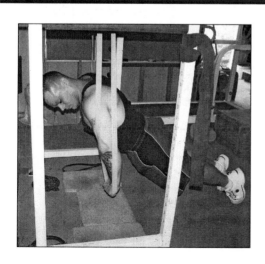

The heavy bands have been attached to the top of the rack and David is leaning forward with his entire weight. David is holding the end of a band in each hand with his arms extended. David can work this exercise a core developer by holding this position for varying lengths of time.

PUSH UPS WITH HEAVY BANDS

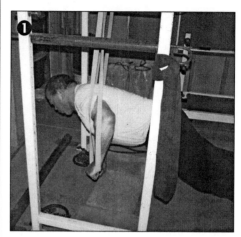

John is using the heavy bands in the rack to perform push-ups. The starting position is with your arms bent at the elbows and body extended and as rigid as possible with your feet on the floor.

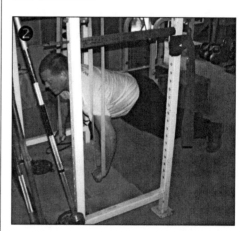

John performs a push-up while holding a band in each arm making sure his body is extended and rigid. This is a tough way to perform push-ups, as all the stabilizers in your upper body have to work extra hard.

PUSH UPS USING CHAINS AND RINGS

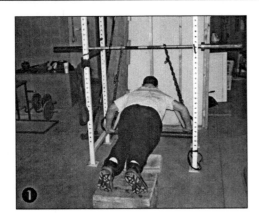

An advanced push-up is performed in a rack. Attach a chain on each side of a bar across the rack. Have a handle or ring to grab onto attached to each chain. Next, loop a heavy band across your back and hold onto it with each hand. Then, prop your feet on a box as John is doing and grab each end of the chain by the handle or ring.

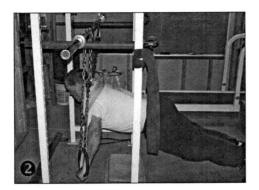

Perform the push-ups from this position. Do as many reps as possible per set and perform multiple sets. This type of push-up using both the chain and heavy bands works your entire upper body and provides serious core training as well because you have to keep your body rigid while performing this exercise. As John Saylor says, "This is a guaranteed butt-kicker."

IRON CROSS WITH STRAPS AND RINGS

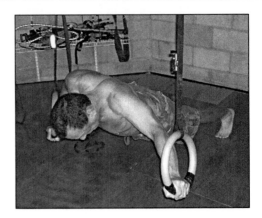

Dan has a set of rings attached to a pair of nylon (non-stretch) cables and performs an Iron Cross. Hold for as long as possible, doing as many sets as you wish. You can also perform push-ups from this position. It's tough to control the swinging of the apparatus and works the stabilizer muscles in your upper body.

LATERAL EXTENSIONS ON CABLES & RINGS

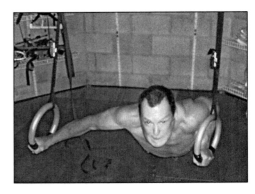

Dan moves from one side to the other, extending his arm full as he does. Rock back and forth, doing as many as possible. This is a really tough exercise and works your shoulder girdle and upper back, as well as your triceps, biceps and forearms.

PUSH UPS WITH FEET AND LEGS IN RINGS

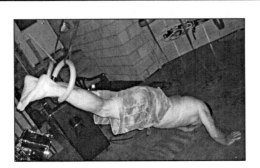

Dan puts his beet in the rings, supports himself with his hands on the floor and performs push-ups. This exercise places a huge amount of stress on your upper body and works your entire upper body really hard.

DUMB-BELL PRESS WITH HEAVY BAND

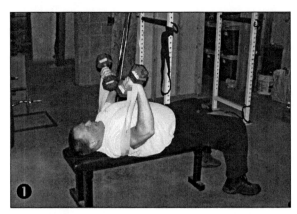

If you think dumb-bell presses on the bench are work now, wait until you try this exercise! Grab each end of a stretch band or heavy band and wrap it around your shoulders as shown in this photo. Have a training partner hand your dumb-bells to you and perform dumb-bell bench presses. The extra resistance from the bands will give you a hard, but great workout.

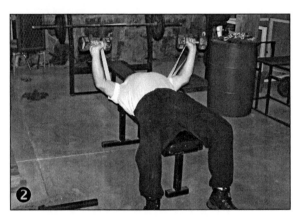

Here's another view of Dumb-bell Press with Heavy Band exercise. The band adds a great deal of additional resistance to this, or any, gym movement.

1-ARM PULLS WITH HEAVY BANDS

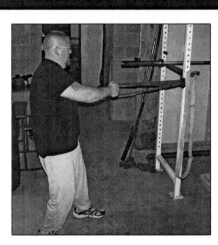

Using a heavy band, Eric pulls with his right hand in the same way he would pull on an opponent's arm when throwing him. This keys in on your shoulders, traps, lats, triceps and forearms, and really gives you a good grip workout. Do as many sets and reps as you wish as a good finisher to your weight room workout.

DECLINE SIT UPS WITH STRETCH BAND

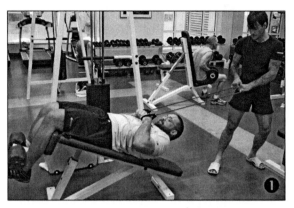

Jake is positioned on a decline bench and holds the end of a band in each hand as shown. Nikolay holds the looped end of the band for support.

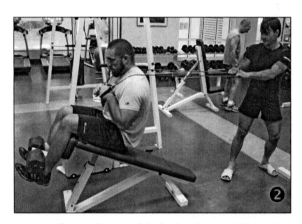

Jake performs sit-ups with the bands providing resistance. Use a moderately heavy band and perform 4 sets of 25 as a good core developer.

USE STRETCH OR HEAVY BANDS TO MAKE ANY LIFTING MOVEMENT HARDER TO DO Adding stretch bands to any exercise you can safely do in the gym will increase the workload and intensity.

STRETCH BAND SIDE STEPS

This exercise is simple and you can do this as a warm-up or cool-down during a workout, either on or off the mat. Go down and back the length of the mat several times or perform this exercise in timed rounds. This works the hip flexors, and is especially good for the inner thighs which are muscle groups necessary for foot sweeps, big throws, squeezing an opponent with your legs in a rodeo ride or fighting in the guard.

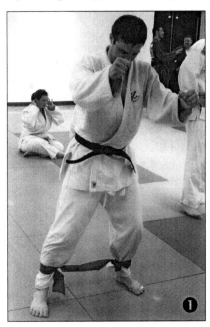
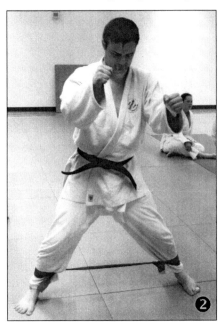
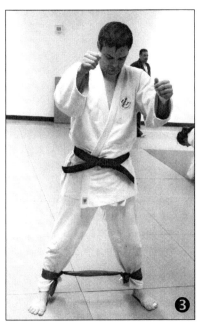

To start, tie a flexible band around your ankles. This is a good auxiliary exercise to develop strength in the adductors and abductors, as well as develop good balance when moving.

Derrick moves sideways, stretching the band. Move with control and fairly slow so that you get more work for your inner thighs, hips and all the stabilizer muscles in your lower body and legs.

As Derrick moves to his side, the tension on the band loosens, and he will continue to perform this exercise down the length of the mat or room.

STRETCH BAND LEG SPLIT FOR THROWING IN THE GYM

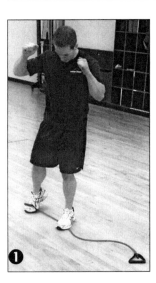
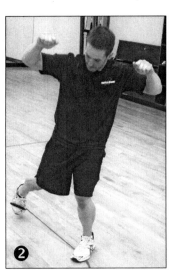
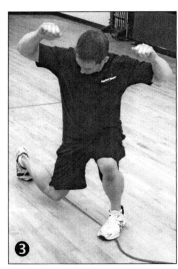

1. Drew has one end of a light band looped around his right foot and is using his left foot to stand on the band, making it taut.

2. Drew slides his right foot back in the same way he would split his legs in a forward throw (Tai Otoshi or Body Drop from judo).

3. Drew fully extends his right leg simulating a throw. He will perform 1 set, doing at least 25 repetitions.

STRETCH BAND LEG SPLIT THROW DONE ON THE MAT

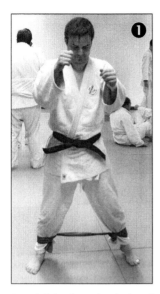

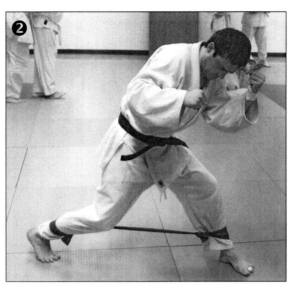

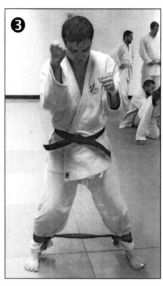

Derrick had an elastic band tied to each ankle.

Derrick splits his legs wide to simulate a Tai Otoshi (Body Drop Throw) on the right side.

Derrick returns to the starting position.

HOW THE SPLIT LEG EXERCISE WORKS

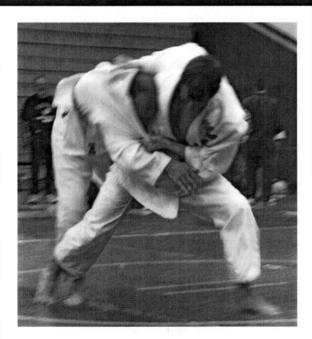

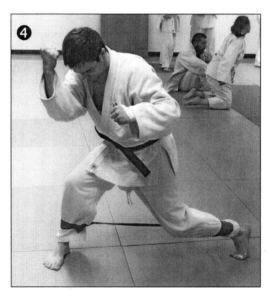

Derrick repeats the exercise, only this time doing it on the left side. Perform 1 set of at least 25 reps as a good auxiliary exercise to develop the muscles in the legs and hips that are used in this and other throwing techniques.

HOW THE STRETCH BAND SPLIT LEG EXERCISE WORKS ON THE MAT

Here's Josh Henges using the Tai Otoshi (Body Drop Throw) in a national judo tournament. This is a powerful throwing technique and is used in all weight categories and by both men and women in a variety of combat sports.

STRETCH BAND FOOT SWEEP

Perform an equal number of reps on each leg to provide balanced training and do a set of at least 25 reps per leg. To develop strong hip and upper leg (primarily adductor) strength, this is a good exercise.

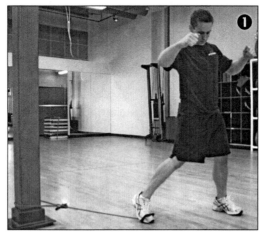

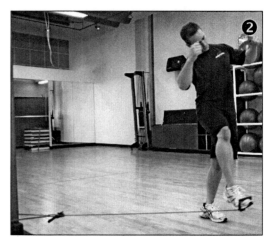

Attach a light to moderately heavy band to a fixed object and loop or attach the other end to your foot as Drew does in this photo.

Drew sweeps his foot forward or across his body, stretching the band. Drew will relax the tension, bring his foot back to the starting position and repeat this exercise.

HOW THE SWEEP DRILL WORKS

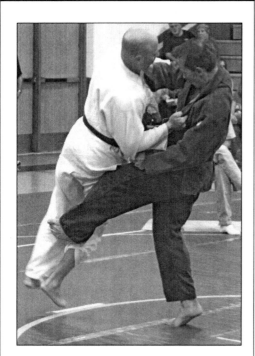

HOW THE STRETCH BAND OR CABLE FOOT SWEEP DRILL WORKS IN ACTION

Here's Drew putting his training to work at the Grand Nationals. Foot sweeps require excellent timing and foot speed, but are also dependent on functional strength

STRETCH BAND KNEE KICKS

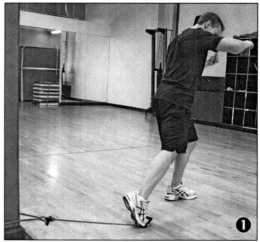

Drew is using a band attached to a pole or fixed object and looped onto his right foot. Perform an equal number of repetitions on each leg to provide balance in your training and do 1 set of at least 25 kicks per leg.

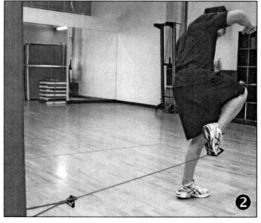

Drew kicks his right knee forward as hard as he can. This develops all the muscles in the legs and hips for explosive strength in kicks and throwing techniques.

STRETCH BAND BREGMAN HOPS

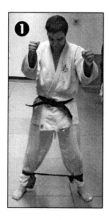

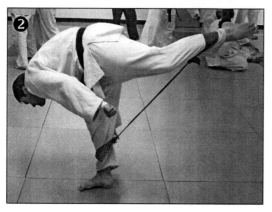

Derrick has an elastic band tied to each ankle.

Derrick leans to his right side and supports himself with his right leg as he lifts his left leg up as shown. Derrick's left leg is pretty straight and his left toe is pointed. Derrick will hop to his left in a complete circle, and then hop back to his right in a complete circle. He will then switch legs and hop on his left leg with his right leg up in the air. Perform 10 repetitions of this exercise for excellent leg strength when throwing an opponent.

POWER DEVELOPED BY THE KNEE KICK EXERCISE

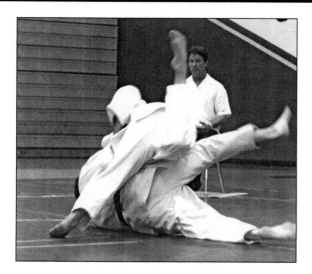

THE DRIVING LEG POWER DEVELOPED BY USING THE STRETCH BAND KNEE KICK EXERCISE

This shows the tremendous power exerted by the legs in the hooking, reaping or sweeping action of a throwing technique. The obvious benefit of this exercise is the development of strong knee kicks, but strong legs are necessary in every combat sport as shown in this photo of a judo tournament.

STRETCH BAND RUN

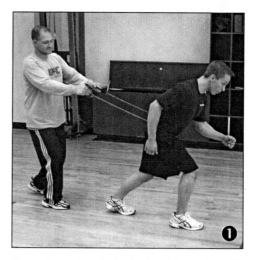

Drew has a band attached to his waist with Bryan holding it to provide resistance. This exercise provides good plyometric training for the legs and hips. A variation of this is for Drew to attach the band (or rope) to a tire or weighted sled instead of having Bryan provide resistance. Drew is ready to start off fast on Bryan's command to start.

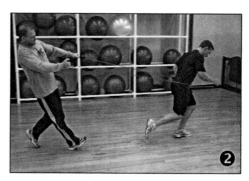

On Bryan's command, Drew starts fast and runs forward with Bryan following to provide resistance.

STRETCH BAND LUNGE STEP

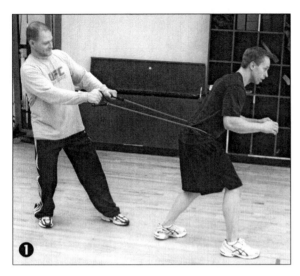

Drew has a band attached around his waist with Bryan holding it to provide resistance.

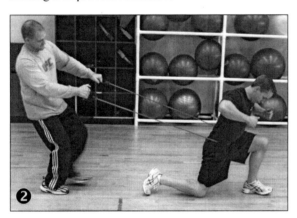

Drew performs a lunge step, dropping low and stepping forward with his left leg. Drew's back is straight.

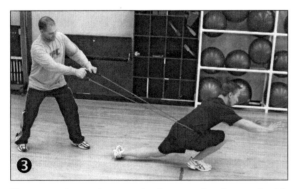

Drew continues the exercise by stepping forward with his right leg. Drew will perform 10 lunge steps to complete the exercise. Perform several sets of 10 for a good workout. This exercise works your legs, hips and back and replicates the low, drop-step used when shooting in for a takedown or throw.

LUNGE STEP POWER IN ACTION ON THE MAT

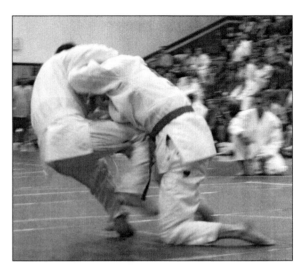

When shooting in for single or double leg takedowns or throws, having power in your lunge (penetration) step is important!

STRETCH BAND WALK

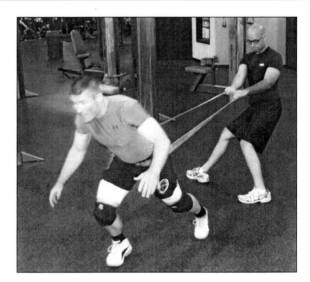

Mike is using a heavier rubber or elastic band and taking slow, deliberate lunge steps. This variation of the exercise places the emphasis on strength in the legs. Perform 3 sets of 10 steps.

STRETCH CABLE CROSS-BODY THIGH LIFT

This exercise is excellent for developing the hips and inner thigh muscles. It's also a good lower back movement because of the controlled twisting action you perform while doing this.

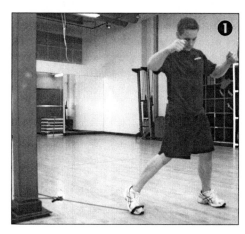

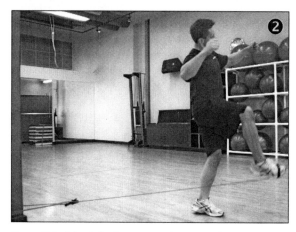

Drew has a band attached to his right foot with the other end of the band attached to a pole or wall. Drew's starting position is as shown here.

Drew lifts his right foot up and across his body, making sure to lift his knee as well. Doing this provides work for the entire leg and hip area. Drew points his right foot as he lifts his leg to provide more work to his calf and hamstring.

STRETCH OR HEAVY BAND BACKWALK

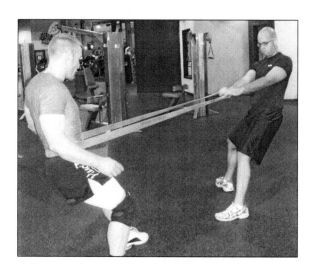

Mike is facing Scott and walking backward. This works the entire lower body and especially the glutes and hamstrings.

HEAVY BAND RESISTANCE AGAINST PARTNER PULL

A variation of this exercise is for Mike to resist when his partner pulls him with the band.

HOW THE THIGH LIFT EXERCISE WORKS

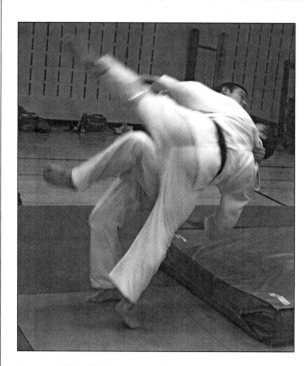

Leg or thigh lift throws or foot sweeps require speed and strength as well as coordination and timing. Specific exercises and drills to increase your speed and strength provide a solid base for skill and technical development.

UCHIKOMI (FIT INS) USING STRETCH BANDS, ROPE OR BELT

This is an old exercise, but one that has stood the test of both time and success. It replicates the movement of an actual throw. You can substitute a judo belt or a rope. The elasticity of the band provides additional resistance making the exercise a bit harder. Perform as many repetitions as your fitness level allows. You can start off by doing 4 sets of 25 reps, and work your way up to 4 sets of 100 reps, then multiple sets with 100 or more reps per set. This is a great cardio exercise in addition to providing good foot-speed training and a good strength workout as well.

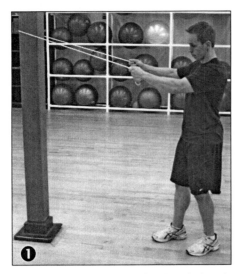
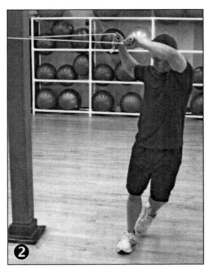
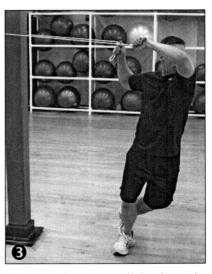

Drew holds the ends of a band that is looped around or attached to a pole.

As Drew steps in with his feet, he pulls the band with his hands.

Drew continues to pull hard on the band as he completes his Uchikomi or fitting movement.

UCHIKOMI (FIT INS) WITH STRETCH BAND RESISTANCE

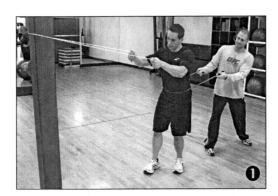
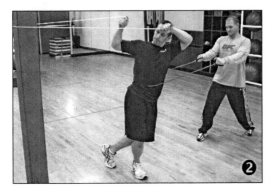
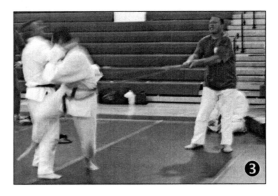

1. Bryan is holding an elastic band looped around Drew's waist in this variation of the Uchikomi Drill.

2. As Drew performs the Fit Ins, Bryan pulls the band, providing more resistance for Drew.

3. Here's the same exercise done on the mat. Author John Saylor is holding a stretch band while Jim does an uchikomi (fit in for a throw) on Mike.

UCHIKOMI WITH A PARTNER HOLDING THE BANDS

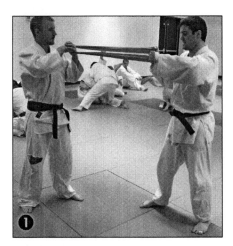
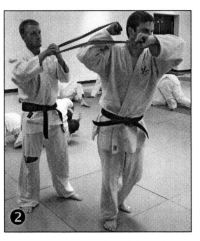
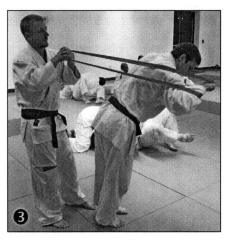

Derrick (right) holds onto each end of the band while Ben holds the other end, stretching the band. Instead of looping the band around a pole or attaching it to a wall, Ben is holding the band.

Derrick fits in for his Uchikomi with Ben providing resistance.

Derrick fits in completely, stretching the band as much as possible. Derrick can hold this position for a 3-count to provide more isometric resistance and increase the workload.

STRETCH BAND UCHIKOMI WALK

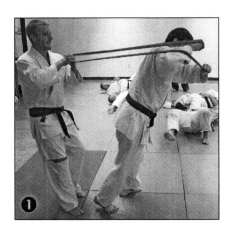
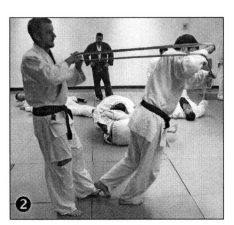
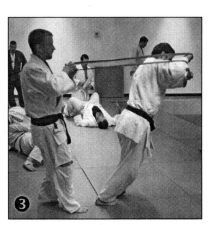

This drill helps develop a strong throwing action and works the lower body as well as the upper body. Derrick fits into a throw holding an end of the band in each hand. Ben lags back and lets the band stretch out as shown.

Ben follows Derrick, but lags behind just enough to keep the band stretched tight and give Derrick resistance.

Walk the length of the mat as Derrick does here. Derrick can walk to one end of the mat and then switch places with Ben and he performs this exercise going back down the mat as well.

The Chest Expander has been around for a long time. Both authors owned Chest Expanders that were made of springs instead of elastic bands as this one is. You can use it in a variety of ways as a supplement to your overall training. It's also handy to pack away when you travel and use to catch a good workout in a hotel room. Chest Expanders are excellent to use as a warm up before a match as well. As you get stronger, add another band. Pull the expander with control and don't let it jerk around.

CHEST EXPANDER

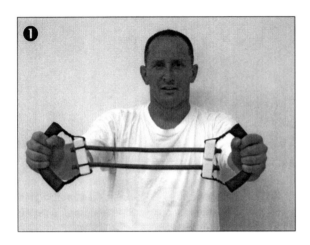

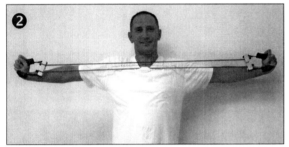

Chad pulls it out as far as possible. This works your shoulders, arms, upper back and pectoral muscles. Perform as many sets as you wish with 10 reps per set.

CHEST EXPANDER BOW AND ARROW

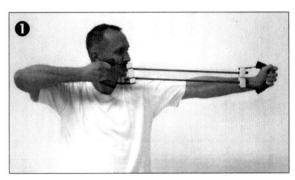

Chad is holding the expander in the same way he would an archery bow. This gives your shoulders a good workout.

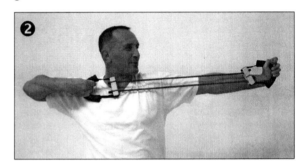

Chad pulls back with his right hand as he keeps his left hand rigid and stable. Perform as many sets as you wish using 10 reps on each arm.

CHEST EXPANDER OVERHEAD

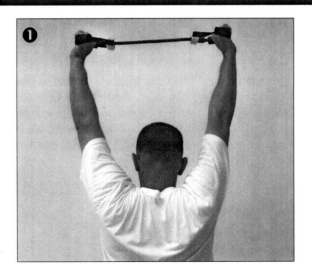

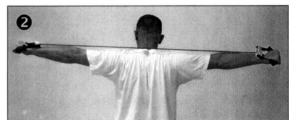

1. Chad has the expander held at arm's length overhead. To get the most out of this exercise, make sure you keep it up at arm's length.

2. Chad pulls the expander out to the side. This works your shoulders incredibly hard. Don't let the expander snap or jerk back, but rather, slowly raise your arms back overhead to finish the rep.

NECK STRENGTHENER LEANING BACK

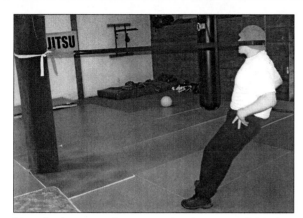

Your body goes where your head goes and it's important to develop strong neck, traps and upper back muscles. Author John Saylor stretches a heavy band on a regular basis as part of his neck strength training. John has looped a band around his head and has attached the other end of the band onto a beam. Notice that John is wearing a cap to keep the rubber band from pulling or tearing out his hair. This works all the muscles in the neck as well as provides work for the trapezius and upper back.

NECK STRENGTHENER AT AN ANGLE

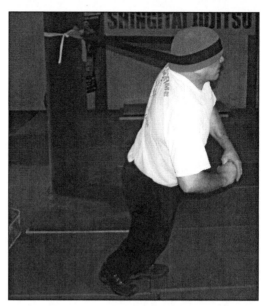

John leans to his right at an angle as shown to insure that every angle of the neck is developed. Hold this position with the band fully extended for a specified time limit or count.

NECK STRENGTHENER FORWARD

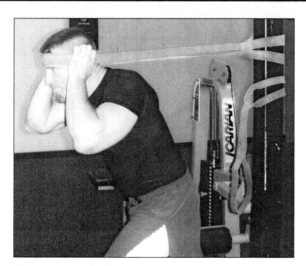

Mike has a band attached to a power rack and has it looped around his head as shown. Mike leans forward to provide training from another angle. This variation places a great deal of the workload on the upper traps.

NECK STRENGTHENER LEANING BACK

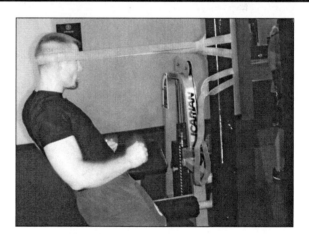

Mike leans directly backward in this variation. As he leans away and when the band is fully stretched, Mike will pull his head backward using only the muscles of his neck to add to the workload.

NECK STRENGTHENER WHILE HOLDING THE STRETCH BAND

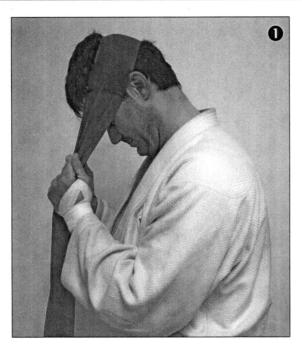

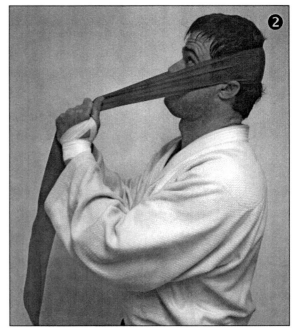

Derrick has looped a band around his head as shown and pulls on it, making it taut. Derrick is looking down.

Derrick straightens his head upright slowly and in a controlled movement. To complete the exercise, he will look down again and repeat the process.

NECK STRENGTHENER - BAND TO THE SIDE

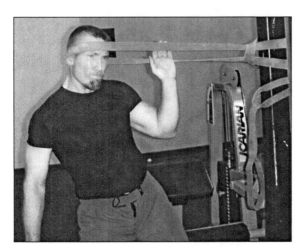

Mike stretched the band directly to his right side. He will do the same to the left side to balance out the development.

TECHNICAL TIP: When working with rubber or elastic bands, you can stretch the band as far as you wish and hold that position for a specified time limit or count. Often, a 3-count is good if you are starting out. You can increase it to a 10-count as you progress in strength.

YOU NEED A STRONG NECK!

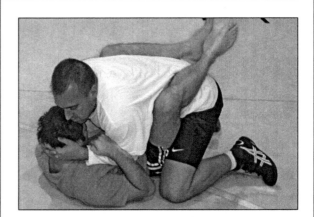

Your neck is a vital link in your body and you use it in a variety of ways. Also, the stronger your neck, the better you can resist chokes or other neck submissions such as this can opener Bret is doing on Chuck. Additionally, you bridge off your head or use it as a "third arm" to control your opponent and need a neck strong enough to get the job done.

TRAINING WITH ROPES AND THINGS YOU PULL

SKIPPING ROPE

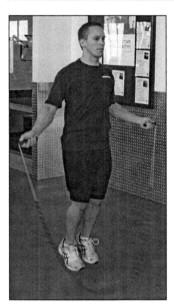

One of the hardest, and least-used forms of cardio development is jumping rope. Use rope jumping as a fantastic, butt-kicking finisher to any workout, either on or off the mat. A great workout is to initially do 3 sets of 30-second rounds, as you adapt to this, increase the workout to doing 3 sets of 1-minute rounds, then add 30 seconds per round as you improve until you get to 3 sets of 3-minute rounds. Jumping rope is hard work and it will vastly improve your cardio capacity! Here's a good example on an exercise that's "so old-fashioned, it's cool." But...there are a lot more exercises you can do with rope.

ROPES GONE WILD

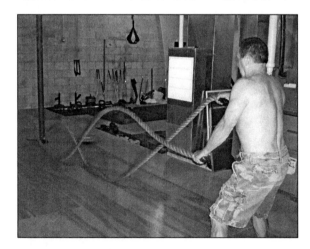

This is an excellent exercise for your grip, but it really works your arms, shoulders, pectorals, upper back and core as well. Dan loops a long rope around a pole and grabs each end of the rope with each hand. Make sure the rope you use is a thick, heavy rope to get the most benefit out of this exercise. Holding the end of the rope in each hand, whip the rope up and down for 30 seconds. Do as many 30-second rounds as you wish. You can whip the rope in other directions as well, back and forth, side to side, or any direction that gives you a workout. Anthony Diluglio in ART OF STRENGTH developed this exercise. More on training with ropes like this can be seen at Dan Rinchuse's web site at www.rinchusemartialarts.com.

ROPE CLIMB

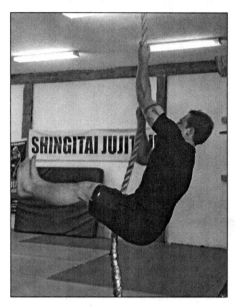

Rope climbing has been around for years as a method of strength development for good reason; it works. Roger is climbing the rope at the Barn of Truth in Perrysville, Ohio. Use this as a great finisher to any workout, whether it's a workout in the gym or in the dojo or wrestling room.

GRIP STRENGTH IS VITAL!

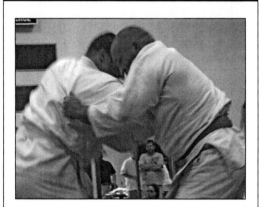

Whether you're in a sport that uses a jacket or not, a strong grip directly equates to success. Before you throw, pin or force your opponent to tap out, you have to grab him first. Then, after you grab him and don't let go of him until it suits you, he's in trouble and that's good for you.

ROPE LEGS RAISE FOR CORE TO ADD CORE WORK

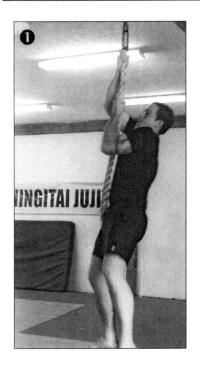

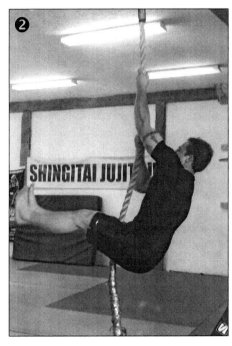

1. Roger holds onto the rope with his legs dangling as shown.

Note: Roger can give himself a tougher workout by climbing the rope with his legs dangling. Roger is pulling his entire body weight as he climbs and this places the entire workload on the arms, shoulders and upper back.

2. Roger continues to hold onto the rope with his hands while he raises his legs. This is a tough core exercise and provides a lot of work to the upper body as well. Perform as many leg raises as possible with the goal of increasing how many you can do each time.

ROPE CLIMB UPSIDE DOWN

Climbing a rope upside down works the muscles from a vastly different angle. To balance out your rope climbing, try climbing the rope upside down. Just remember, if you fall, land safely or have a partner or crash pad under you.

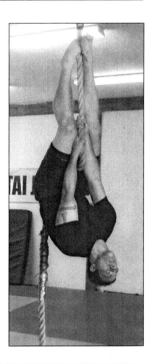

TECHNICAL TIP: Wear a weighted vest, ankle weights or belt attached with weights to make climbing the rope more difficult.

ROPE PULL UPS

Your grip strength will vastly improve if you do this exercise on a regular basis. Pull-ups are far more difficult when you have to grab a rope with each hand! You can do pull-ups with both hands on one rope, but in either case, make sure the rope is thick and heavy. A thicker rope is harder to hold and that makes it tougher for you to grip it. Doing this repeatedly will increase the strength in you hands, arms, upper back, shoulders and every other part of your body.

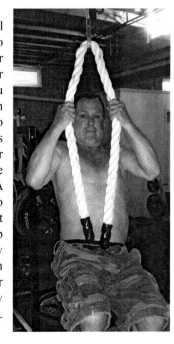

PULL UPS USING A TOWEL

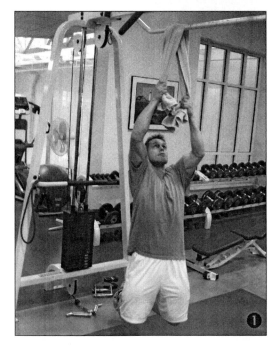

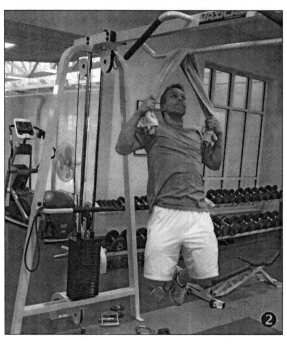

Use a towel to hold onto when doing a variety of exercises, in this case, pull-ups. Drew loops a towel over the pull-up bar and starts the exercise by holding onto the towel with each hand.

This is especially useful for those who compete in sports that require a jacket such as judo, jujitsu or sambo. If you don't want to cut up an old gi jacket, you can use a towel instead.

USE A TOWEL, JUDO BELT, JACKET OR ROPE

JACKET PULL UPS (USE LAPEL OR SLEEVE)

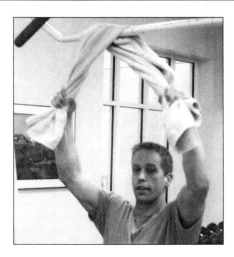

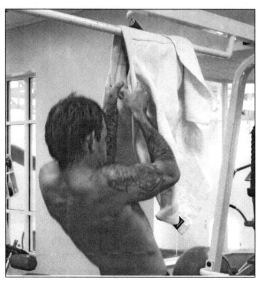

Drew performs the pull-up by gripping onto the towel instead of the bar. This is a fantastic grip workout and highly recommend for anyone competing in a sport where a gi is used. Even if you don't compete in a sport where a gi is used, this exercise really works your entire arm structure, especially your forearms and hands. It also works many of the stabilizer muscles in your upper body and forces yu to perform a stricter pull-up.

Nikolay is performing pull-ups using a judogi jacket. In this photo, he is holding onto the lapels, but he can also hold onto the sleeves or any part of the jacket. Holding onto the lapels give Nikolay a realistic feel since the lapel is often used to grip.

TOWEL BENT OVER ROWING

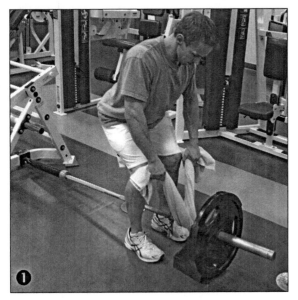

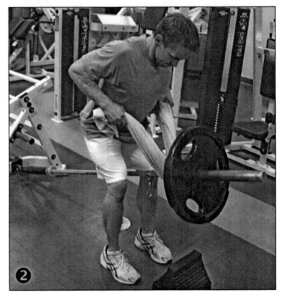

Drew uses a towel wrapped under the bar when performing Bent Over Rowing. Holding the towel replicates the feel of actually grabbing an opponent's jacket.

Drew pulls up with both hands on the towel competing the exercise. Use a towel, judo jacket, rope or judo belt to hold onto when performing many exercises from time to time. This breaks up the monotony of doing the exercises the regular way and concentrates on an essential part of grappling; grip strength.

PALM DOWN GRIP

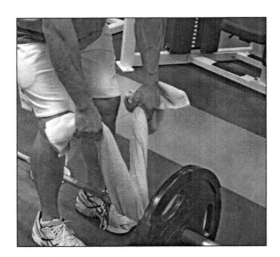

Drew holds the towel with his palms down in this first variation of the Bent Over Rowing with a towel. This is the most often used grip when doing this exercise and it emphasizes the work on the brachioradialis (the muscle on the upper part of the forearm near the elbow joint), which is important for grip strength.

PALM UP GRIP

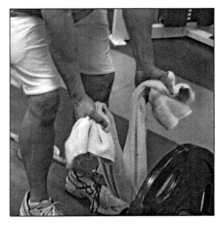

Drew is holding the towel with his palms up. When performing Bent Over Rowing, this grip works the lats, teres major in the upper back, the traps, rhomboids and the entire arm structure.

WRIST CURLS VARIATION

Drew can perform wrist curls from this position and get even more work in for his grip. Simply curl your hands upward, making sure not to make the lift into a biceps curl with the emphasis of the work on the forearm.

LAT PULLDOWNS USING A GI SLEEVE

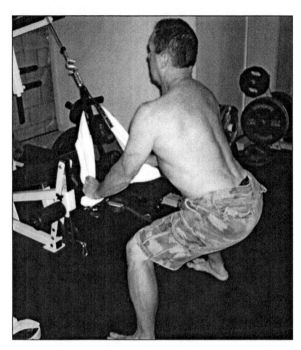

To improve your gripping power and work the stabilizers and smaller muscle groups in your arms, shoulders, back and chest, use a towel, judo belt, rope or piece of a uniform sleeve (or heavy collar) as a handle. Dan is doing pull-downs with a cable machine using a gi sleeve. You may not use as much weight in your triceps pushdowns using a towel instead of a regular handle, but it really strengthens your grip.

LAPEL CHOKES REQUIRE A STRONG GRIP

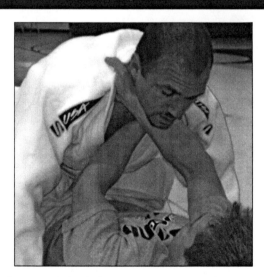

Grip strength is vital to every grappler or fighter. This photo shows how working with a towel, judogi jacket, rope or judo belt when performing strength exercises can be valuable when choking an opponent.

ROPE KETTLEBELL SWING

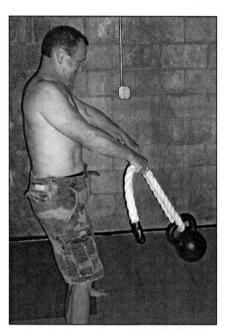

Swing a Kettlebell on a rope forward and back through your legs, in a circle around your body or anyway that will give you a workout. The dual benefit of holding firmly onto the rope for grip strength and the total body workout of swinging the implement makes this exercise a good one to include in your training.

SLEEVE, TOWEL OR ROPE KETTLEBELL CARRY

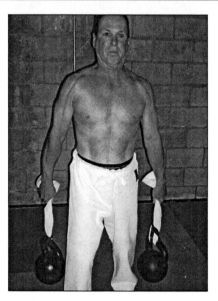

In this variation of the Farmer's Walk, Dan ties the sleeves of a gi or a towel on a pair of kettlebells and goes for a walk with them. Dan can also do curls, lateral raises or any movement he would with a kettlebell or dumb-bell. This is a terrific grip workout, but it also is a good workout for your traps, shoulders and arms.

HAMMERS AND SWINGING THINGS

The hammer has been used as a tool to build things and hit people with since the dawn of time. Mankind also discovered along the way that swinging a heavy hammer around makes you stronger. Remember, when training with a hammer, follow safety precautions and make sure no one is anywhere near you when you start swinging it. Also remember that hammer swings are extremely hard on your lower back, so swing the hammer with control, and don't let go of it. A flying hammer can hit someone and cause serious damage or death, so be careful!

HITTING A TIRE WITH THE HAMMER

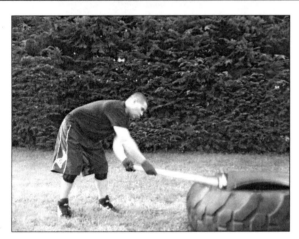

Go to the hardware store and buy an eight or ten pound hammer and get a good workout.Hitting your hammer onto a tire or any object that won't break or splinter will give you a workout you won't soon forget. Old-time boxers used to chop wood, and some fighters still do, to work the muscles used for punching. Swinging a hammer and hitting a tire does the same thing, but you don't have to worry about a sharp axe or splinters of wood flying all around. If you don't have a huge tire as shown in this photo, use a tire of any size. Hammer swings are hard work, so use hammer swings as the last exercise in your routine. A good way to intensify this exercise is to get on both knees and swing the hammer onto the tire. This intensifies the workout for your upper body. Something to seriously think about is that you should always wear sturdy boots, preferably high-top boots to protect your feet and support your ankles when working out with a hammer. Hit the tire with your hammer from a variety of angles to work as many muscle groups as possible.

TWO TIRE HAMMER SWINGS

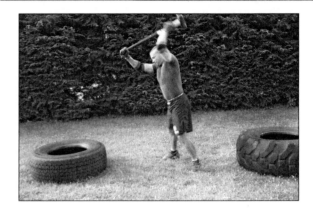

For some variety in this exercise, use two tires. Hit one tire with your hammer, then on the rebound from the first tire, spin around and hit the other tire. Make sure the tires are close enough to each other (and you) so that you can make a good turn with your body without injuring your lower back, knees or ankles.

RUN AND HIT THE TIRE

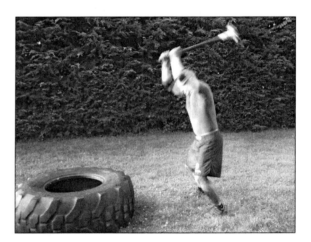

Mike starts by standing about 10 feet away from the tire and firmly holding the hammer by the handle with both hands straight up over his head. Run forward holding the hammer over your head and when close enough to the tire, swing the hammer and hit the tire with it. This exercise really works the stabilizers in your entire upper body, but especially in your shoulders, upper back and arms. Do this as a change of pace in your training routine.

TECHNICAL TIP: To avoid boredom in your training routine, every so often, use different things to lift, carry, throw or add to your training to make it fun and more interesting. Get outside and do some stone lifting, tire flipping or other unusual exercises. You and your training partners can challenge yourselves with different exercises and drills using implements you don't normally handle. This makes your body constantly adapt and grow. Not only that, there's definitely something to be said for the bragging rights when telling people about how many times you did an overhead press with a big anvil!

HEAVY CLUB OVERHEAD SWING

You can make your own heavy club with a solid thick wood like hickory by getting a woodcarver to make it into a big club. A wood ball bat will do if you don't have a heavier club, but however you make it, swinging a club is a good workout.

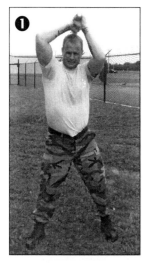

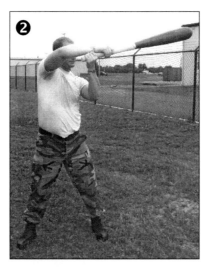

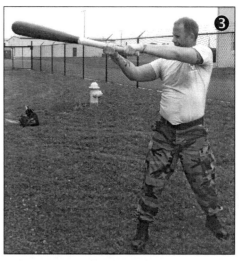

Sean starts the exercise by holding the club over his head as shown. Make sure you have a solid footing on the ground with a fairly wide stance for stability.

Sean swings the club to his left, keeping his body erect.

Sean continues to swing the club around his body as shown. He will perform 10 swings, then switch the direction he swings the club.

HEAVY CLUB OVERHEAD CHOP

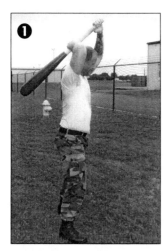

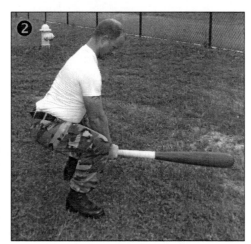

TECHNICAL TIP: You can use a sledgehammer instead of a heavy club. Also, if you chop wood with an axe or hatchet, be careful; they're sharp!

Sean holds the club overhead in the same way he would hold an axe when chopping wood.

Sean swings the bat down in a chopping motion. Perform 10 repetitions. This is a good upper body exercise, emphasizing all the muscles in the upper back and shoulders.

CLUB 1 HAND SWING

CLUB 1 HAND FIGURE 8 SWINGS

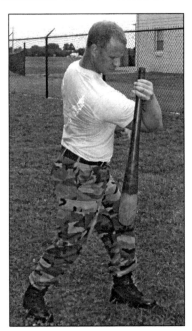

Sean swings the club in a figure 8 pattern with each arm, performing a complete figure 8 with one arm, and then doing the same with his other arm. This offers some variety and works the entire shoulder.

A variation of the Club Swing is to swing the implement with one hand instead of two. Perform an equal number of swings with each arm.

BOTH HANDS HAMMER SWINGS (FIGURE 8 PATTERN)

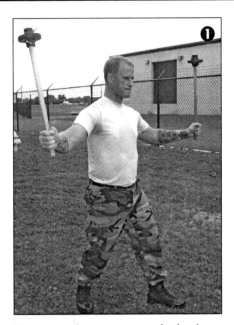

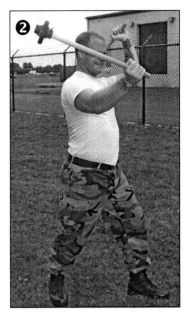

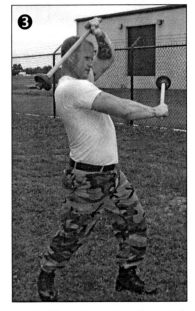

You can make your own swinging hammers by purchasing a dowel stick at any hardware store, or even a heavy gauge PVC pipe. Use some barbell collars with a 10-pound barbell plate locked on the handle. To start, Sean holds a hammer in each hand as shown.

Sean swings the hammers in a figure 8 pattern, swinging each hammer in an opposite direction.

Sean will perform 10 swings with each arm, and then switch directions on each arm swing for a second set. This exercise is useful for functional shoulder strength. Use no more than 10 pounds on each hammer.

BOTH HANDS HAMMER HOLD TO FRONT

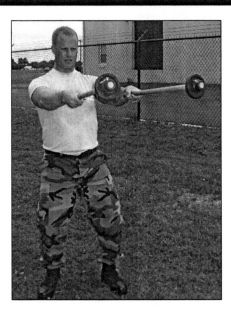

A tough isometric exercise is to hold a pair of hammers in front of you. Even light weight gets heavy when you hold it straight out in front of you (or to each side) for an extended period. Perform 2 or 3 sets, holding the hammers as long as possible each set. This works your entire upper body, but especially your back, shoulders, arms and traps.

BOTH HANDS HAMMER WINDMILL SWINGS

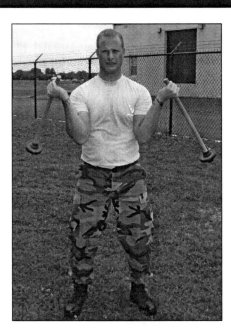

Another variation of training with the hammer is to hold a hammer in each hand and swing it in circles. Sean keeps his elbows in close to his side, emphasizing the workload to his shoulders. Use a pair of light hammers as a good warm-up for heavy lifting. For safety, make sure that the weights are firmly attached to the hammer handles.

SCOTTISH HAMMER

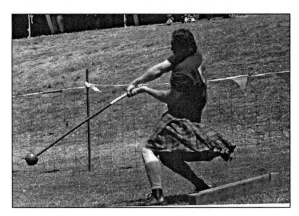

Swinging a hammer on a long handle develops serious strength. The hammer throw is a standard event in Scottish Highland Games. The Scottish hammer is a 16 (or 22) pound metal ball attached onto a rattan wood or PVC pole 50 inches in length. You can check on the Internet where to buy equipment for the Highland Games and get yourself a Scottish hammer. This photo shows author Steve Scott more than a few years ago swinging the hammer in the Highland Games.

There are some hammers marketed under different names that are similar to the Scottish hammer and are effective training tools as well, but swinging a hammer with a flexible handle (the rattan wood or PVC is the best) really makes a tough way to train. If you swing too fast, the hammer will bring you off your feet, so you have to work hard to control it, and most importantly, don't let go if it unless you intend to throw it as done in the Scottish Highland Games.

A good workout using the Scottish hammer is to stand with a fairly wide stance and hold the hammer at the end of the handle as shown in this photo. Swing the hammer to your left for 10 full swings circling the weight over your head and body. Take a 30-second break before swinging the hammer to your right for 10 full swings. This exercise works the entire body, but is great for the back, shoulders, traps, arms, pectorals and provides a really though core workout. For more information on the Scottish hammer or the Highland Games, go to any of the many web sites on the Internet.

SWING STICK TRAINING BLOCKING DRILL

While certainly not anywhere as heavy as some of the other things we swing in this book, the Swing Stick is a good tool for fighters. Wrap each end of a long PVC pole with foam for padding. The momentum of the long pole simulates the force of a punch to a partial degree.

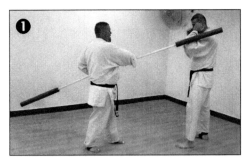

Eric swings the stick high and Greg blocks it with his left arm.

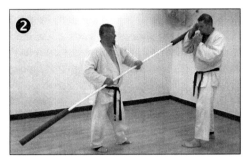

Eric immediately swings the other end high, forcing Greg to block with his right arm.

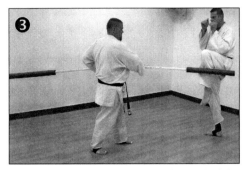

Eric immediately swings the other end of the stick low and Greg blocks it with his leg.

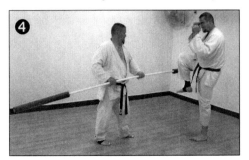

Eric swings the other end of the stick low and Greg uses his right leg to block .

SWING STICK TRAINING MOVEMENT DRILL

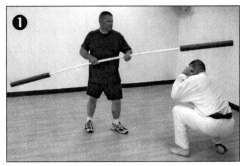

Eric swings the stick at Greg, who is forced to duck under it as shown. Eric can move around the room swinging the stick, with Greg ducking it or they can stay in one place and perform the drill.

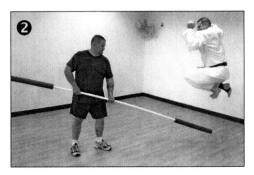

Eric swings the stick low with Greg jumping to avoid it. This is a good drill for plyometric jump training. Perform 10 swings as part of a workout.

SHORT SWING STICK BLOCK

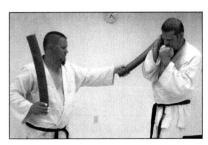

Purchase a foam "noodle" and cut it in lengths that you can use as a Swing Stick. Eric swings the stick at Greg's head and Greg blocks it.

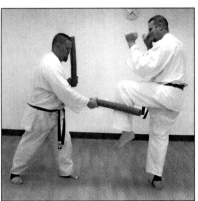

Eric uses the stick to swing low, allowing Greg to practice his low blocks with his leg or arm. Swing as fast or as slow as you wish, depending on your level of skill and your training goals.

SLED TOWING, PULLING AND PUSHING

Towing, pulling or pushing heavy objects is a test of strength as well as a means of developing it. This type of training is especially useful for fighters and grapplers as it develops tremendous lower body strength, as well as an extremely strong lower back area. Before the word "extreme' became overused, this type of training exemplified what extreme training was all about. Used in Strongman contests for many years, towing and pulling a sled is a real test of hardcore strength and endurance.

Sled Towing is when you attach the sled to your body in some way and walk forward, towing the sled behind you. **Sled Pulling** is when you face the sled and pull it toward you, either by moving or walking backward or remaining stationary and pulling the sled to you. **Sled Pushing**, obviously, is getting behind a sled and pushing it.

Towing, pulling or pushing a sled is hard work and doing it develops a gritty, hardcore attitude about your development as an athlete and fighter. Doing this type of training isn't for everyone and performing this heavy-duty type of training really does toughen you up. If you're willing to tow, push or pull a heavy sled around on a regular basis, taking a beating (and dishing one out) from another human being isn't so intimidating.

LUNGE STEP SLED TOW

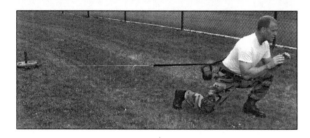

Sean does a drop step or lunge step as he tows the sled. This develops power when shooting in for a takedown on an opponent.

TECHNICAL TIP: You can also tow or pull a tire if you don't have access to a sled. In fact, you can pull or tow anything heavy (a wheelbarrow filled with rocks, a car or any object) simply by connecting a rope or chain from it to you! Towing a heavy object provides tremendous lower body training for strength, and is a total body workout. Towing heavy things also requires a gritty, tough attitude in training and this translates to having that same attitude when fighting or grappling an opponent.

SLED PULLING AND TOWING

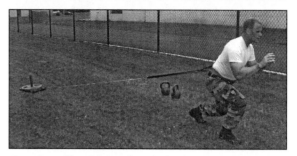

Sean is pulling his towing sled using the basic pulling technique. Tie or affix the towrope or chain to your leather weight belt and pull the sled as shown. Pull the sled on grass, dirt or a track where you have less resistance than concrete or gravel. The softer surface allows you to get a better footing and provides a safer pulling action. Sometimes, concrete surfaces can cause the sled to tip over.

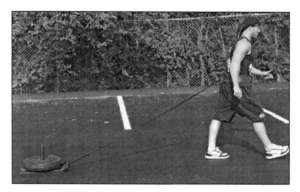

John Kerr is walking with this sled, taking normal steps with the emphasis on keeping his body upright. An upright body when towing a sled works your lower back, abs and hips a great deal, giving you excellent core strength.

OVERHEAD HANDLE HOLD WHILE TOWING

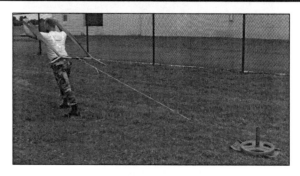

Sean holds a bar or handle over his head as he tows the sled as shown in this photo. This places the workload on the shoulders.

SLED TOW WITH HEAVY BANDS

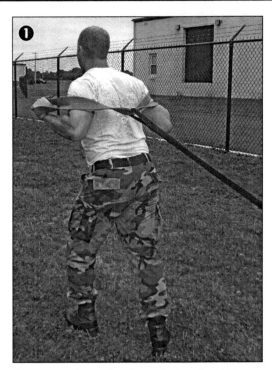

Sean uses a heavy band attached to the sled rope with the bands wrapped around his shoulders as shown to start this exercise.

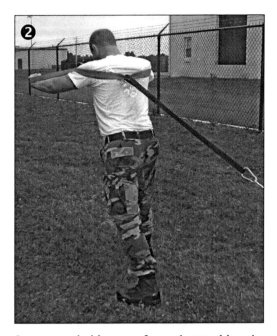

Sean extends his arms forward, stretching the heavy band as he does. This is a good deltoid exercise. As Sean walks, he straightens and bends his elbows, making this a difficult way to tow a sled.

OVERHEAD KETTLEBELL HOLD TOWING

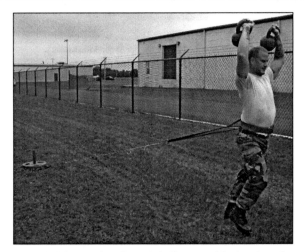

Sean holds a pair of kettlebells over his head as he tows the sled.

SLED TOW KETTLEBELL PRESS WITH BANDS

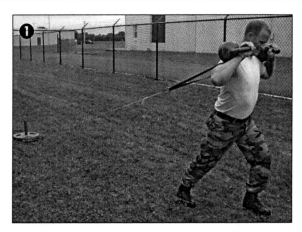

Sean starts this exercise by holding a pair of kettlebells (or dumb-bells) at his shoulders as shown.

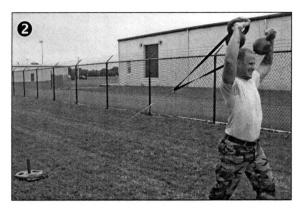

As Sean walks forward to tow the sled, he presses the kettlebells overhead, performing 10 reps and then taking a break before continuing.

TWO BANDS ON BAR TOW SLED

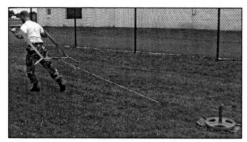

Sean tows the sled by holding onto a pair of heavy bands that are attached to a bar behind him. The bar is attached to the tow sled rope.

SLED PULL WHILE HOLDING MEDICINE BALL

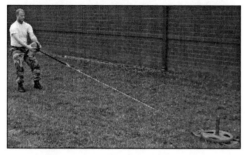

Sean walks backward while holding a medicine ball that is attached to the towrope. This focuses on grip strength as well as pectoral and deltoid strength.

SLED PULL MEDICINE BALL OVER SHOULDER

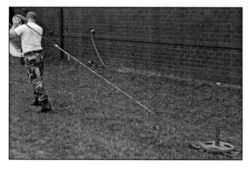

Sean holds the medicine ball over his left shoulder as he tows the sled. He will tow the sled for a specific distance and then hold the ball over his right shoulder on the way back.

SLED PULL CHOKING MEDICINE BALL

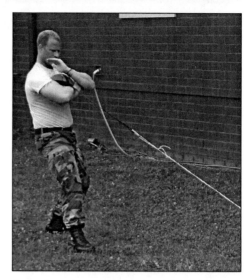

Sean has the medicine ball in a figure 4 rear naked choke as he pulls the sled. This strengthens all the muscles necessary for this choke.

SLED TOW W/MEDICINE BALL OVERHEAD

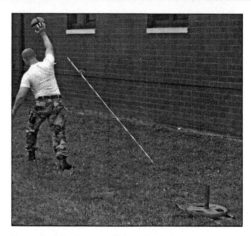

Sean holds the medicine ball with one hand over his head as shown as he tows the sled.

SLED PULL MEDICINE BALL RUSSIAN TWIST

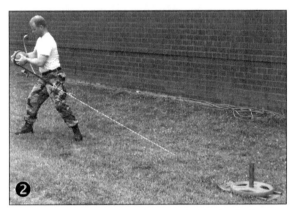

Sean starts the exercise by holding a medicine ball with both hands at his waist as shown.

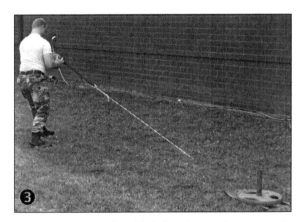

Sean rotates to his right while holding the ball as he steps backward, pulling the sled as he does.

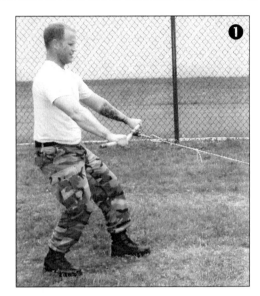

Sean rotates the ball to his left as he continues to walk backward. This is a tough core exercise in addition to the grip work it takes to hold and control the medicine ball.

SLED PULL WITH HANDLE

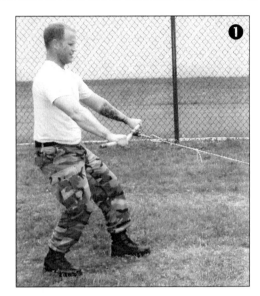

Walking backwards and pulling the sled works you from a different angle. Sean is using a lat pulldown bar as his handle.

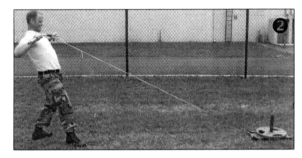

As Sean walks backward, he pulls the handle to his chest to make the sled move and providing extra upper body work. Your glutes, lower back and legs, in general, get a great workout by doing this.

SLED PULL SNATCH USING BAND

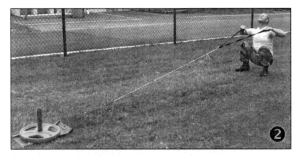

Sean starts the exercise by squatting low and holding a towrope in each hand as shown.

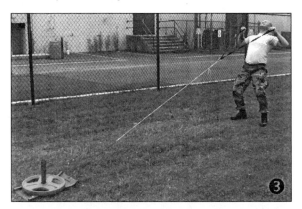

Sean pulls each rope handle high to his chest in the same way he would perform a Snatch with a barbell.

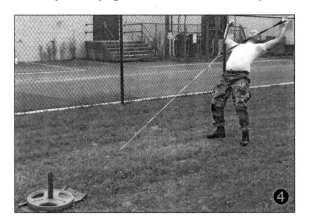

Sean explodes upright as he snatches the towrope.

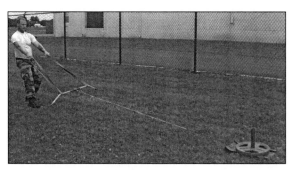

Sean completes the exercise by expanding his arms up and outward as shown. Perform a set of 10 reps. This exercise is great for grapplers who want to develop explosive power in their throws.

SLED PULL USING DOUBLE HEAVY BANDS

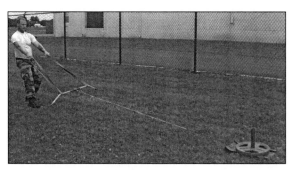

Sean holds a pair of heavy bands attached to a handle that is attached to a towrope. Sean walks backward pulling the sled as he does.

SQUAT LOW WALK BACKWARD

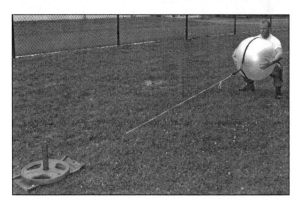

Sean squats and holds an exercise ball in his arms that is attached to a towrope. Sean jumps backward as he holds the ball that is attached to the rope. Sean can also squat walk backward as he pulls the rope. This exercise is a hard one and works the lower body very hard.

SLED PULL SUPLEX WITH EXERCISE BALL

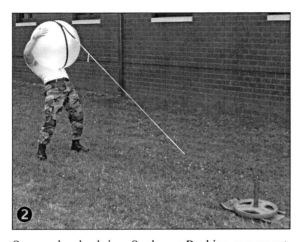

Sean holds the exercise ball as shown.

Sean arches back in a Suplex or Bucking movement. This pulls the sled. After each Suplex, Sean steps backward and starts another Suplex. Perform 10 Suplexes.

SLED PULL EXERCISE BALL RUSSIAN TWIST

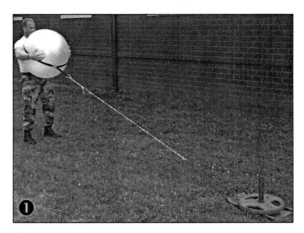

Sean holds the exercise ball that is attached to the sled towrope.

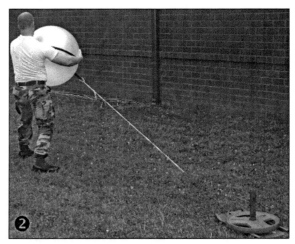

Sean rotates to his left and then to his right as he walks backward, towing the sled as he goes.

PULL WITH ONE HAND USING A BAND

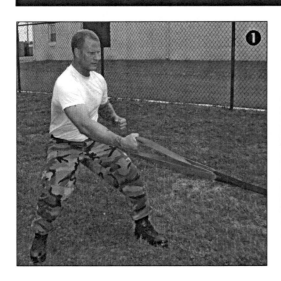 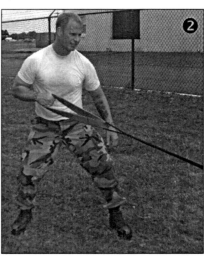

1. Sean increases his pulling power for his throwing techniques by using one hand to pull on an elastic band that is affixed to the rope.

2. Sean pulls the sled with the heavy band. This really develops your upper back, deltoids and general shoulder area. It also provides heavy work for your entire arm.

SLED PUSH

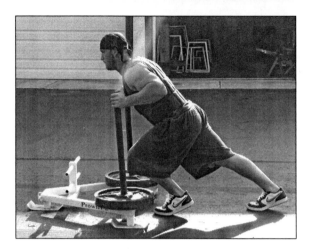

John pushes the sled in this basic application. The idea is to provide enough resistance that you develop driving power for your throws, takedowns or punches. A good routine is to use enough weight so that you can push the sled for at least 100 feet without stopping. Depending on your fitness level and the time in your training cycle, perform about 3 to 5 sets.

SLED PUSH AND A WEIGHTED VEST

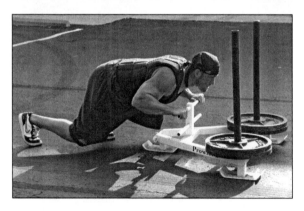

A good way to develop a deep lunge step when shooting in for a takedown is to push the sled in this low position. Look at the weighted vest John is wearing as he pushes the sled.

LEVERAGE LIFTS, CATCHING THE SHOT AND HAND-HELD IMPLEMENTS

CATCHING THE SHOT

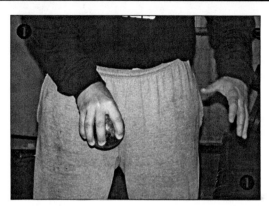

This is a fantastic finish to any workout and really develops a strong grip! Hold an 8 or 10 lb. shot (like in track and field), with your palm down. Make it a point to grip the shot firmly in a claw-like fashion and wrap your fingers around the shot as far as possible. Do this exercise over a rubberized floor or a surface that won't be damaged when you drop the shot.

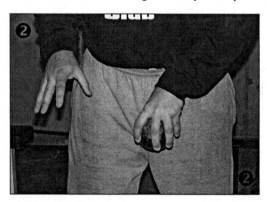

Steve lets go of the shot with his right hand and quickly catches it with his left hand.

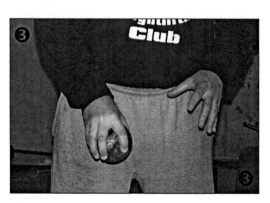

Switch back to your right hand and do as many catches as possible without stopping. Eventually, you'll drop the shot. Author Steve Scott has done 661 shot catches with a 10 pound shot before dropping it.

DUMB-BELL GRIP PASS

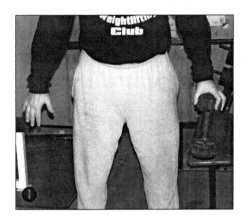 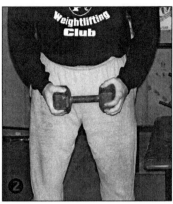 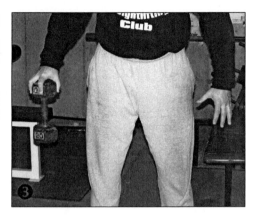

Use a light dumb-bell and preferably one that is in the "hex" shape. Hold the end of the dumb-bell in your left hand at your left side as shown.

Swing the dumb-bell in front of your body as shown and grab the other end of it with your right hand.

Quickly let go with your left hand and move the dumb-bell to your right side. Repeat this back and forth. This is harder than it looks and is a good way to strengthen your grip.

KAMI JAR GRIPPING

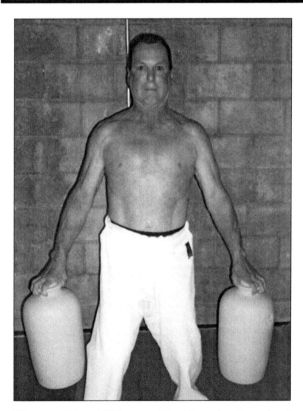

These traditional Okinawan Kami jars give Dan a hard grip workout. He's grabbing the top of each jar and can carry them, lift them or perform hand and arm movements used in karate or striking arts. You can use a heavy vase or jar that has no lip on the top, making it harder to pick up. You can also fill the jars with water or sand, making them heavier.

PICKING UP A HUMAN BEING

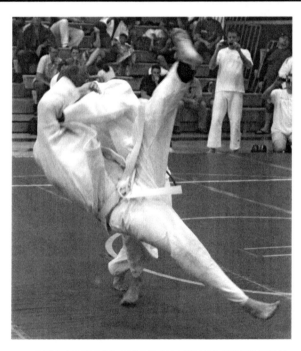

**THERE'S NOTHING MORE AWKWARD THAN PICK-
ING UP A HUMAN BEING**

Picking up heavy and awkward objects offers a similar "feel" to actually throwing an opponent. Many of the same muscles you need to lift stones, anvils or other big objects are used in lifting and throwing opponents. While technical skill is a major factor in throwing an opponent or taking him to the mat, you need the physical strength necessary to make that technical skill work.

LEVER LIFTS FOR FOREARM STRENGTH

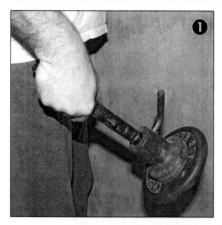

Holding a dumbbell bar on one end with a weight on the other end and lifting it up and down offers a good workout for your forearm and hands. Start by lowering the weight.

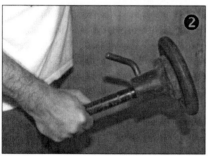

Lift the weight upward to complete the movement. Use moderate weight and perform several sets of 25 to 50 repetitions as a finisher to your workout.

LEVER LIFT (REAR DIRECTION)

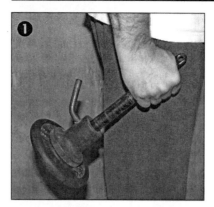

To start, hold the implement in the lowered position.

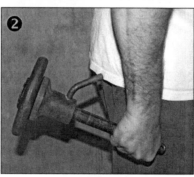

Complete the movement by lifting the dumb-bell. This works the inside and back of your forearm; not an area that usually gets a lot of work.

EXTENSIONS USING HAND WHEELS

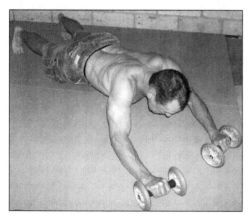

Using Hand Wheels gives your abs, chest, arms and shoulders a good workout. This is a good warm-up exercise before a lifting session. Dan starts with his buttocks high in the air and rolls the wheels forward and straightens out as shown. He will arch back up, rolling the wheels back in. This works your abs hard. Do as many reps as you wish as a great warm-up.

EXTENSIONS WITH ALTERNATING ARMS

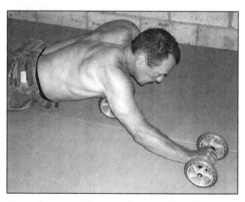

Dan changes this exercise, making it harder, by alternating his arms as he does it.

CARRYING AND MOVING HEAVY AND AWKWARD THINGS

Walking is harder than you think! You can get a fantastic strength workout, or an equally tough cardio workout, simply by picking something heavy up and taking it for a walk.

Moving, rolling, lifting or pushing heavy objects may not be something you do everyday in your training program, but taking a day every once in a while to move heavy stuff provides a tough, but fun, day of training. Depending on where you are in a training cycle, you might want to schedule in a "day in the park" once a week or once a month to do some stone or barrel lifting, pushing or pulling vehicles, stone throwing, log lifting or caber tossing, hammer swings or other heavy work that not only works your muscles in different ways, but is really a lot of fun to do.

STONE CARRY

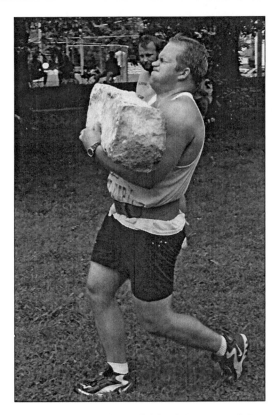

Chad Ullom, world-class Highland Games and Strongman athlete, is carrying a heavy stone. Athletes in ancient Greece as well as the gladiators in Rome lifted, carried and threw stones to increase their strength and stamina. When carrying heavy stones or objects, walk, don't run. Running increases the chance of injuries to the ankles, knees or other parts of your body.

INMAN MILE

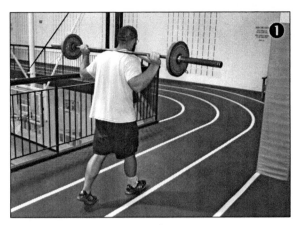

Strongman Mike Inman invented this tough workout years ago. In fact, Bill Clark included this as an event in his annual "Weightlifter's Weekend" for many years. Load a barbell with your body weight. If you weigh 240, put 240 pounds on the bar. Make sure you use good locks to keep the plates on the bar.

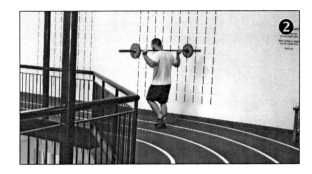

Place the bar across the back of your shoulders as shown and take the barbell for a walk. Don't run. Use good lifting form when you walk. The reason it's called the Inman Mile is that its inventor could carry his body weight for a full mile before dropping the weight or stopping. Not many people can replicate this and it's advised that you be in tremendous shape before attempting this. However, you can load the bar up with any poundage you wish and take it for a walk. You don't have to go a mile, but if you can walk around the track with a poundage that makes you work hard, then this exercise will be a great addition to your training program. This not only works every muscle in your body, but it kicks your butt from a cardio standpoint as well! We're not exaggerating when we warn you that you will need several days to rest after doing this exercise.

TECHNICAL TIP: The odd shape of a large stone makes you work muscles that you don't use if you work with only barbells, dumb-bells or kettlebells.

ANVIL CARRY

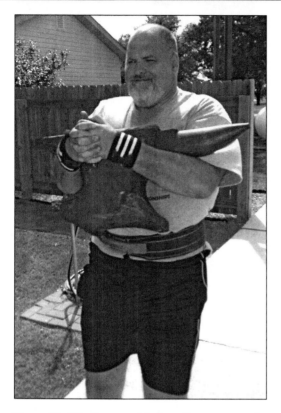

Thom VanVleck, a world-class Strongman athlete and national champion in the Highland Games, takes his 190-pound anvil out for a walk. Actually, you can carry any odd-shaped, heavy object as shown earlier in the Stone Carry. The idea is to force your body to adapt to a heavier workload under more stressful conditions. You can also carry a barrel or beer keg filled with water or sand (to make it more difficult to balance when carrying). Remember, safety is important when carrying odd shaped objects. Walk, don't run. Wear shoes and if you have to drop the object, make sure your feet and legs are clear of the object when you let go.

FARMER'S WALK HOLDING AN ANVIL

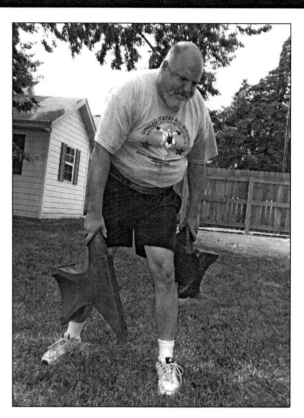

Thom holds a 110-pound anvil in each hand as he walks, and makes his walk extremely tough by holding each anvil by the horns (narrow part of the anvil). Not only is this a tough workout for your entire body, it will develop a very strong grip. This is the type of training that gives you hard, thick, strong hands; the kind of hands that grip hard and punch hard in a fight. If you live in an area where you might find anvils, make it a point to buy some and use them as a great addition to your training.

TRAINING TIP: Another way to use the Farmer's Walk is as a finish to a lifting session or on-mat workout. A "finish" is doing a tough exercise or gym movement immediately after you have completed your training routine for that workout. Grab a pair of heavy dumb-bells and take them for a walk around the building or parking lot after any workout. The authors would set a specific day of the week and choose a tough finish exercise to do that day and the Farmer's Walk was one of the toughest. For example, on Mondays, we might finish up by doing as many dips as possible for one set. On Wednesdays, we might carry a pair of 100-pound dumb-bells around the building in the Farmer's Walk, and on Friday, we might do as many Hindu Squats as possible without stopping as a finish.

TIRE FLIP

Flipping a big, heavy tire over provides you with a hard workout. Make sure to use good lifting form whenever possible, but the odd size of the large tire makes it hard to handle. Depending on the size of the tire, you can alter your workout to your strength level and interest.

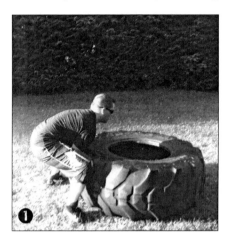
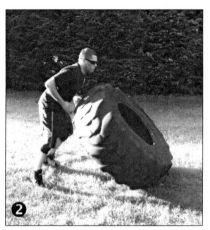
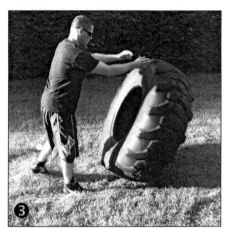

Mike starts the exercise by using good lifting form with a straight back and squatting low, allowing his legs to handle the load.

As you lift the tire off the ground, keep pushing forward to get it to flip over.

Push the tire over and make sure you are out of the way if it bounces on the ground in a weird way.

TIRE OVERHEAD PRESS

OVERHEAD ANVIL PRESS

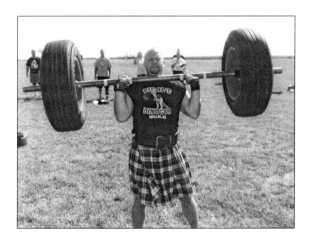

World All-Round Lifting Champion Chad Ullom performs the Overhead Press using a barbell loaded with heavy tires and wheels. This implement weighs 200 pounds and is awkward, making it feel like a lot more than what it actually weighs, and giving Chad a more challenging workout. Additionally, Chad is using a 2-inch thick bar, making the bar hard to grab and making the lift even more difficult.

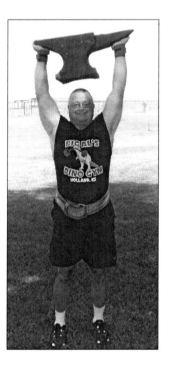

World All-Round Lifting Champion Al Myers lifts a 220-pound anvil overhead in a Strongman contest. Lifting objects that are unusual in shape forces you to work muscles that you wouldn't normally work if you lifted only barbells, dumb-bells or kettlebells. There are several good reasons that you should lift or train with odd-shaped objects, but picking an opponent up and taking him down to the ground or mat is one of the most obvious reasons for training with odd-shaped objects.

STONE LIFTING

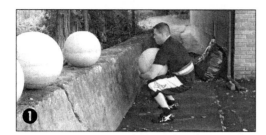

Mike starts the exercise by squatting low and holding the stone with his hands and arms. Mike is using round stones in this exercise.

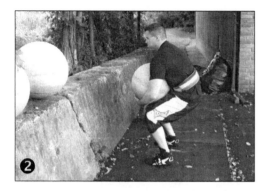

Mike lifts the stone as shown here.

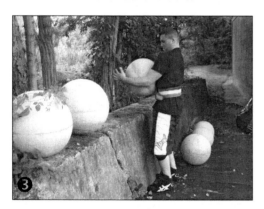

Mike lifts the stone and places it on the ledge to complete the exercise. You can use stones of any size or shape when performing this exercise.

ANVIL LIFTING

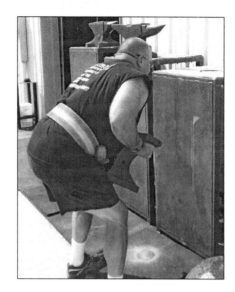

Al is lifting anvils instead of heavy stones. Picking up unusually shaped objects such as stones, anvils, logs, barrels or anything else forces your body to work in unusual positions.

1 ARM ANVIL PRESS

Here's one of the reasons why blacksmiths were such strong guys. Anvils provide a different way of lifting weight and if you can get one, use it every so often as a fun (and really hard) addition to your training.

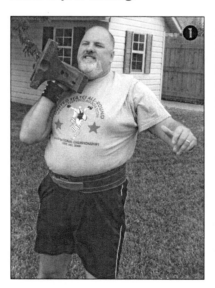

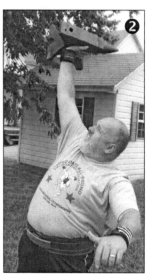

World-class Highland Games athlete Thom VanVleck is one of the strongest men in the world in Anvil Lifting. Thom is shouldering a 110-pound anvil in this photo.

Thom lifts the anvil with his right hand. Notice how his right palm is pressed against the anvil. This requires a great deal of strength, especially in the hands, because of how Thom balances the anvil as he lifts it.

SECTION TWO: PART 6: EXERCISE BALL TRAINING

● ● ● "Core strength is important. It the important link connecting your lower body to your upper body." **Bob Corwin**

Working with the Exercise Ball might have a less than macho reputation, but it shouldn't. This piece of equipment works the heck out of your core and makes your entire stabilizer muscles work overtime. Regularly working with the Exercise Ball will definitely produce positive results in your strength level. There are many exercises using this piece of equipment, and we've included some that we believe work best for fighters and grapplers. The extreme workload that the Exercise Ball forces on your core, hips area and legs is ideal for grappling and fighting. What Bob Corwin said is true. Your core (the lower back, abdominals, hips and all the stabilizing muscles from your hips to your chest) is the link connecting your lower body to your upper body. Core strength is fundamentally important in all combat sports. Using an Exercise Ball is one of the most effective ways of developing core strength ever invented. Additionally, training with weights, the medicine ball or other strength implements is made significantly more difficult when you do it on an Exercise Ball.

EXERCISE BALL PLANK

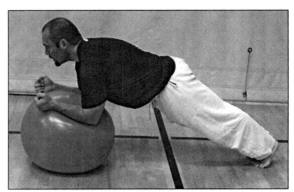

This is a good core exercise. Chris leans on the ball with his forearms as shown, making sure to keep his body as straight as possible. Doing this forces your core muscles to work hard to maintain the position.

PALMS UP TO MAKE THE PLANK HARDER

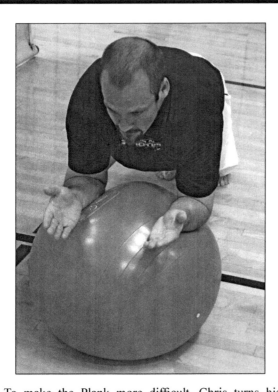

To make the Plank more difficult, Chris turns his palms upward as he leans on the ball. In addition to working your core, your shoulders and arms have to work hard to stabilize your body on the ball. Perform this exercise by time, using the clock or simply counting to 30 as you hold the Plank position.

EXERCISE BALL PLANK WITH FEET ON BALL

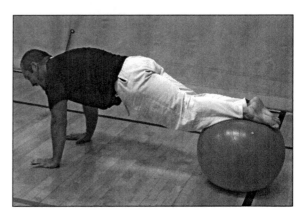

Chris places both of his feet on the ball as shown, as he straightens his body into the Plan position and supports himself with his hands as shown on the floor. Hold this position for 30 seconds or a 30 count. This really works your hips, and entire leg structure as well as providing a good workout for your arms and shoulders.

EXERCISE BALL PLANK EXTENSION

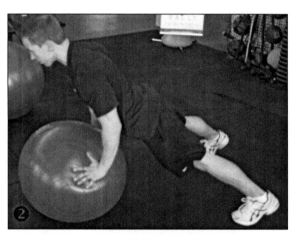

Holding the Plank position on a ball with your arms straight adds to the workload. Drew starts the exercise by leaning over the ball with his body rigid and feet spaced wide on the floor.

Drew rolls the ball downward in the direction of his feet to add to the stress of the exercise. This is an excellent shoulder, triceps and upper back exercise as well as a tough workout for your core.

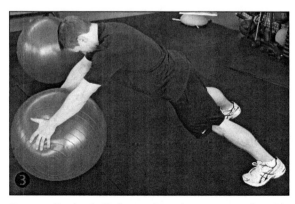

Drew rolls the ball forward as shown, extending his body. This focuses in on the upper back and rear deltoids along with increased workload to the entire core area. Repeat this back and forth rolling of the ball for 10 repetitions.

PLANK ROLL FORWARD EXTENSION

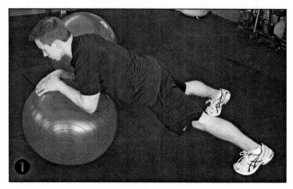

Drew holds the Plank as shown, making sure his chest area is directly over the ball and his arms are bent.

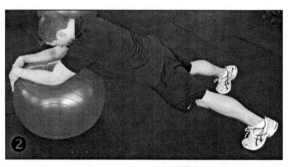

Using his arms, Drew rolls the ball forward, extending his arms and shoulders as shown. This works the upper back, entire shoulder area and core really hard. Repeat this back and forth rolling for 10 repetitions.

HIP AND LOWER BODY STRENGTH

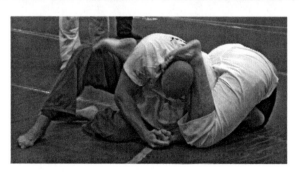

HIP AND LOWER BODY STRENGTH IS DEVELOPED BY USING THE EXERCISE BALL

Using the Exercise Ball also develops leg and hip strength. This attempt for a rolling armlock at the AAU Freestyle Judo Nationals show how lower and middle body strength is necessary in any combat sport.

PLANK SWIM (PALMS DOWN)

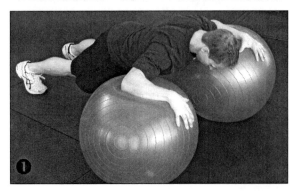

Drew assumes the Plank position with one arm on each ball. The balls are wide enough so Drew can lower his body between them. Perform 10 reps.

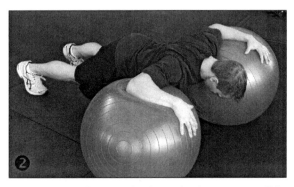

Drew lowers his upper body as far down as possible between the balls each time. This is an excellent exercise for your pecs and front deltoids.

CORE AND HIP STRENGTH

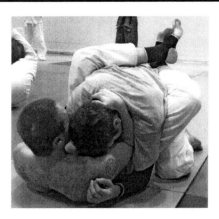

CORE AND HIP STRENGTH ARE VITAL FOR SUCCES IN ANY GRAPPLING SITUATION

Core strength is important when working out of the guard (or any position). Controlling your opponent's movement and aggressively dictating the position requires skill, but it takes functional strength to develop and refine that skill so you can use it against a resisting, fit and skillful opponent.

PLANK SWIM (MAKE A FIST)

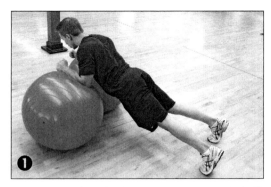

Drew starts by placing one arm on each ball, making a fist in each hand to increase the tension. The balls are close together on the floor.

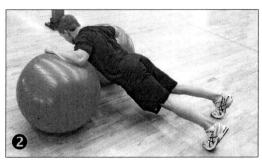

Drew moves his elbows outward, which rolls the balls to the side, as he lowers his body.

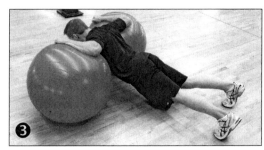

Drew lowers his body as low as possible between the balls, keeping his body as rigid as possible.

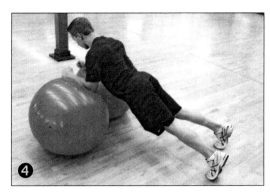

To finish, Drew uses his arms to roll the balls together and raises his body in the Plank position. This is a tough exercise for the core, and works your entire upper body, especially your pecs.

EXERCISE BALL PLANK TWISTS ON BENT KNEES

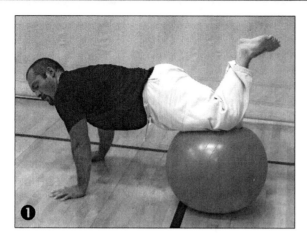

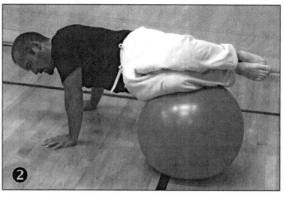

This is an excellent core movement and is great for lower body control. Chris starts by assuming a Plank position with his knees bent and resting on the ball.

Chris turns his knees to his left, making sure to keep his knees bent, toes pointed and control his entire lower body as he turns. Chris will turn back to the starting position, and then turn to his right to complete the movement. Perform 10 reps of this exercise.

EXERCISE BALL PLANK HIP TWISTS

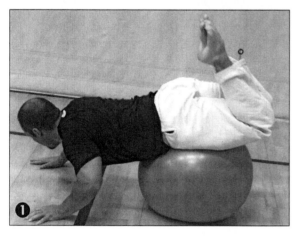

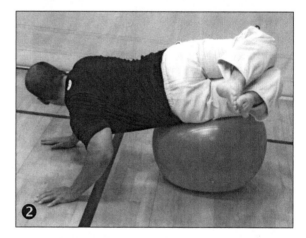

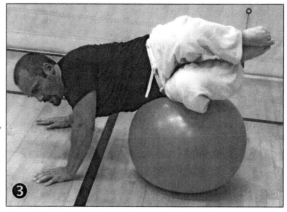

1. Chris makes this exercise a bit harder by placing his hips on the ball as shown to start. Notice that his knees are bent with toes pointed to make the exercise harder and to add more workload to his core and lower body.

2. Chris keeps his knees bent as he turns to his right, making sure his left hip is on the ball. He will turn back to the starting position after performing this movement.

3. Chris turns to his left as shown, to complete the exercise. Perform 10 reps of this for a tough core and lower body workout.

EXERCISE BALL JACK KNIFE ON KNEES

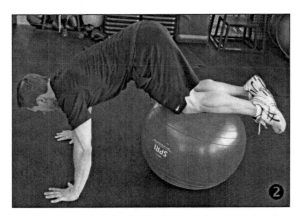

Drew places both knees on the ball as shown, making sure his rear end is pointed to the ceiling.

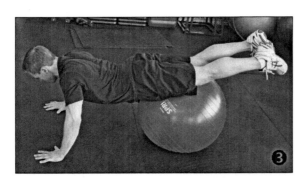

Drew rolls the ball backward, gradually straightening his body as the ball rolls back.

Drew extends his body as he rolls the ball back as far as it can go. To complete the exercise, Drew will roll the ball forward, back up to the starting position. This is a tough exercise for your core and 10 reps should do you.

EXERCISE BALL JACK KNIFE ON LEGS

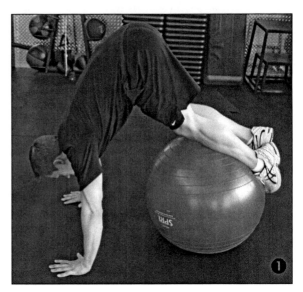

To add to the workload, Drew arches his back as shown with his legs straight, making sure his shins are on the ball. It helps to point your toes as Drew is doing.

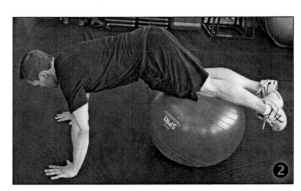

Drew extends his body as he rolls the ball back as far as it can go, gradually straightening his body.

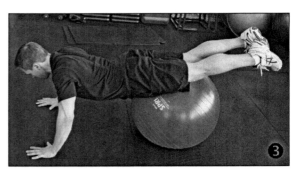

Drew extends his body as shown and will roll the ball forward to complete the exercise. This is not an easy exercise and 10 reps will give you a good workout.

HOLD BALL WITH FEET AND HIP TWISTS

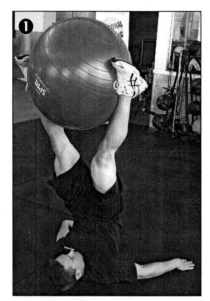

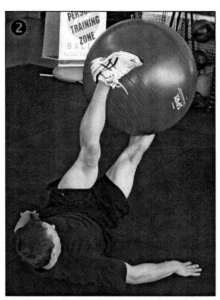

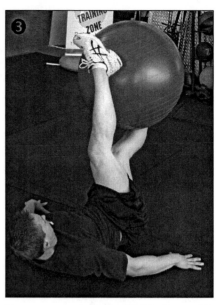

Drew holds the ball between his feet while lying on his back. This is a tough trunk rotation exercise and really works your legs. Do it slowly to get the most benefit form it.

Using his feet to hold and control the ball, Drew rotates the ball to his right.

Drew rotates the ball with his feet to his left to complete the exercise. As with most of theses exercises, 10 reps will give you a good workout.

POSITION TO GET THE TAP OUT

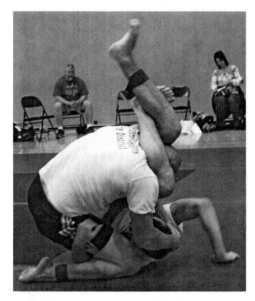

YOU NEVER KNOW WHAT POSITION YOU MAY HAVE TO BE IN TO GET THE TAP OUT

Core, hip and leg strength are effectively developed through regular use of the Exercise Ball. The definition of "functional" strength is being able to use your strength in realistic, and often unexpected situations.

EXERCISE BALL CHEST TO FLOOR PLANK

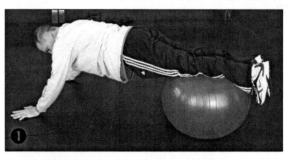

Bryan holds a Plank with his knees and shins on the ball. Bryan's hands are spaced wide apart on the floor.

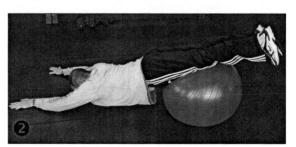

Bryan lowers his upper body to the floor, making sure to keep his body rigid as he does. Bryan will raise his body up and perform 10 repetitions of this exercise. It's a lot harder than it looks!

EXERCISE BALL SIT THROUGHS

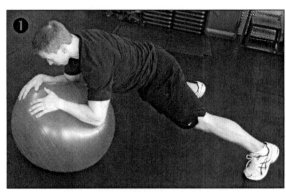

A good way to simulate a movement used in grappling is to practice sit-throughs on an Exercise Ball. Drew places his arms on the ball as shown, with his feet spaced wide apart on the floor.

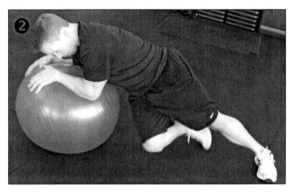

Drew controls the ball with his arms and upper body as he starts his sit-through by swinging his right leg to his left.

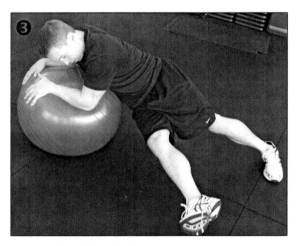

Drew swings his right leg through as shown. To complete the exercise, Drew will swing his right leg back to the starting position and repeat this movement using his left leg. Perform 10 reps on each leg.

SIT THROUGH WITH LEGS ON BALL

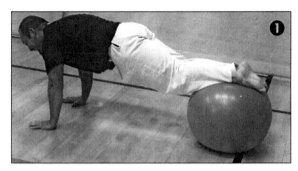

To develop excellent lower body control and give your entire core a great workout, do this exercise. Chris places his feet and shins on the ball as he assumes the Plank position with his hands on the floor as shown.

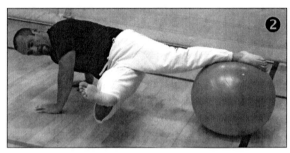

Chris swings his right leg through and turns his body to his left while keeping his left lower leg on the ball.

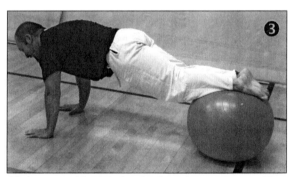

Chris moves his right leg back to the starting position and takes a quick rest before continuing the exercise.

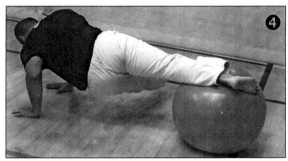

Chris swings his left leg through in the same way he did his right leg. Chris will move his left leg back onto the ball to complete the exercise.

EXERCISE BALL AROUND THE WORLD WITH MEDICINE BALL

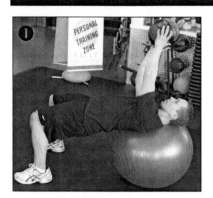

Drew supports his body with his upper back resting on the ball. His body is straight and his feet are wide apart. Drew holds a Medicine Ball above him and will move it in a complete circle above his body.

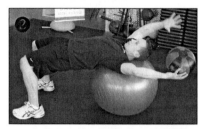

Drew holds the Medicine Ball in his left hand, moving it to his hip.

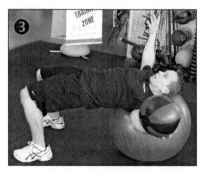

Drew continues to move the ball in his left hand down toward his hip.

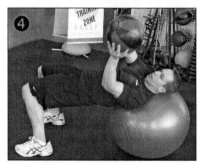

Drew moves the ball over the left side of his body and grabs it with his right hand above him as shown.

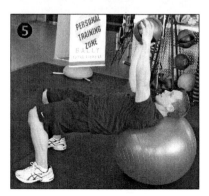

Drew holds the ball above his body in the starting position.

This is a good core exercise and gives some added work to your shoulders. Perform 10 repetitions.

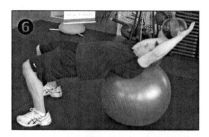

Drew continues with the ball in his right hand, moving it up and over his head, with his arms are extended.

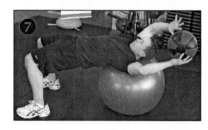

Drew moves the ball from his right hand to his left hand to complete the circular movement.

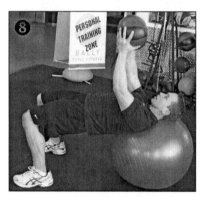

Drew finishes, coming back to the starting position.

TECHNICAL TIP: A good way to use the Exercise Ball is to perform a circuit. Do 1 set of 10 reps on one exercise, and then move to another exercise performing 10 reps, and then on to another exercise, doing as many exercises as you wish in the circuit. You can add to the intensity of the workout by moving to each exercise with a minimum of rest between the different exercises. Doing a circuit of anywhere from 5 to 10 different Exercise Ball movements isn't for the feint of heart.

EXERCISE BALL DUMB-BELL PRESS

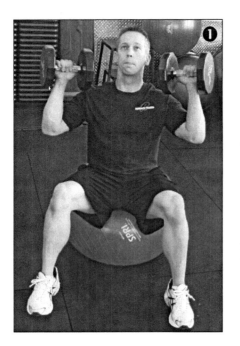
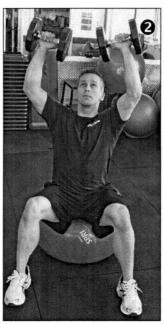

1. Drew sits on the Exercise Ball while he holds a dumb-bell in each hand.

2. Drew balances himself while sitting and presses the dumb-bells over his head. Drew will perform 3 to 5 sets of 10 repetitions, using a light to moderate dumb-bell or kettlebell. You can also use a barbell, but make sure that you have a spotter for safety. Another good way to use this exercise is to use a pair if light dumb-bells and perform 15 to 25 reps per set to increase your muscular endurance.

EXERCISE BALL DUMB-BELL PRESS (LEGS CLOSE)

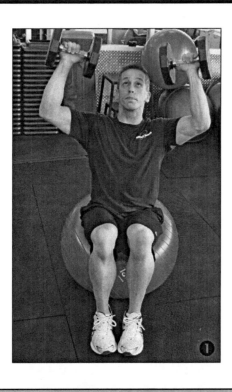
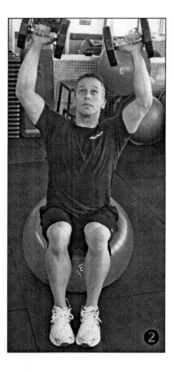

1. A good way to make this exercise more difficult is to sit on the ball with your legs close together as shown here. Sitting with your legs and feet close doesn't give you're the stability you had with your legs wide for the base. This forces your core stabilizer muscles to work harder.

2. Drew completes the exercise. It's a good idea to use light weight on this exercise, as it's a tough core workout and you can get the added benefit of some muscular endurance for your shoulders. As said before, use light weight and perform 3 to 5 sets of a high rep count of anywhere from 15 to 50 reps per set.

TECHNICAL TIP: Lifting dumb-bells, medicine balls, kettlebells, barbells or any object is a lot harder to do when you are balancing yourself on an Exercise Ball. To add intensity to most any lift, perform it on an Exercise Ball. Safety is important, so make sure to perform any exercise with control and it's always a good idea to have a training partner nearby to assist you.

EXERCISE BALL DUMB-BELL "BENCH" PRESS

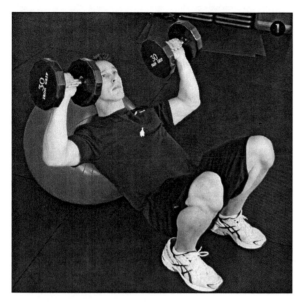

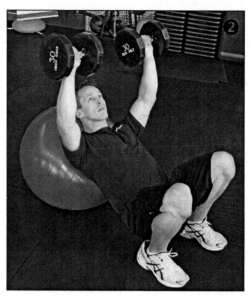

Drew balances his upper body on the Exercise Ball with his back straight and body rigid. Look at how his hips are low and almost touching the floor. Drew holds a dumb-bell in each hand.

Drew presses the dumb-bells upward, making sure to balance his body on the ball.

EXERCISE BALL ARCH HIPS DUMB-BELL PRESS

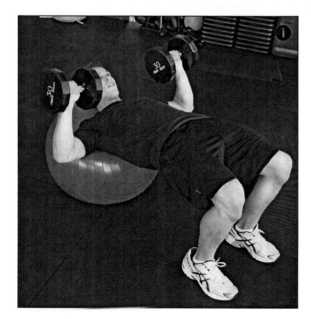

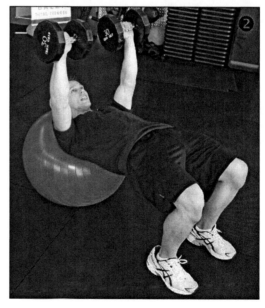

To make this dumb-bell press more difficult, Drew starts the exercise with his upper back on the ball, making sure his body is straight and hips are elevated as shown. This is a tough exercise as balancing your body on the Exercise Ball and pressing dumb-bells works just about every stabilizer muscle in your body.

Drew presses the dumb-bells and performs 3 to 5 sets of anywhere from 10 to 50 reps for each set. A good routine author Steve Scott often followed on this exercise was to perform 5 sets, doing as many reps as possible on each set and using a fairly heavy pair of dumb-bells.

EXERCISE BALL DUMB-BELL FLYS

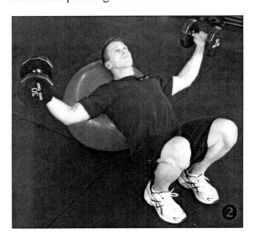

Performing dumb-bell flyes is a good variation of the pressing movement shown before.

Drew uses a light to moderate amount of weight and makes sure to use strict and correct lifting form when performing this exercise. Use the same set and rep count as any of the above-listed pressing movements.

1 ARM DUMB-BELL "BENCH" PRESS

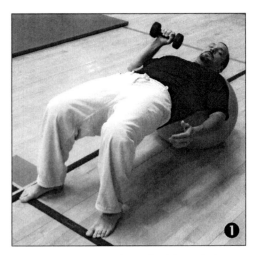

Chris uses only one hand in this variation of the dumb-bell press on an Exercise Ball. The advantage of this in your training is that this exercise places your body in an unbalanced position on the Exercise Ball and really forces you to work on balancing your entire body on the ball as you press the weight.

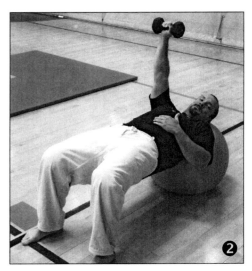

Chris extends the dumb-bell over his head. Perform 10 or more reps on each arm and do 3 to 5 sets.

DUMB-BELL PRESS EXTENDED ARM

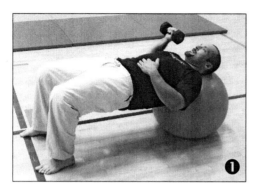

Chris holds the dumb-bell at his chest as he places his upper back on the Exercise Ball and balances his body.

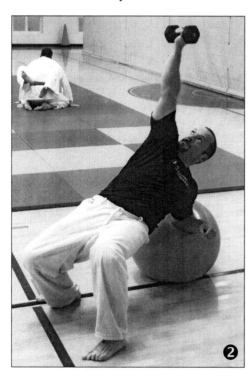

Chris presses the dumb-bell upward with his right hand and, as he does this, places his left elbow on the ball and balances himself on it. He fully extends his right shoulder as he performs the movement. This is a tough exercise and works your entire upper body, with special emphasis on your core stabilizers that support you while doing this movement. Use light weight and perform 6 to 10 reps for anywhere from 3 to 5 sets.

DUMB-BELL PULLOVERS

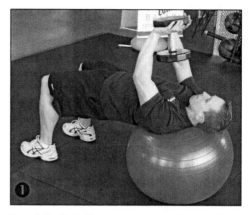

Dumb-bell Pullovers are great, but doing them on an Exercise Ball makes it even better. Drew balances his body on the ball as shown and holds a dumb-bell above him.

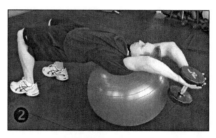

Drew performs a pullover while balancing his body on the Exercise Ball.

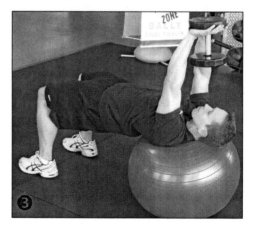

Drew returns to the starting position and readies himself for another repetition. You can use almost (but not quite) as much weight on this as you would use if you were on a bench. Make sure you have a spotter for safety who can hand the weight to you at the start of the exercise and take the weight form you at the finish. Use your normal rep and set count. You can use this in place of your normal Dumb-bell Pullover routine.

EXERCISE BALL 1 ARM DUMB-BELL ROWING

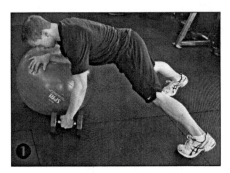
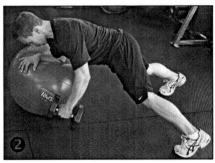
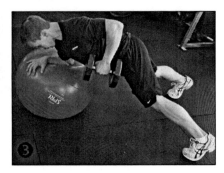

Bent-over Rowing is another staple of athletes and Drew performs this movement on the Exercise Ball. He places his right arm on the ball and has his feet placed wide apart on the floor. Drew holds the dumb-bell (or kettlebell) in his left hand on the floor.

Drew performs a 1-arm row as he stabilizes himself on the ball.

Drew lowers the dumb-bell and will continue on, performing your normal routine for this exercise.

EXERCISE BALL BALANCE STAND AND SQUAT

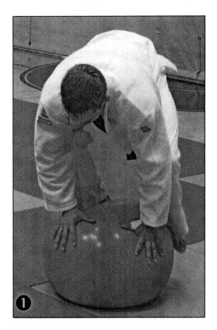
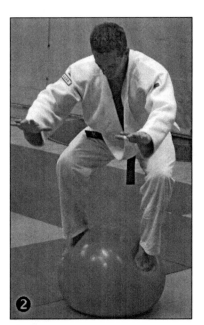
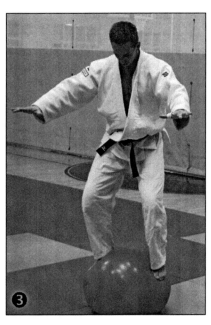

If you have good strength and skill when using the Exercise Ball, here's a tough exercise that will challenge you. Drew carefully climbs on the Exercise ball making sure to stay balanced as he steps onto the ball. He holds onto the ball with his hands to stabilize himself as he steps onto it.

Drew balances his body on the ball and gradually takes his arms off the ball and assumes a semi-squat. Take your time to balance yourself on the ball.

There are different sizes of Exercise Balls, all varying in strength. Use a heavy-duty ball for this exercise.

Drew stands upright, balancing himself. He can hold this position for as long as he wishes, or when he becomes more advanced in this exercise, Drew can also perform as many squats on the ball as possible (usually no more than 10 reps will be enough). This exercise is terrific for working your entire body, but especially your hips and legs, forcing all the stabilizer muscles to work overtime.

EXERCISE BALL DUMB-BELL SQUATS

An advanced variation of this Ball Squat is to perform it while holding dumb-bells or kettlebells. Usually, 10 reps are enough, but if you want to do more, go for it! This is a tough, advanced exercise and works your entire body, especially your lower body and core.

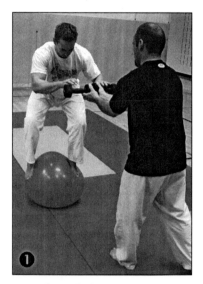

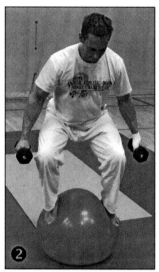

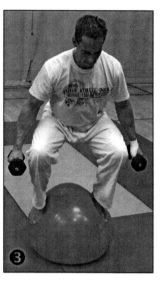

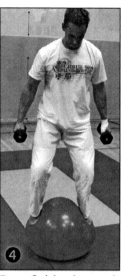

Drew has climbed onto the Exercise Ball and Chris hands him a pair of light dumb-bells.

Drew gradually balances himself on the ball with a dumb-bell in each hand.

Drew performs a squat, going as low as possible while maintaining his balance.

Drew finishes by standing upright.

EXERCISE BALL WALL SQUATS

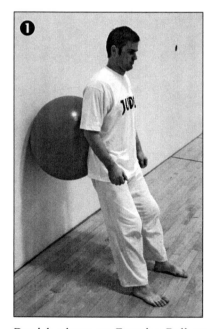

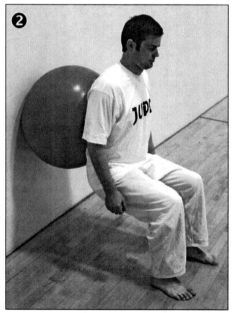

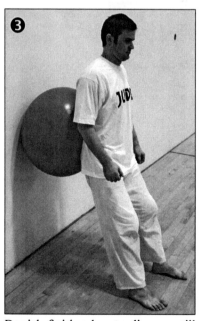

Derrick places an Exercise Ball on the wall and leans into it at about the middle of his back. His feet are forward, but not very far. If your feet are too far forward, the exercise isn't as challenging.

Derrick performs a squat; all the while, leaning into the ball. You can squat as low as you wish, but make sure not to bounce at the bottom of the squat. Perform the squat gradually and with control.

Derrick finishes by standing up still leaning into the ball. This is a good exercise to use to break the monotony when working your legs. Perform 3 to 5 sets, doing as many reps as possible per set.

EXERCISE BALL 1 LEG WALL SQUATS

The good thing about this exercise is that you maintain constant stress on your muscles when performing it because you are leaning into the ball to hold it against the wall.

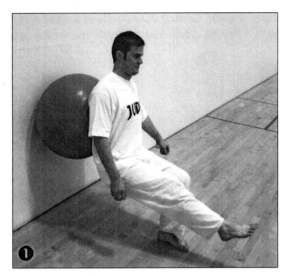

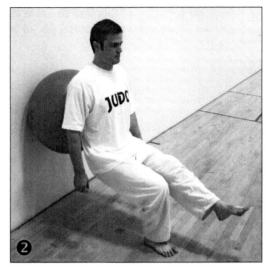

Derrick makes the Ball Wall Squat more difficult by lifting and extending one leg forward and using the other leg to perform the squat.

Derrick will do a set of 10 on one leg, and then switch and do a set of 10 on his other leg.

EXERCISE BALL WALL UCHIKOMI

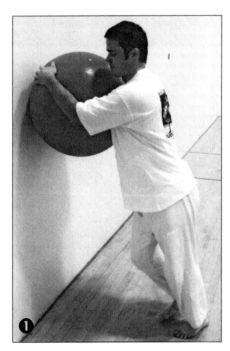

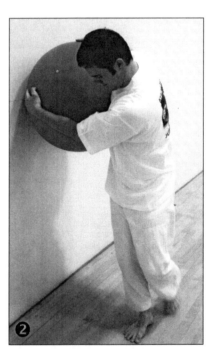

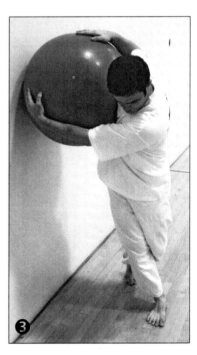

Using an Exercise Ball when training on your fit-ins (Uchikomi or Butsukari) is a fun way to get some extra work in for your throws. Derrick holds onto the ball and leans into it. His chest is pressing the ball against the wall.

Derrick starts the exercise by stepping in, all the while holding the ball against the wall.

Derrick finishes by fitting in all the way into his Uchikomi, still pressing the ball against the wall. Perform a high number of repetitions, working up to sets of 100 reps. Perform as many sets as you wish, but do at least 3 to 5 sets of 100 reps.

SECTION TWO: PART 7: MEDICINE BALL TRAINING

● ● ● "Be strong and let us fight bravely..." 2Samuel 10:12

MEDICINE BALL LOW SQUEEZE

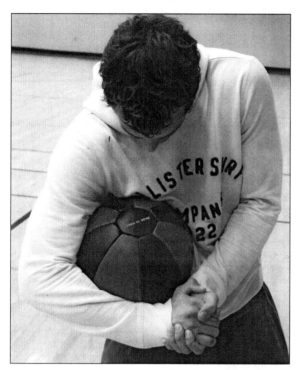

Josh holds the ball at his side, cradles it in his arms as shown and locks his hands together in a square grip. Josh squeezes the ball as hard possible for a 10-count and does several sets like this. Josh can also perform 1 set of 10 squeezes, squeezing the ball for a 3-count on each rep.

HOW SQUEEZING A MEDICINE BALL WORKS

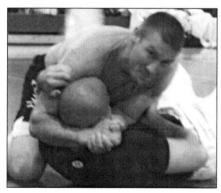

Mike shows how a strong grip can translate into success on the mat by squeezing Scott's head in this neck crank.

For years, the Medicine Ball was a staple in boxing gyms, or sometimes found in a corner at the local public lifting gym. They didn't often appear in many commercial gyms, as most people thought these heavy, leather balls were only good for pounding on boxers' guts to harden them for withstanding a punch. Then, sometime around the mid to late 1980s, people rediscovered how useful these heavy round balls were in all aspects of training. Medicine Balls now come covered in a variety of materials and have proven to be a useful, durable and versatile training tool for fighters and grapplers in all combat sports. Using the Medicine Ball works the many stabilizer muscles in your entire body. This is especially useful when performing the many small muscle movements that are so critical in all phases of combat sports. This part of Section 2 presents how we like to train with Medicine Balls. Use your imagination in making up drills, games and exercises.

MEDICINE BALL HIGH SQUEEZE

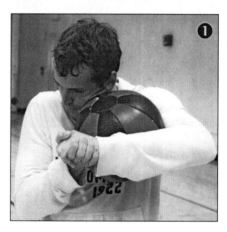

Josh squeezes the ball with it cradled at his shoulder. Josh holds the ball in his left shoulder, squeezing for a 10-count and then switches the ball to his right shoulder.

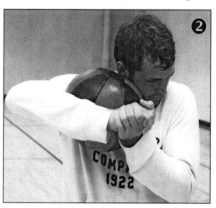

Josh switches the ball to his right shoulder and squeezes for a 10-count. Josh will switch back and forth, performing about 5 sets on each shoulder.

CONDITIONING FOR COMBAT SPORTS

MEDICINE BALL HEAD & ARM PIN SQUEEZE

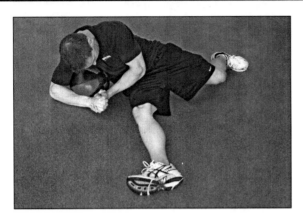

Drew holds the ball in a Kesa Gatame (Scarf Hold or Head and Arm Pin), squeezing it in the same way he would if he were holding an opponent.

STRONG HEAD CONTROL

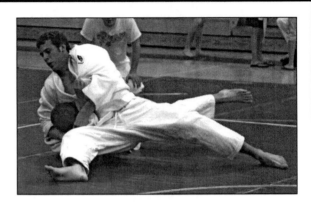

STRONG HEAD CONTROL KEEPS OPPONENTS FROM GETTING UP

A common hold-down in all grappling sports is the Head and Arm Pin or Kesa Gatame. Putting a hard squeeze on your opponent's noggin makes him much less willing to escape.

MEDICINE BALL SHRIMPING

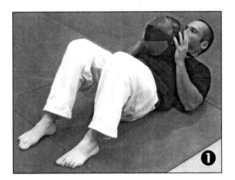

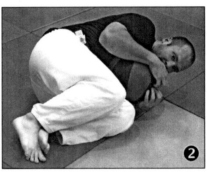

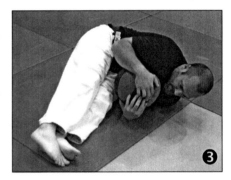

The "Shrimp" movement is an important skill in all forms of grappling and groundfighting. Chris holds the ball at his chest while lying on his back.

Chris shrimps to his left side while cradling the ball in his arms and torso.

Chris continues to hold the ball as he extends his legs, pushing on the mat to complete the shrimping movement.

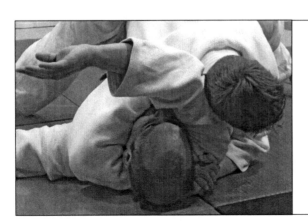

ARM TRIANGLES AND SHOULDER CHOKES REQUIRE A STRONG GRIP

Squeezing a medicine ball uses the same muscles required for controlling and choking your opponent with a variety of chokes and strangles.

MEDICINE BALL CATCH

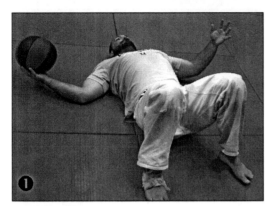

Jake lies on his back holding a ball in his extended right arm.

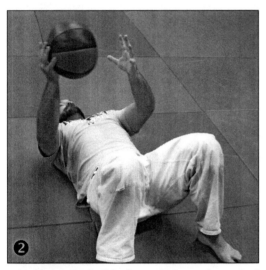

Jake moves the ball in front of him as shown and transfers it to his left hand.

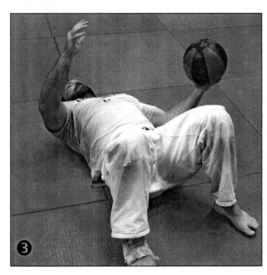

Jake continues this drill for anywhere from 10 to 50 reps. This exercise is good for shoulder and arm strength, isolating yourself in this position.

ARM STRENGTH AS DEFENSE

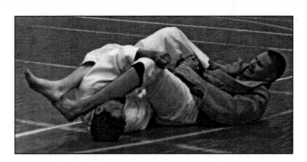

ARM STRENGTH MAY BE YOUR LAST DEFENSE WHEN YOU'RE CAUGHT IN AN ARMLOCK
John, on the bottom attempts to pull his arm free from Jeff's armlock in this freestyle judo match. Your arm strength may be your last chance to avoid getting armlocked.

MEDICINE BALL CRUNCHES

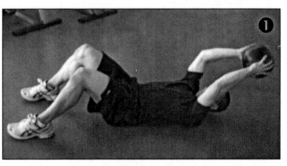

Here's a great core exercise that works your arms, shoulders and back as well. As Drew lies on his back, he holds the ball in his hands with his arms extended above his head.

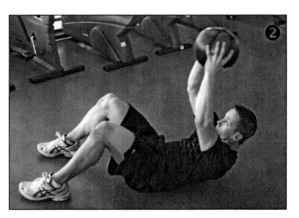

Drew curls up, crunching his abs while holding the ball overhead as shown. Perform at least 10 reps, with the goal being about 50 reps per set.

MEDICINE BALL FIGURE 8 WITH LEGS UP

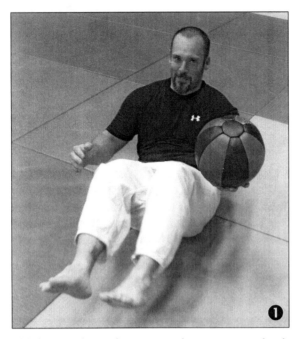

This is a good exercise to strengthen your core, shoulders and arms. Chris sits on his buttocks with his legs and feet raised off the mat or floor as shown while holding a medicine ball in his left hand.

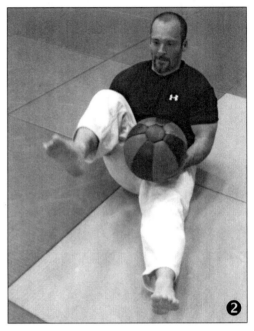

Chris lifts his right leg and moves the ball under his right leg and exchanges it to his right hand.

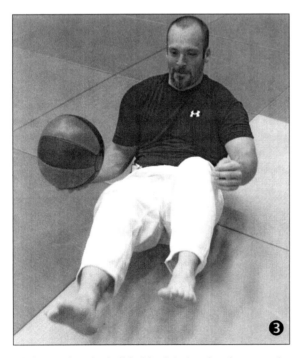

Chris now has the ball in his right hand and crosses the ball over his right thigh as he lifts his left leg.

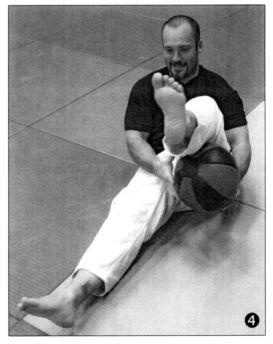

Chris passes the ball under his left leg and transfers the ball to his left hand, forming a "figure 8" pattern. Chris does this for 10 reps.

MEDICINE BALL CORE ROTATION

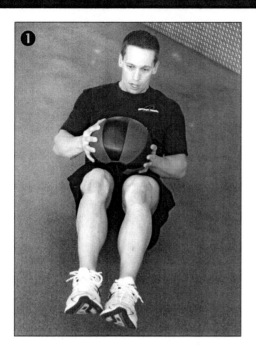

This is an excellent drill for core strengthening and used in all aspects of groundfighting, especially when fighting in the Guard position. Drew holds a medicine ball, making sure that his knees are bent and his feet are not touching the mat or floor.

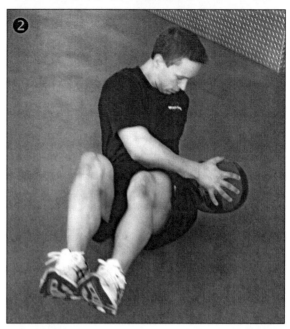

Drew rotates to his left and moves the ball to his left hip as shown.

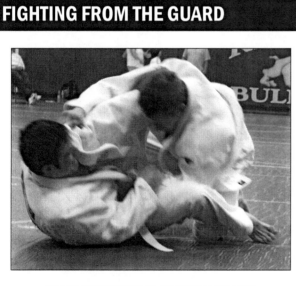

FIGHTING FROM THE GUARD

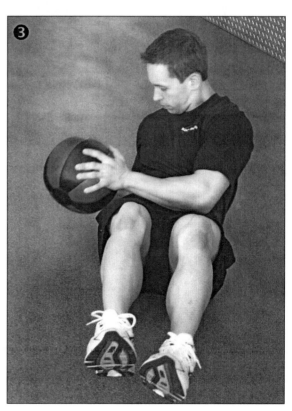

CORE STRENGTH IS NECESSARY FOR FIGHTING FROM THE GUARD

Core strength is vital when fighting from the Guard, or for that matter, fighting in any position.

Drew rotates to his right, moving the ball to his right hip. Perform 10 to 50 reps, depending on the weight of the medicine ball, your fitness level and your needs.

MEDICINE BALL TOSS FOR DISTANCE

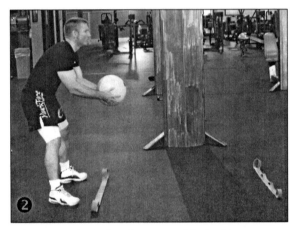

A good exercise for total body strength is to toss a heavy medicine ball as Mike does here.

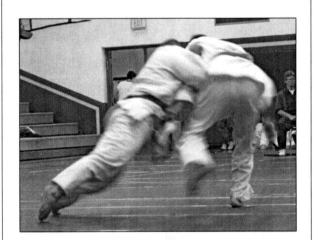

Mike tosses the ball as far as possible, in this case tossing the ball over a heavy band he uses as a goal.

USING EXPLOSIVE POWER ON THE MAT

Here's a photo of Jake driving his opponent over in a freestyle judo match. Explosive power is necessary for all phases of grappling or fighting and sometimes, as shown here, you just have to push your opponent over and get him to the mat!

MEDICINE BALL TOSS FOR HEIGHT

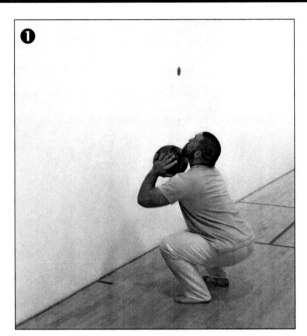

Here's a good exercise that develops explosive power. It's a good plyometric drill engaging Jake's lower body as well as his upper body. Jake squats low as he holds a heavy medicine ball as shown.

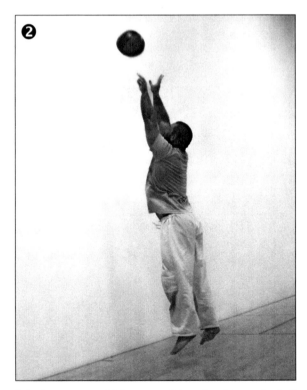

Jake jumps up as high as possible as he throws the ball upward as high as possible in an explosive, plyometric movement.

MEDICINE BALL BACK ARCH

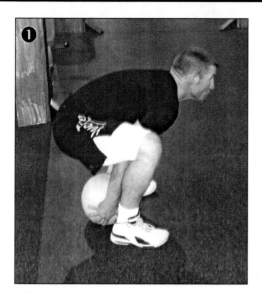

Mike holds a heavy medicine ball in his arms as shown while bending over as shown.

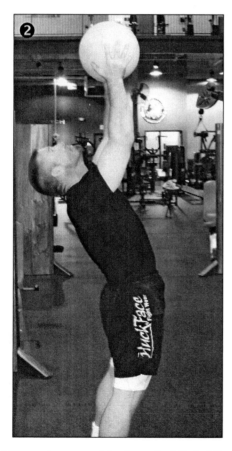

Mike arches up and backward while holding the ball making sure to arch back as far as possible. This is a good exercise for lower back strength and flexibility as gives your shoulders a good workout as well.

MEDICINE BALL HEAD LEAN (FRONT)

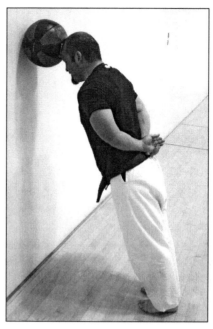

This exercise strengthens your neck and trapezius. Chris holds a heavy medicine ball to the wall with his head, leaning into the ball with his entire body weight. Chris can hold this for time, roll the ball up and down the wall vertically or move it sideways. He can also roll his head side to side giving his neck a full range of movement.

MEDICINE BALL HEAD LEAN (SIDE)

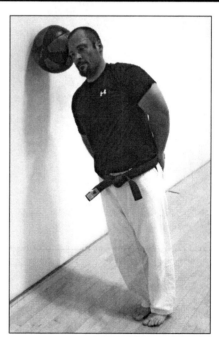

Chris can also hold the ball to the wall with the side of his head. Move it vertically up and down or sideways.

PARTNER PLAY CATCH

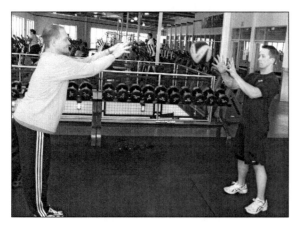

Bryan and Drew are playing catch with a heavy medicine ball. As you catch the ball with both hands, allow it to come to your chest, and then use both hands to toss it back to your partner in the same way you would pass a basketball. This is a good warm-up before a lifting session.

TOTAL BODY STRENGTH

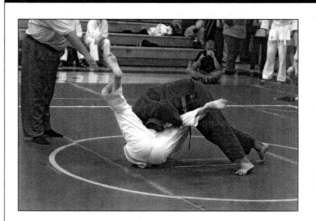

IT TAKES TOTAL BODY STRENGTH TO PIN AN OPPONENT

Total body strength, including all the small muscles that support and stabilize your joints and larger muscle groups, is necessary when grappling in any sport.

MEDICINE BALL WALL THROW

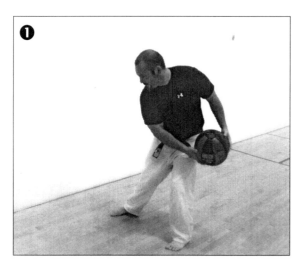

If you have a sturdy wall, this explosive strength drill is fun to do and strengthens your core and hips. Chris rotates as he throws the ball at the wall.

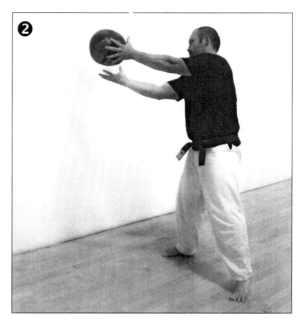

Chris throws the ball at the wall at hard as he can. Chris doesn't need a wall to throw the ball at, but it allows him to get in more reps because he doesn't need to chase the ball each time he throws it.

MEDICINE BALL THROW, SPRAWL AND CATCH DRILL

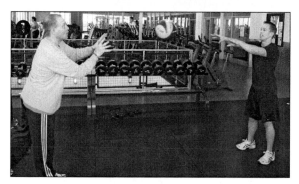

This is a good drill simulating a sprawl, and provides a cardio workout as well as an explosive strength exercise. Drew starts the drill by tossing the ball to Bryan.

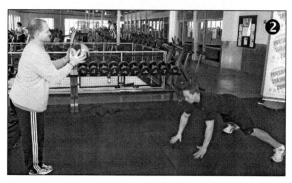

As soon as Drew tosses the ball to Bryan, he drops to the floor to start his sprawl.

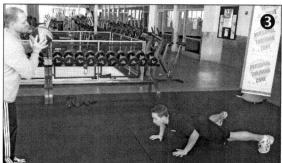
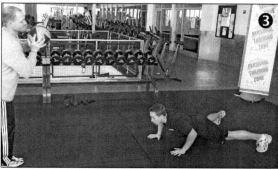

Drew sprawls and immediately jumps back up.

A STABLE BASE

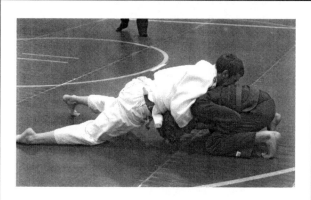

**A STABLE BASE FROM THE LEGS
PRODUCES WINNING RESULTS**

In much the same way you support your hands on a medicine ball, A.C. uses his legs as a wide base as he chokes his opponent with a Guillotine.

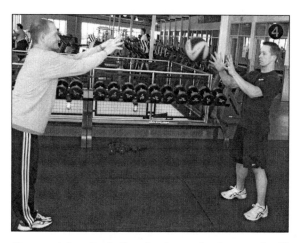

Drew catches the ball as he jumps back up and will continue the drill performing at least 10 reps, and working toward about 50 reps.

MEDICINE BALL SINGLE BALL PUSH UPS

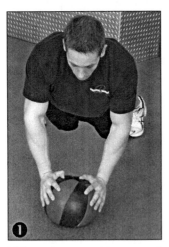

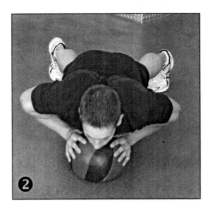

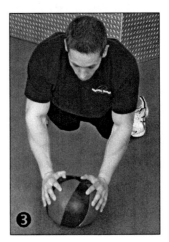

This push up provides strength and balance training. Drew uses both hands on the medicine ball supporting the weight of his body as shown.

Drew performs a push up. Look at how his feet are wide providing a good base. He can also have his feet close together, depending on his goals.

Drew completes the push up and performs at least 10, with the goal of doing a lot more. A good routine is to perform 5 sets of as many push ups as possible.

MEDICINE BALL PUSH UPS

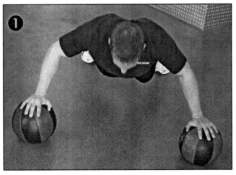

This push up forces you to use the many stabilizer muscles in your body to balance yourself as you perform it. Drew has one hand placed on each medicine ball.

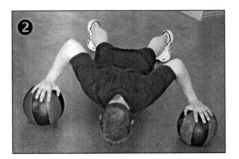

Drew has a wide base with his arms and performs a deep push up as shown.

MEDICINE BALL 1 ARM PUSH UPS

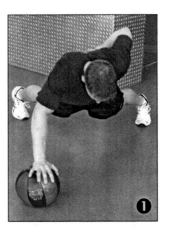

A great 1-arm push up is to balance your hand on a medicine ball (or even a basketball). This works all the smaller stabilizer muscles in the shoulder in addition to the work it provides as a 1-arm push up.

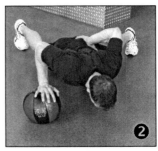

Drew performs his 1-arm push up supporting his body weight on the ball.

MEDICINE BALL TO FLOOR PLYOMETRIC PUSH UPS

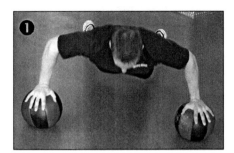

Drew places each hand on a medicine ball as shown using a wide base.

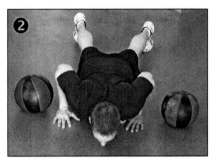

Drew drops his body to the floor, moving his hands under his shoulders.

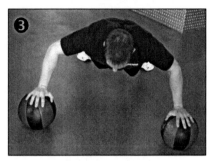

Drew explodes back up and immediately places his hands on the balls. This requires excellent coordination and develops strength and balance.

MEDICINE BALL FORWARD AND BACKWARD DRILL

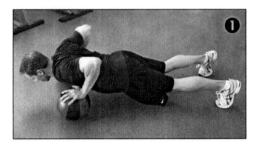

Drew starts this exercise by placing each hand on a medicine ball as shown.

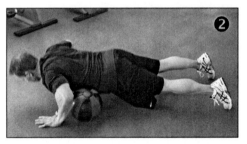

Drew moves his entire body forward and catches himself on the floor with his hands placed immediately in front of each ball.

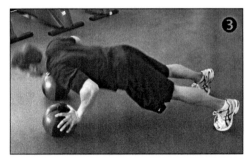

Drew quickly pushes off the floor with his hands and pops up and back onto each ball. Drew places his hands briefly on the balls.

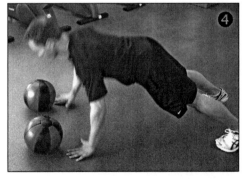

Drew quickly pushes off with each hand on each ball and moves backward landing on the floor with each hand. This is a great drill for coordination as well as strength development. The shoulders, triceps and upper back obviously get a lot of work, but holding yourself in this Plank position also works your core.

MEDICINE BALL POP UP DRILL

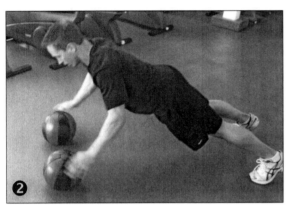

This exercise is a good explosive strength developer. Drew balances himself on the medicine balls as shown.

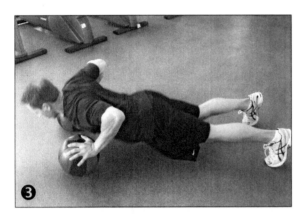

Drew pops up, pushing off each ball with his hands as high as possible.

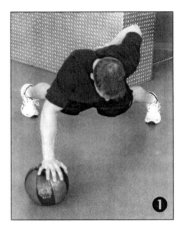

Drew comes down and lands with one hand on each ball.

MEDICINE BALL 1 ARM PUSH UPS

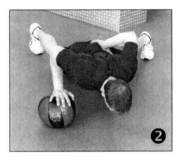

A great 1-arm push up is to balance your hand on a medicine ball (or even a basketball).

Drew performs his 1-arm push up supporting his body weight on the ball. This develops excellent work for all the smaller stabilizer muscles in the shoulder in addition to the work it provides as a 1-arm push up.

MEDICINE BALL ALTERNATING 1 ARM PUSH UP DRILL

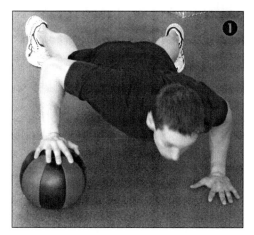

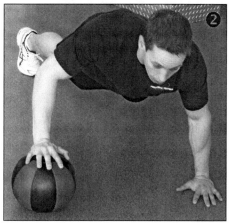

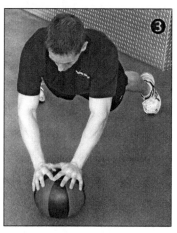

Another great drill is to alternate arms when doing push ups. Drew has his right arm on the ball while in a push up position to start.

Drew performs a push up with his right hand on the ball and his left hand on the floor.

Drew quickly moves to his right and places both hands on the ball as he moves his body to his right.

MEDICINE BALL BRIDGES

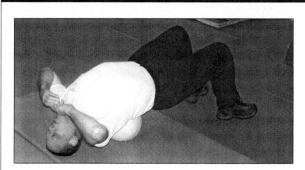

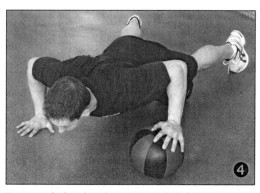

John Saylor bridges with a Medicine Ball placed under the middle of his back. This allows him to roll up onto his shoulders higher and get a better arch or bridge.

Drew switches hands and has his left hand on the ball and his right hand on the floor as he performs a push up.

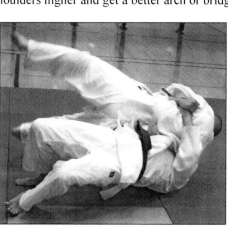

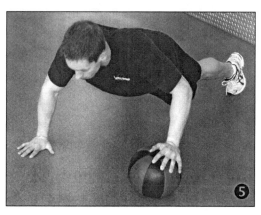

BRIDGES CAN IMPROVE YOUR PIN ESCAPES

This Bridge and Roll escape from the Head and Arm Hold (Kesa Gatame or Scarf Hold) is the result of a lot of drilling, but just as important, a strong bridge!

Drew completes the push up and will perform at least 10 reps, with the goal to perform a lot more.

SECTION TWO: PART 8:
JUMPING, EXPLOSIVE POWER & PLYOMETRIC TRAINING

● ● ● "Faster than a speeding bullet and able to jump tall buildings in a single bound..."
The Introduction to the "Superman" Television Show from the 1950s.

TRAINING IN PLYOMETRICS WILL ENABLE YOU TO SHORTEN THE AMOUNT OF TIME YOU NEED TO APPLY MAXIMUM FORCE.

TECHNICAL TIP: Plyometrics training produces fast, powerful movements. The muscle is initially lengthened, followed by a short rest, then a rapid contraction. When the stretch nerve receptors are stimulated, there's a reflex that causes an automatic contraction of the muscle. Jumping, hopping and other explosive movements and exercises develop power.

EXPLOSIVE POWER ON THE MAT

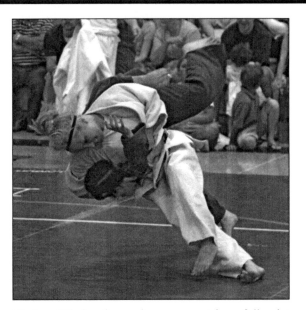

Chelsea Whaley throws her opponent for a full point using tremendous explosive power. The plyometric chain of movement goes from Chelsea's legs to her hips, then to her upper body, through her arms and into her opponent to produce a successful, and powerful, throw.

Jump and Plyometric training develops power. Power involves strength (force) as well as speed (distance divided by time). It's a vital element in any type of combat sports or martial arts. Another way of putting this is to say that muscle power is determined by how long it takes for strength to be converted into speed. Plyometrics is effective in increasing the speed and/or force of a muscular contraction. Plyometrics allows you to shorten the amount of time you need to apply maximum force, and this is what we mean by power. Throwing an opponent with skill and force requires power. Punching or kicking an opponent requires power. Pulling an opponent's arm free to apply an armlock requires power.

Before you start any training in plyometrics or explosive strength training, you must have a solid foundation of strength and fitness. Plyometric training isn't for novices. Plyometrics are exercises that you use to develop power. Used along with strength training, the explosive movements of plyometrics build strength and the elastic recoil that provides more power for throwing, striking or performing a sudden movement on an opponent. In other words if you are doing a High Jump where you stand still and jump straight up in the air as high as possible, you bend your knees and squat down a bit, putting a short stretch on the muscle prior to a powerful contraction to propel you up. The theory is that it recruits more muscle fibers to perform this task. Plyometrics increase strength up to 10% and improve elastic recoil.

TECHNICAL TIP: Jump Training and Plyometric Training aren't easy. Before starting a program of plyometric or jump training, you must have a good base of overall strength, especially in your legs and hips. If you have any type of injury, especially a joint injury, don't perform plyometrics. This type of training will be too hard on your joints and any injury you may have will only get worse. Plyometric Training is intense and we don't recommend that you perform it more than once per week, even if you're a strong, experienced athlete.
IMPORTANT: Before you start training in plyometrics, make sure you have a solid foundation of strength and fitness. We recommend that you be able to perform 5 repetitions of the Squat at 60% of your own body weight before starting a program of Plyometric training.

HIGH JUMP

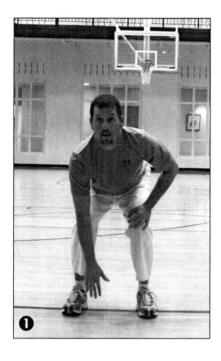

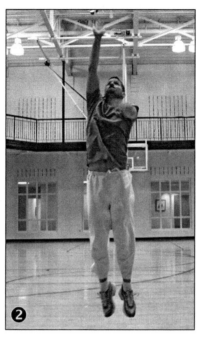

1. This is a great exercise and can be used as an excellent warm-up before going on to more difficult plyometric drills or Box Jumps. Ron squats down, touching the gym floor with one hand.

2. Ron immediately jumps up as high into the air as possible. If you're in a basketball gym, try to touch the rim.

HIGH JUMP WITH DUMB-BELLS

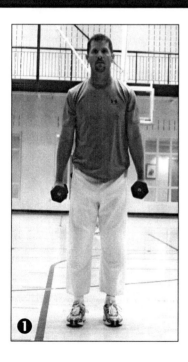

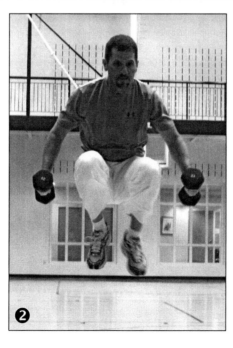

1. Ron holds a dumb-bell or kettle-bell in each hand as shown.

2. Ron jumps as high as possible, making sure to try to tuck his knees up to his torso as much as possible as he jumps. Ron will land, and take his time, then perform another jump as high as possible.

TECHNICAL TIP: This is a great plyometric jump because holding a dumb-bell in each hand forces you to work a lot of stabilizer muscles as well as increases the workload in the jump.

LONG JUMP

This exercise develops explosive power in the hips and legs, which is necessary for all aspects of fighting or grappling, but especially throwing and takedowns. Since the goal of this exercise is to develop speed and explosive leg power, don't turn it into a cardio drill. Keep your reps per set in the 3 to 5 range and perform 3 to 5 sets.

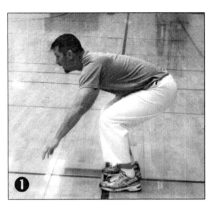
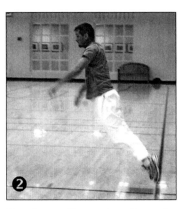
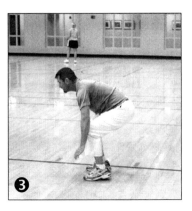

Ron squats low as shown and rocks forward and back swinging his arms to gain momentum.

Ron jumps forward as far as he can.

Ron lands on both feet simultaneously, gets set and will perform another jump.

TECHNICAL TIP: On shots such as the double leg or single leg takedown, you are often shooting in on a horizontal plane. Because of this, it's smart to rotate into your Jump Training exercises like Long Jumps and other exercises that develop explosive forward leg drive. Nationally renowned wrestling coach Joe DeMayo has said that once you are close enough to touch your opponent with your hands, it's a "2 to 3 foot race" to the takedown. Exercises like Long Jumps and Lunge Steps with an added stretch band for resistance will go a long way in helping you win that race!

LONG JUMP WITH DUMB-BELLS

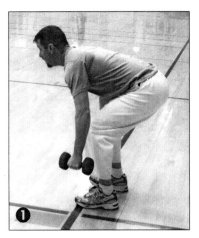
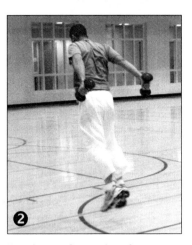
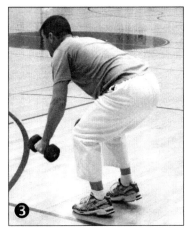

Using a dumb-bell or kettlebell in each hand makes the Long Jump harder and provides a tougher workout.

Ron jumps forward as far as possible, making sure to not drop the weights.

Ron lands on both feet at the same time, and gets set to perform another rep. Perform this exercise using the same set and rep count as in the Long Jump.

LONG JUMP WITH MEDICINE BALL

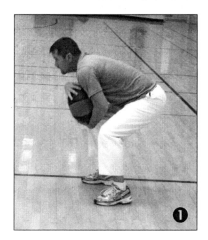

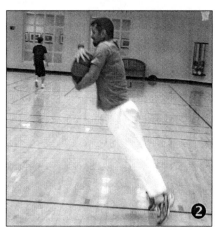

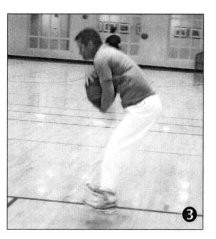

Ron tucks the Medicine Ball in tightly to his body and readies himself to perform a Long Jump.

Ron jumps forward as far as he can holding the Medicine Ball.

Ron lands, and then readies himself to continue to jump forward across the gym.

TECHNICAL TIP: When doing jump or plyometric drills, you will often jump as high as possible rather than in rapid repetition. Make each jump count and jump as high as possible or as high as the drill calls for. Plyometric training develops power and explosive strength, and while you get some cardio benefit from doing it, the primary purpose of jump training isn't aerobic or cardio in nature.

FRONT JUMP WITH MEDICINE BALL

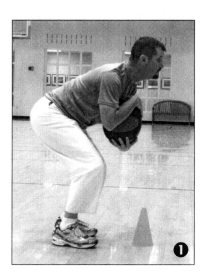

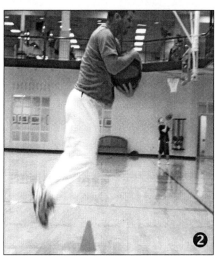

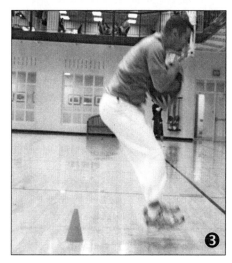

Ron tucks the ball in tightly to his body and readies himself to jump over the cone.

Ron jumps as high as possible over the cone holding the Medicine Ball.

Ron will land, and then turn around and jump back over the cone.

CONDITIONING FOR COMBAT SPORTS

1 LEG LONG JUMP

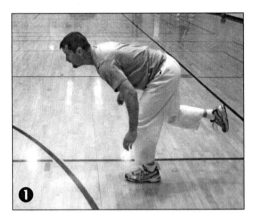 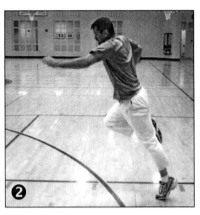 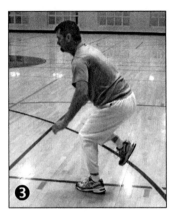

A great way to develop explosive power for 1-legged throws is to perform this drill. Ron stands on his left leg and will jump forward.

Ron jumps forward as far as possible, driving off his left leg and foot as shown.

Ron lands on his left foot and leg and will continue to jump forward across the gymnasium. After a brief rest, Ron will jump back across the gym on his right leg.

TECHNICAL TIP: Your safety is important when doing Plyometric or Jump Training exercises. We don't recommend this type of training for athletes that haven't reached puberty or 13 years of age. Your weight is a consideration as well. If you weigh more than 220 pounds, you should be careful and if you perform Jump Training or Plyometrics use a low intensity approach. Make sure you wear good athletic shoes and the surface you jump on has some softness or spring to it. Never jump on a concrete or tile floor. Use good jumping form when doing these exercises. Don't rush through Plyometric exercises; take your time and perform them correctly. Make sure that you use good technique when jumping, bounding, leaping or hopping.

SIDE 1 LEG OBSTACLE HOPS

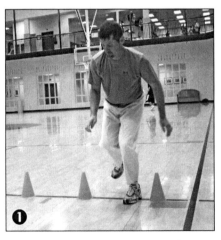 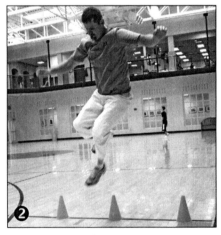 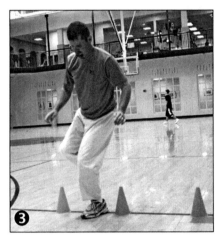

Set a line of cones on the gym floor as shown. Ron balances on his left leg.

Ron hops to his right over the cone, springing off his left leg.

Ron lands on his left leg as shown. Ron continues to hop over the line of cones, then switch to his right leg and hop back the other way.

SIDE OBSTACLE HOP WITH MEDICINE BALL

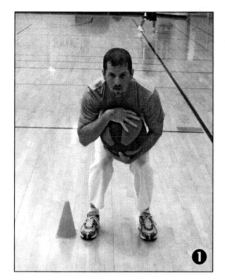
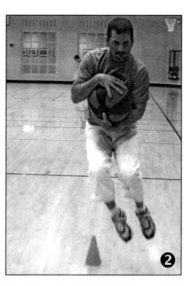
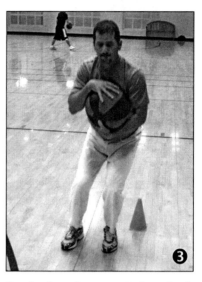

Ron holds a Medicine Ball as he readies himself to hop sideways over the cone.

Tucking the ball tightly to his body, Ron hops over the cone.

Ron lands and prepares to jump back over the cone.

BOUNDING

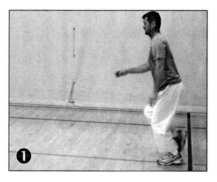
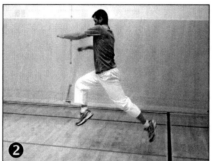
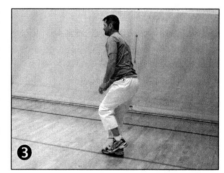

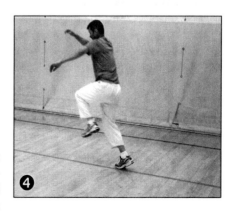

1. Ron starts his bound.

2. Ron bounds as far as possible each time.

3. Ron lands firmly on the floor or ground before he starts to bound again.

4. Ron continues on with the Bounding exercise.

Bounding is running and jumping combined. Actually you jump more than run, so make sure to get a good, firm landing before you start your second rep when bounding. This exercise is excellent for developing forward explosive strength and is useful for throwing techniques. Bounding is an excellent warm-up Plyometric drill before you go on to some more intense Plyometric training.

BOX JUMPS

When people think about Plyometric Training, the first thing that usually comes to mind is the Box Jump. This exercise develops tremendous explosive power and speed in the hips and legs. It is useful for all throws, takedowns, power in punching, kicking and for use as a solid base in all phases of grappling and groundfighting.

A few months prior to the writing of this book, author John Saylor was training in Louie Simmons' gym, the Westside Barbell Club. While there, John met John Kerr, the former linebacker for the Minnesota Vikings who was out with a back injury. Since the time of his injury, he has strengthened his back and had just completed a 650-pound Sumo-style Deadlift. Even more impressive was his 60-inch Box Jump. No kidding—60 inches for a Box Jump! It's no surprise that in a recent training camp, John Kerr scored the fastest time ever recorded in the NFL in the L-Drill (where the player sprints out a set distance and cuts to the left or right). Obviously, John's hard work with the Westside Barbell Club paid off and his prospects of playing professional football again appear very good.

The point of this narrative is to pose this question: Do you think an explosive Box Jump like that demonstrated by John Kerr would help with your throws, takedowns, striking skills or other fighting skills? If your answer is "yes," you've been paying attention to what we're trying to convey in this book. Box Jumps, along with a variety of Squat variations, built on a solid foundation of lower body strength, should be an integral part of your training program.

Recommended Sets and Reps: There are a large number of possible set and rep schemes, depending on your goals, but start out with 5 sets of 5 jumps. Later, you might try 6 sets of 3 jumps. Remember, the goal is explosive power and not cardio or aerobic training. Make each jump a separate and explosive event in and of itself.

> **TECHNICAL TIP: To add difficulty and increase the training effect, you can wear a weighted vest, hold a dumb-bell or kettlebell in each hand, strap ankle weights around your ankles or arms or hold a heavy medicine ball when performing Box Jumps.**

FRONT JUMP ON SHORT BOX

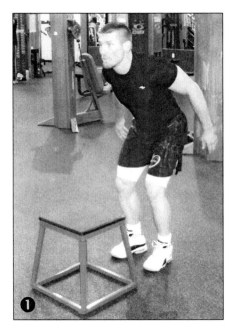 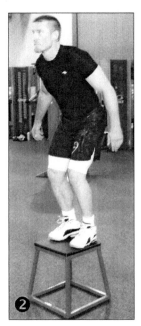

Mike stands in front of his short box, ready to jump onto it.

Mike jumps onto the box, balances himself, and then hops back down, readying himself for another jump.

LOWER BODY POWER IS IMPORTANT

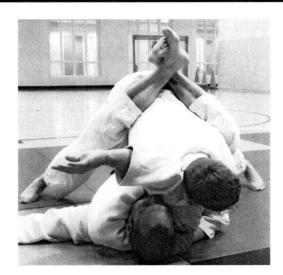

LEG AND LOWER BODY POWER IS IMPORTANT IN GROUNDFIGHTING AS WELL
All effective chokes rely on controlling your opponent with your legs. Explosive leg power helps set up and control your opponent do that you can better make him tap out or hold him for time to get the win.

FRONT JUMP ON TALL BOX

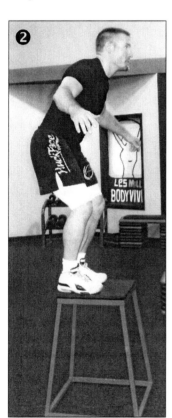

Mike uses good body mechanics to ready himself for the jump onto the high box. Look at the flexed legs and body lean into the direction of the jump.

Mike makes a maximum effort to jump onto the box. He will steady himself, and then hop back down, getting ready for the next jump.

FRONT JUMP FAST REPS ON TALL BOX

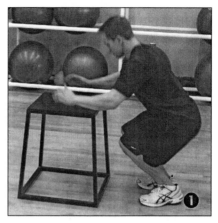

Drew demonstrates this Box Jump drill that incorporates a fast, explosive jump and a quick hop back down, followed by an immediate ready position, then another jump.

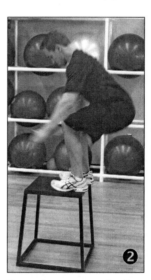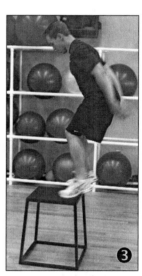

Drew jumps onto the box and gets a good landing.

Drew immediately hops back down, exploding backward with power.

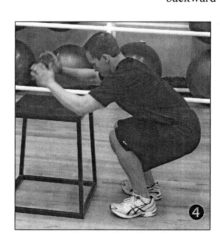

Drew makes a solid landing, flexing his knees to serve as a "spring" landing for safety.

DOUBLE JUMP TALL TO SHORT BOX AND TURN AROUND JUMP SHORT TO TALL BOX

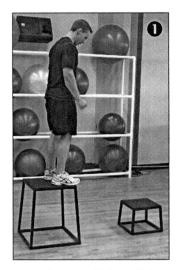

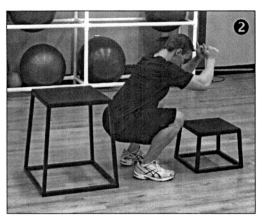

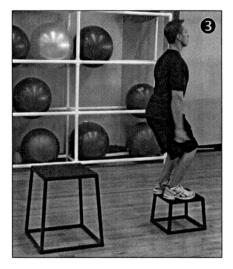

Drew jumps off the tall box onto the floor.

Drew lands in this flexed position, readying himself for the next jump to the smaller box.

Drew jumps up onto the smaller box.

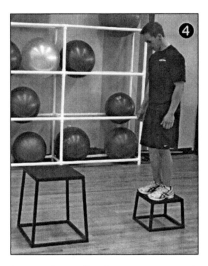

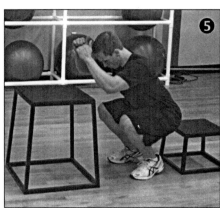

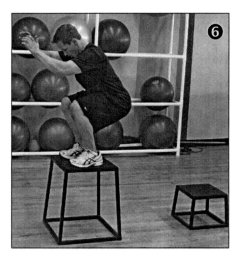

Drew immediately turns around, readying himself to jump off the small box to the floor.

Drew lands in the flexed position as shown and readies himself to jump up on the tall box.

Drew completes the exercise by jumping up on the tall box. Drew will continue this drill until he completes a set of 3 to 6 jumps.

STRADDLE JUMPS

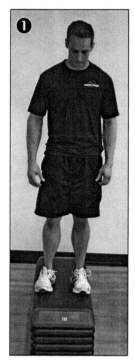 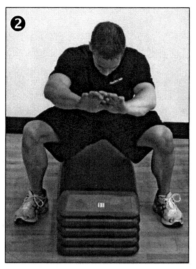 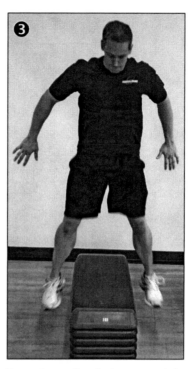 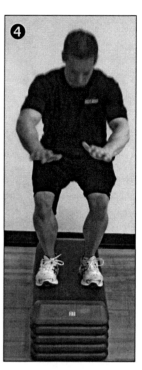

Drew stands as shown on a narrow box. As you see, you can use cardio steps or any short box that is stable.

Drew widens his stance and lands on the floor as shown.

Drew immediately jumps straight up as shown.

Drew lands on the box and will prepare himself for another rep.

SUCCESSFUL THROWING TECHNIQUES REQUIRE POWERFUL SPRINGING ACTION FROM THE LEGS

Look at how David Fortin uses his right leg to spring up powerfully from the ball of his foot to throw his opponent with this Tai Otoshi (Body Drop) throw. Developing a solid foundation of leg strength and power produces winning results on the mat.

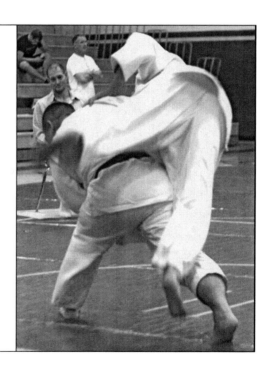

SIDE HOPS OVER A SHORT BOX

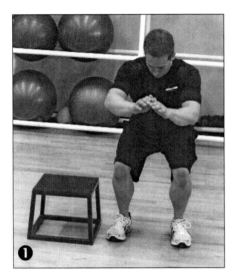

Drew prepares himself to hop sideways over the small box.

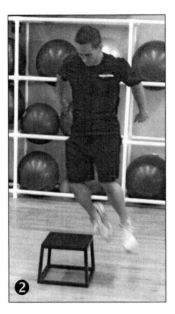

Drew hops to his right over the small box.

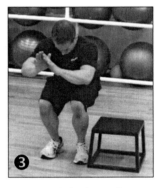

Drew lands in the spring position and immediately prepares himself to jump back over the box.

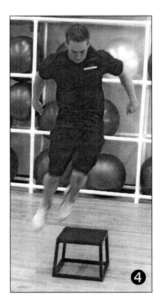

Drew Jumps to his left over the box.

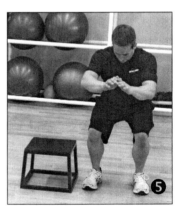

Drew lands with his legs flexed as shown and prepares to perform another side hop.

SIDE HOPS ONTO SHORT BOX

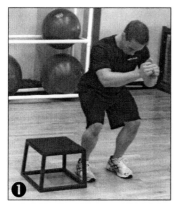

Drew prepares to hop to his right onto the short box.

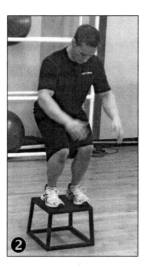

Drew hops onto the short box as shown, gets a stable footing very quickly and prepares to jump to his left to the floor.

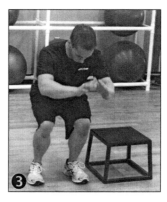

Drew jumps to the floor, landing in the spring or flexed position. He readies himself to jump to his left back onto the short box.

TECHNICAL TIP: Occasionally, to test your explosive strength, jump up on as high of a box as possible. Rest between attempts until you're completely recovered. Keep adding height to the box until you can't jump any higher. Record the height of your best jump and keep this number in your records. Try for a new record every month to 6 weeks.

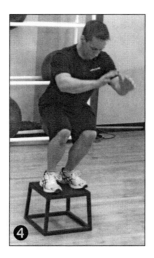

Drew jumps onto the short box, pauses, gets a stable footing and readies himself to jump onto the floor to his left.

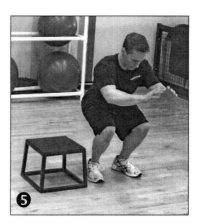

Drew completes the exercise by landing on the floor as shown.

SECTION TWO: PART 9:
AGILITY LADDER, STAIRS AND BALANCE TRAINING

● ● ● "You have to 'feel' your judo." Old Japanese Judo Axiom

Coordination is one of the most difficult skills to learn, and then master. What is known as Proprioception: balance, timing, foot speed, knowing where your body is in relation to your opponent, ability and movement are all factors that make up and are necessary for what we perceive to be "skill." Skill is the practical application of technique and is entirely dependent upon all the physical, mental and emotional factors that we possess and how we apply them.

This part of Section 2 features how you might be able to develop your coordination skills to a higher level. An elite athlete or fighter possesses that "feel" for his craft. It's a kinesthetic awareness that only comes from serious, intense training. It's that ability to sense where your opponent's body is in relation to yours and then take advantage of the situation. Using an Agility Ladder, Balance Board, Balance Beam and other tools to enhance your balance, coordination and kinesthetic awareness can make that 1% difference that may be the difference between winning and losing.

The authors vividly remember, back in the early 1980s, when Bob Corwin included the use of agility training and balance board training into his judo team's training program. Bob, a top coach from Yorkville, Illinois, had tough guys, but when he began including the use of agility training, his athletes moved to another level; and it was a successful one! Naturally, we did everything we could to tap into what Bob was doing and this part of Section 2 includes some of what Bob was doing, as well as what we learned from others.

After you've developed (1) Functional Flexibility and Mobility, and then (2) Cardio and Muscular Endurance, followed by (3) Strength, you must have (4) Proprioception, or the ability to have balanced, coordination movement and awareness of where your body is. In other word's, develop a "feel" for what you do. Specific Skill Development on an elite level can only be achieved if you've developed the physical and kinesthetic abilities listed above. Using the exercises in this part of Section 2 can help you achieve a higher level of Proprioceptive ability.

BALANCE, AGILITY & COORDINATION

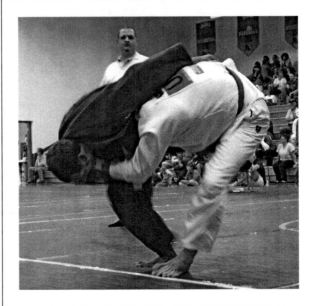

BALANCE, AGILITY AND COORDINATION ARE VITAL TO ELITE LEVEL PERFORMANCE
Both athletes in this photo are hopping on one leg, each with very different reasons. The attacker is hopping on his right leg finish his Uchi Mata (Inner Thigh) throw attack while the defender is hopping on his left leg to avoid the throw.

BALANCE BOARD (BOTH LEG BALANCE)

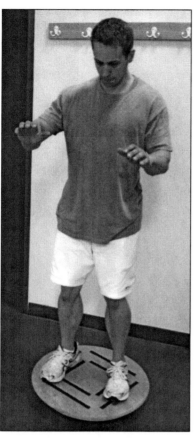

BALANCE BOARD (1 LEG BALANCE)

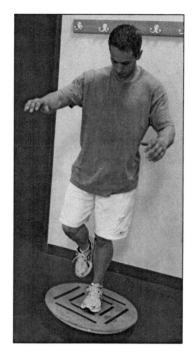

When you can stand on both legs, try to stand on 1 leg for an extended period of time.

BALANCE BOARD 1 LEG SQUATS

After being able to stand on 1 leg perfectly balanced, go on to performing 1-legged squats on the Balance Board. If you can perform 10 1-legged squats, you have excellent balance!

The "K Board" as Bob Corwin called it back in 1981 is the Balance Board of today. Basically, it's a board on a round bottom that you can stand on to improve your balance and kinesthetic awareness. Drew shows how you stand on the board and balance yourself. Balance Board training is effective when used while not in a heavy training cycle for a big fight or tournament. Use the board about 30 minutes a day and perform as many feats of balance as possible on it. We're showing only a few drills you can use on the Balance Board.

BALANCE BOARD SQUATS

After you've mastered being able to stand on the board with little trouble, go on to performing Hindu Squats on it.

BALANCE BOARD BALL HOLD

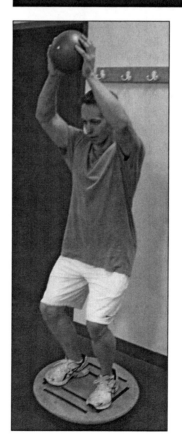

As you master standing perfectly balanced on the board, hold a ball at chest level, and then eventually, hold it above your head. Holding the ball above your head requires a great degree of coordination and balance. Initially, hold a light ball, then move on to holding a heavier ball like a Medicine Ball.

> **TECHNICAL TIP: Keep a Balance Board around the house or apartment and play on it when you're not at the dojo or gym training. It's a great way to improve your balance and a fun "toy" to have around. It's a good way to have some fun while improving your balance!**

BALANCE BOARD PLAY CATCH

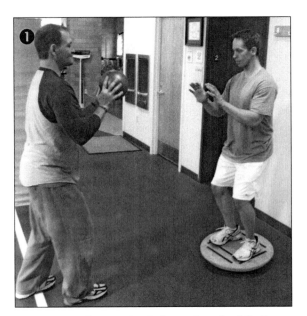

Drew is standing on the Balance Board while Bryan tosses a ball to him.

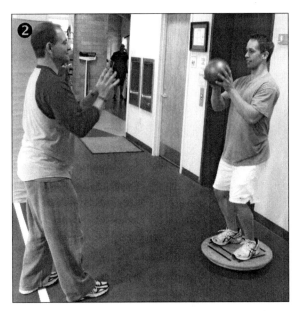

Drew catches the ball without losing his balance or falling off the board. Eventually, Bryan will toss the ball faster to Drew, forcing Drew to work harder at balancing himself on the board.

AGILITY LADDER TRAINING

There are agility ladders available commercially, but you can always use athletic tape or duct tape to make your own agility ladder on the floor or even on your mat. The idea of an Agility Ladder is to increase your foot speed and explosive power and to know where your feet are and whether they are doing what they are supposed to be doing.

SHORT FORWARD JUMPS

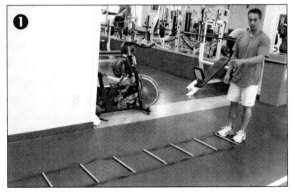

Drew stands at one end of the ladder.

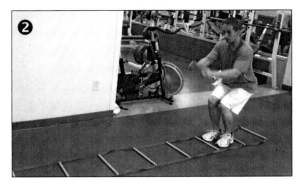

Drew quickly hops forward with both feet into the next rung of the ladder.

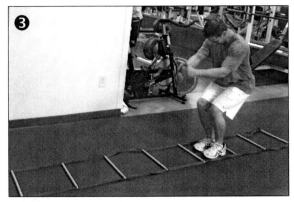

Initially, Drew will perform these hops slowly, but as his skill improves, he will be able to hop quickly. This drill improves your foot speed dramatically!

1 LEG FORWARD JUMPS

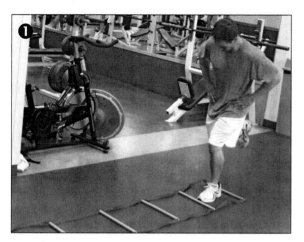

Hopping on 1 leg is more difficult than hopping on both legs, so try this after you become skilled at hopping on both legs. This drill is excellent for doing forward throws or supporting a kicking leg.

1 LEG JUMPS CAN ALSO BE DONE AS SIDE HOPS Perform 1 leg hops moving to the side for a different training experience.

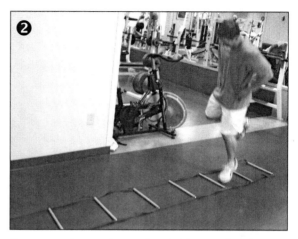

Drew continues down the ladder performing the 1-legged hops. Initially, he will perform them slowly, but as his coordination improves, he will increase the speed of his hops.

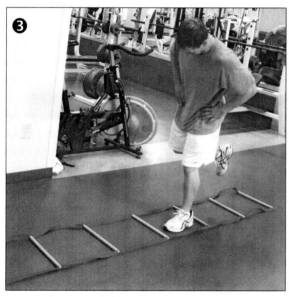

As in all ladder drills, hop down the length of the ladder, and then back again for a complete set.

BALANCE AND COORDINATION

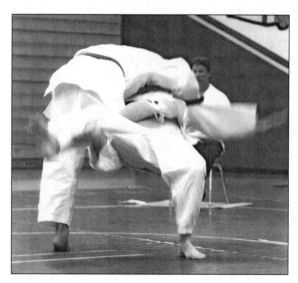

BALANCE AND COORDINATION RESULT IN A SUCCESSFUL THROW

Many throws rely on having one leg posted or positioned on the mat. This base leg, or "driving" leg is Mark Lozano's support when he throws his opponent in this photo from the AAU Judo Grand Nationals.

LONG JUMP

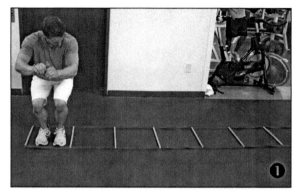

To develop explosive power, but also add the increased skill of controlling that explosive power, perform long jumps on the Agility Ladder. Drew stands at the end of the ladder.

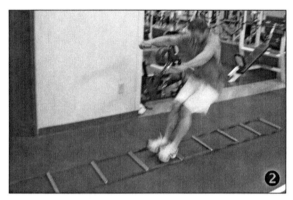

Drew hops as many rungs as possible, making sure he lands between the rungs. In this jump, Drew has jumped over 5 rungs.

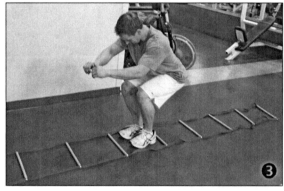

It's important for Drew to land perfectly balanced and keep his feet within the confines of the ladder.

SIDE LONG HOPS

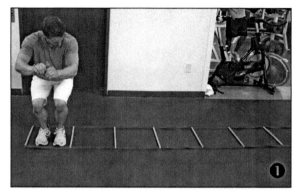

This is a good plyometric drill that also develops co-ordination and body control. Drew stands in the space between rungs as shown.

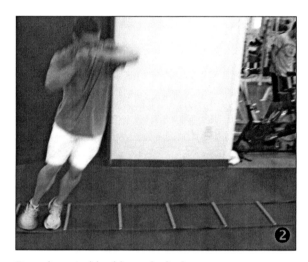

Drew hops to his side explosively.

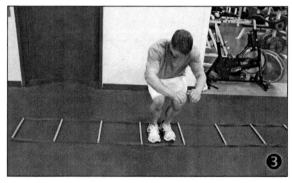

Drew hops to his side over as many rungs as possible and lands in a space between rungs.

SHUFFLE STEP

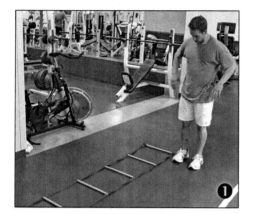

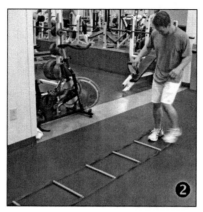

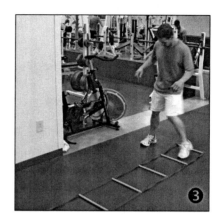

To develop coordination and foot speed, Drew will perform a shuffle from side to side while moving forward down the length of the ladder.

Drew moves into the initial space between rungs.

Drew completes the side shuffle.

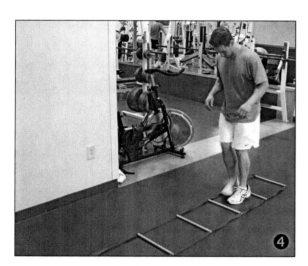

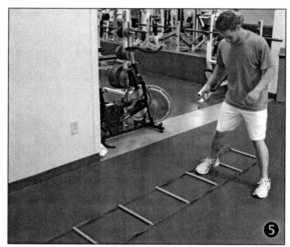

Drew starts back the other way in the side shuffle as he moves to the next space between the rungs.

Drew completes the second shuffle in the drill and will continue on like this until he has moved down the entire length of the ladder.

SHORT SIDE HOPS

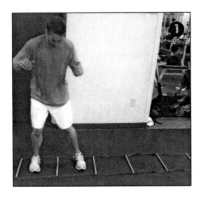
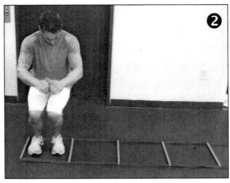
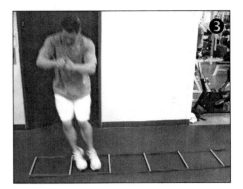

Drew will hop to his side as quickly as possible into the next space, jumping over 1 rung as a time.

This is an excellent drill for lateral movement and controlled foot speed.

As soon as Drew lands, he immediately hops to the next space. Hop over each rung without hitting on a rung, down the length of the ladder.

TECHNICAL TIP: If you don't have access to a commercially produced Agility Ladder, make your own Agility Ladder by taping some duct tape or white athletic tape on the gym floor or even on a mat.

LADDER SIDE STEP

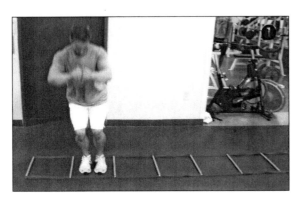
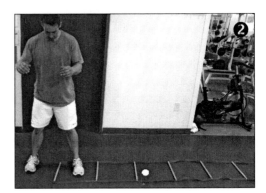

Drew steps one rung at a time sideways as quickly as he can. This is an excellent foot speed drill and develops your coordination.

It's important to keep a good, upright posture to develop your balance and foot speed more effectively. Drew steps sideways down the length of the ladder as shown.

BALANCE BEAM TRAINING

A good way to develop balance is to work on a narrow beam. Abundance of Strength also applies to balance. If you can perform a kick while standing on a balance beam, you will certainly be able to perform a kick with more skill when standing on a floor.

If you don't have a portable balance beam (and who does?), you can make your own by sanding down and painting a 4" by 4" piece of lumber.

BALANCE BEAM FARMER'S WALK

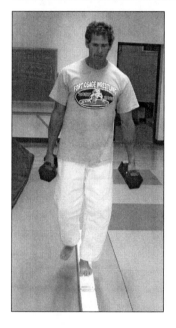

Kelvin walks down the length of the beam holding a pair of dumb-bells (or kettlebells).

BALANCE BEAM WALK WITH DUMB-BELLS

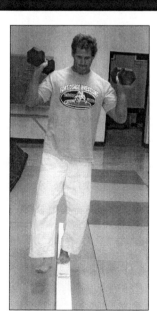

Kelvin increases the difficulty of walking on the beam by holding a pair of dumb-bells up at his shoulders as shown.

BALANCE BEAM WALK

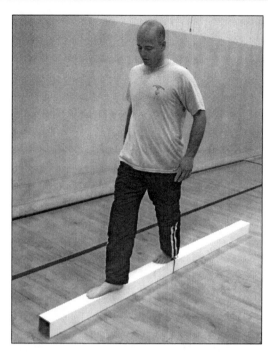

Brian performs the basic skill on the Balance Beam by walking down the length of the beam with good control and balance. Initially, you will walk slowly, but as you improve, you will be able to walk quickly. This is a basic skill and one that is necessary before moving on to the other balance beam drills.

BALANCE BEAM 1 LEG BALANCE

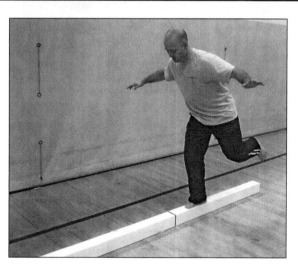

Brian balances himself on 1 leg as shown. Try to hold this position as long as possible. When you are comfortable doing this, lean forward and extend your leg up higher in the air to increase the difficulty.

BALANCE BEAM FRONT KICK

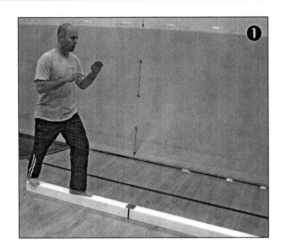

Brian readies himself so he can perform a front snap kick while on the beam.

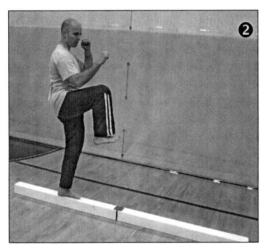

Brian balances on one leg as he lifts his kicking leg. A good variation of this drill is to simply hold this position for as long as possible.

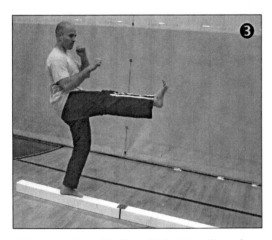

Brian completes his front kick. He will perform another kick down the length of the beam and then kick with the other leg on the way back.

1 LEG HOP ON BALANCE BEAM

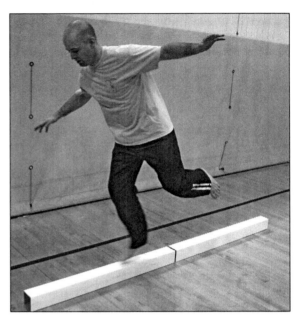

Brian hops on 1 leg down the length of the beam. He will hop on his other leg on the way back.

TECHNICAL TIP: Make this exercise more difficult by strapping on ankle weights around your ankles or wearing a weighted vest.

BALANCE BEAM TENNIS BALL CATCH

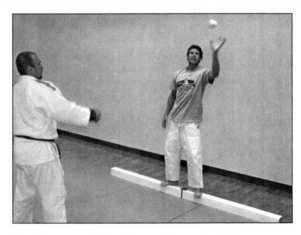

Catching a small ball is really tough. Mike tosses a tennis ball to Kelvin while Kelvin is balanced on the beam. To make this drill harder, Mike will throw several balls to Kelvin in rapid succession, forcing Kelvin to catch all the balls while balanced on the beam.

SIDE KICK ON BALANCE BEAM

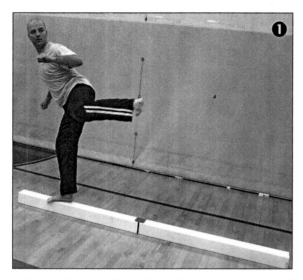

Brian performs a side kick on the beam as shown. If you can perform a kick while balancing on a narrow beam, kicking on a flat surface is considerably easier.

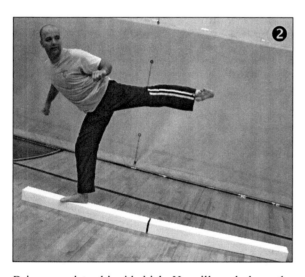

Brian completes his side kick. He will work down the length of the beam, kicking with the same leg. On the way back, he will kick with the other leg.

TECHNICAL TIP: Another good drill with tennis balls is for your partner to throw the balls at you while you are standing on the beam. His job is to hit your chest with the ball and your job is to swat it away. If you don't want to use tennis balls, and want to have a slower object thrown at you, use wadded up pieces of paper as balls. The paper balls move through the air slower than a tennis ball and don't hit as hard.

SIDE STEP ON BALANCE BEAM

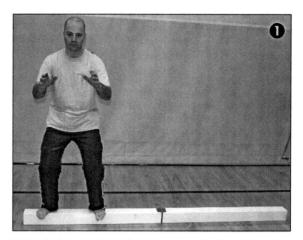

Brian balances himself as shown on the beam.

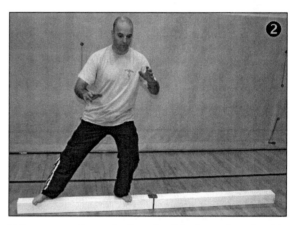

Brian moves down the length of the beam keeping his balance as he moves.

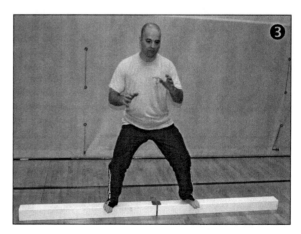

Brian completes his side step and will move down the length of the beam. This is a basic skill and one that is necessary before moving on to the following drills.

BALANCE BEAM SQUAT

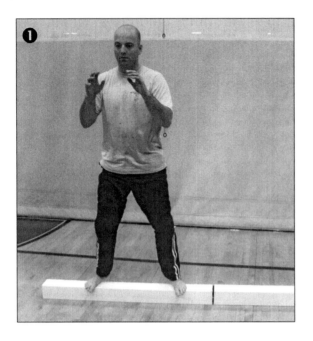

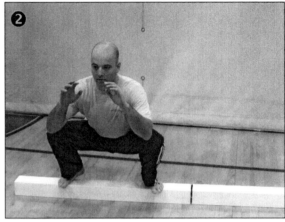

1. Brian will do a full squat balanced on the beam.

2. Brian squats on the beam. He can perform repetitions of squats like this, or stay in the squatting position and move sideways down the length of the beam.

BALANCE BEAM PUNCHING

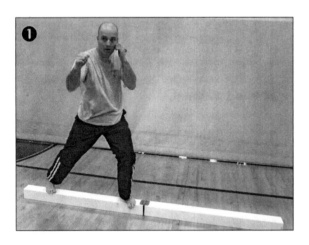

1. Brian balances himself on the beam and moves sideways down the length of the beam as he throws punches.

2. Brian can also perform quick punches as he balances himself on the beam as shown.

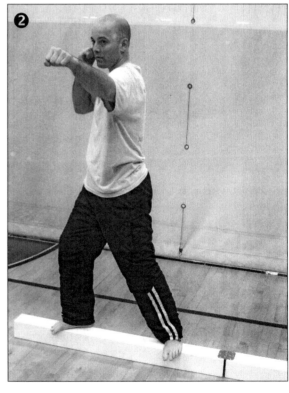

BALANCE BEAM DUMB-BELL SQUATS

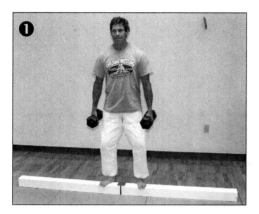

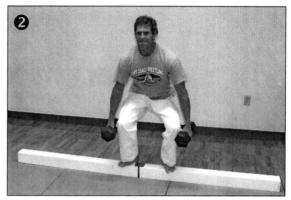

Kelvin holds a pair of dumb-bells or kettle-bells as he balances on the beam.

Kelvin performs a squat while holding the dumb-bells. He will perform a set of 10 squats.

BALANCE BEAM BALL HOLD

BALANCE BEAM SQUAT BALL OVERHEAD

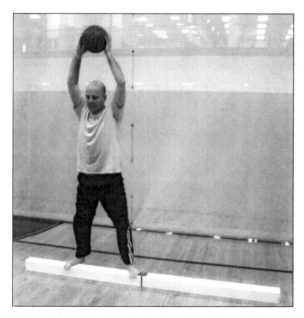

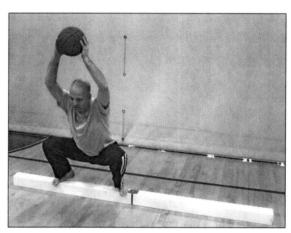

Brian holds the ball over his head and performs squats. Performing 10 squats is tough, but make this your goal. As Brian improves, he can move sideways in a squat position down the length of the beam.

Brian initially holds the ball at his chest and as he improves his skill, he will hold the ball over his head as shown. He can either hold this position for time or move sideways down the length of the beam holding the ball.

BALANCE BEAM BALL CATCH

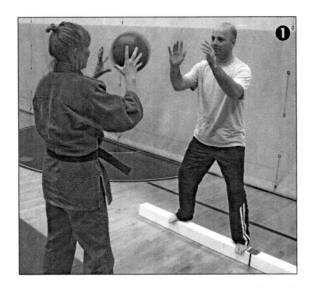

Sharon tosses the ball to Brian as he balances himself on the beam.

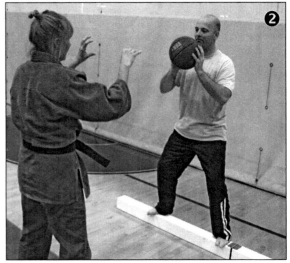

Brian catches the ball. He can perform 10 catches with his partner, or to make it more difficult, move sideways down the length of the beam as Sharon tosses the ball to him.

BALANCE BEAM SIDE CATCH

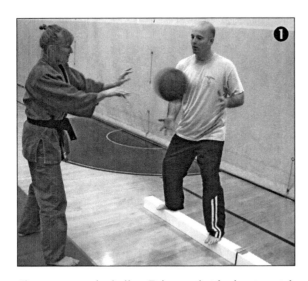

Sharon tosses the ball to Brian so that he has to catch the ball at his hip. This forces Brian to work harder holding his balance on the beam.

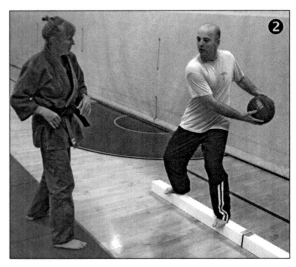

Brian catches the ball as shown and tosses it back to Sharon.

STAIR RUNNING

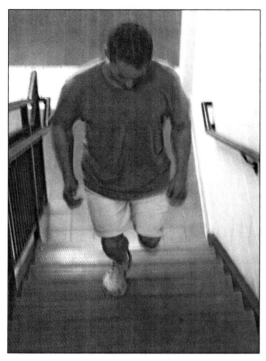

Running stairs may be an old exercise, but it still works! Running up and down stairs is a tough cardio workout, but it also teaches excellent coordination and foot speed skills. Moving your feet up each step while running develops coordination, plain and simple. A good stair workout is to run the stairs after a hard workout on the mat for a specified number of sets or for a specific time period.

1 LEG STAIR JUMP

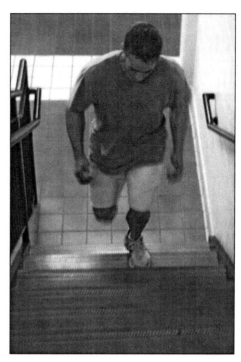

When you are comfortable with stair jumping on both legs, perform stair jumps on 1 leg. We recommend that you go 1 step at a time, making sure you land safely on each step. Initially, you will perform this drill slowly, but as you become used to it, you will perform it more quickly. This is an advanced method of Stair Jumping; so make sure you are skilled at jumping with both feet before attempting this.

STAIR BOUNDING

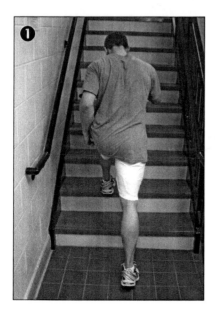

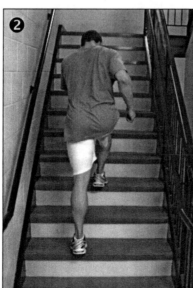

1. Bounding is part running and part jumping. Run up the stairs several steps at a time...or at least more than one step at a time. This adds to the stress of the cardio workout and really increases your leg strength as well.

2. Bounding up the stairs can replace simply running up the stairs and provides for a very tough leg and hip workout!

STAIR SHORT JUMP

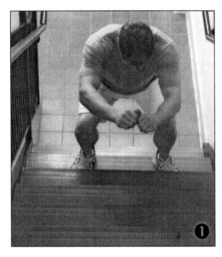

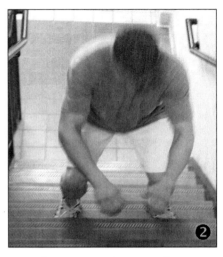

Using the stairs for developing explosive power is a good way to improve your athletic ability. This drill is performed by quick, short jumps 1 step at a time. Drew shows how to prepare for the initial jump.

Drew jumps up each step, going 1 step at a time, as quickly as possible. When he reaches the top step, he pauses, gets a much-needed rest for about 60 seconds, and then walks down the steps to start his second set.

AGILITY & BODY MOVEMENT

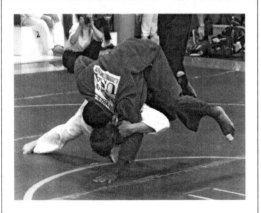

AGILITY, COORDINATION AND BODY MOVEMENT

Elite level performance in any combat sport results from a combination of many different types of training. This Shoulder Throw from the AAU Freestyle Judo Nationals shows how truly difficult it is to get an edge on an opponent. Combat athletes have to be excellent in many different aspects of athletic performance.

STAIR LONG JUMP

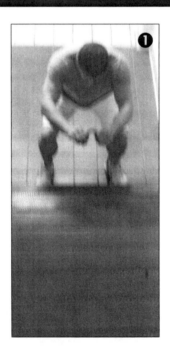

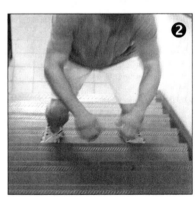

1. Drew jumps up as many steps as possible in each jump. This is an excellent plyometric drill that is similar to Box Jumps.

2. Drew jumps up several steps, gets his balance and readies himself for another jump.

ABOUT THE AUTHORS

JOHN SAYLOR

John Saylor began judo and jujitsu training at the age of 14 under Korean War Veteran Sgt. Doug Grant, and Jim Nichols. Immediately after graduating high school Saylor left home and trained under 2-time World Judo Medallist Kil Soon Park from 1972 through 1975. Following his time with Kil Soon Park, Saylor spent a couple years on the Ohio State University Judo Team. From 1978 through 1980 Saylor moved to New Jersey and trained under former All-Japan College Champion and 2-time U.S. Olympic Coach, Yoshisada "Yone" Yonezuka. John also trained for many years at Camp Olympus, the great summer training camp founded by 1964 Olympic and 1965 World Medallist, Jim Bregman. Here John worked with many great instructors including Olympians Jim Bregman, George Harris, Ben Campbell, Jim Wooley, World and Olympic Champion Anton Geesink, Hayward Nishioka, Paul Maruyama, Geoff Gleeson, Bill Montgomery, and many others.

Especially influential in John's career was 1976 Heavyweight Olympic Medallist, Allen Coage, who later wrestled in WWF as "Bad News Brown." Allen took Saylor under his wing and for several years served as a mentor, training partner, and friend. Allen Coage, who before entering the WWF wrestled for Antonio Inoki in Japan, was also the first to teach John the system of body weight exercises advocated by the great professional submission wrestler Karl Gotch. These are exercises John still incorporates in his training today.

Throughout his competitive career Saylor, as a member of various U.S. Judo Teams, trained and competed throughout Europe, Japan, South America, Canada, and South Africa. In 1979, while staying at Tokai University in Japan, Saylor was able to train with and observe some of the best judoists in the world, including the great Heavyweight Olympic and World Champion, Yasuhiro Yamashita, 1980 Light Heavy Weight Olympic Champion Robert Van de Walle of Belgium, and 2 complete Soviet Teams. Most of the Soviets were not only world-class judo fighters, but top SOMBO wrestlers as well.

John went on to win the National Collegiate Championship in 1974, the U.S. National Championship in 1978 and 1980, and was a two-time medallist in the Pan American Judo Championships in 1976 and 1979. Saylor also won the gold at the 1978 National Sports Festival (now called the U.S. Olympic Festival), which served as the U.S. Judo Team Trials, the United States Judo Association National Championship in 1978, and was twice a member of the U.S.J.A. Team to South Africa (1977 and 1979), which went undefeated in '79. In 1978 Saylor was voted First Team All-American. Saylor also won a bronze medal at the 1980 Pacific Rim International Judo Championship, where his only loss

STEVE SCOTT

Steve Scott first stepped onto a mat in 1965 as a 12-year-old boy and has been training, competing and coaching since that time. He holds advanced black belt rank in both Shingitai Jujitsu and Kodokan Judo and is a member of the U.S. Sombo Association's Hall of Fame.

Steve is the head coach and founder of the Welcome Mat Judo, Jujitsu and Sambo Club in Kansas City, Missouri where he has coached hundreds of national and international champions and medal winners in judo, sambo, sport jujitsu and submission grappling. Steve served as a national coach for USA Judo, Inc., the national governing body for the sport of judo as well as the U.S. Sombo Association and the Amateur Athletic Union in the sport of sambo. He also served as the coach education program director for many years with USA Judo, Inc. He has personally coached 3 World Sambo Champions, several Pan American Games Champions and a member of the 1996 U.S. Olympic Team. Athletes who trained with Steve at his Welcome Mat program in Kansas City have also competed in World Championships in judo, sambo and submission grappling in addition to numerous international judo, sambo and grappling events such as the Pan American Championships, World University Games, Pacific Rim Championships and other tournaments. He served as the national team coach and director of development for the under-21 national judo team and coached U.S. teams at several World Championships in both judo and sambo. He was the U.S. women's team head coach for the 1983 Pan American Games in Caracas, Venezuela where his team won 4 golds and 6 silvers and the team championship. He also coached numerous U.S. teams at many international judo and sambo events. Steve conducted numerous national training camps in judo at the U.S. Olympic Training Centers in Colorado Springs, Colorado, Marquette, Michigan and Lakes Placid, New York. He also serves as a television commentator from time to time for a local MMA production.

As an athlete, Steve competed in judo and sambo, winning 2 gold medals and a bronze medal in the National AAU Sambo Championships, as well as several other medals in smaller national sambo events and has won numerous state and regional medals in that sport. He was a state and regional champion in judo and competed in numerous national championships as well. He has trained, competed and coached in North America, South America, Europe and Japan and has the opportunity to train with some of the top judo and sambo athletes and coaches in the world.

Steve is active in the Shingitai Jujitsu Association with his friend John Saylor (www.JohnSaylor-SJA.com) and has a strong Shingitai program at his Welcome Mat Judo, Jujitsu

ABOUT THE AUTHORS

JOHN SAYLOR

was by koka (smallest score in judo) to Haruki Uemura, the 1976 Open Weight Olympic Gold Medallist.

After a serious shoulder injury in 1982 John retired from competitive judo. Since then he has devoted himself to coaching and teaching judo, jujitsu, submission grappling and self-defense. He served as Coach of the U.S. National Judo Training Squad at the Olympic Training Center from 1983 through 1990 that produced, or served as a temporary home, for many National, Pan American, World and Olympic medallists and champions. Shortly after leaving the OTC, John completed his B.A. at Colorado Christian University. After completing his degree Saylor helped train 3-time Olympian Grace Jividen. He accompanied her to the 1992 Barcelona Olympics where she narrowly missed a bronze medal in a hard-fought, scoreless decision loss against the Cuban.

In 1987 John was voted Coach of The Year by the United States Judo Association. During his tenure as Coach of the U.S. National Judo Training Squad at the OTC, John was selected by the governing body of judo, along with his good friend Steve Scott, to attend the U.S. Olympic Committee Coaches College. John and Steve completed this program several times, and for 2 years John was asked to present a segment on training for combative sports. It was during these coaches' college sessions that John developed a life-long friendship with outstanding coach and co-author Steve Scott.

In 1985 John Saylor founded the Shingitai Jujitsu Association, and has remained active as director to this day. John holds advanced black belt rank in Shingitai Jujitsu and Kodokan Judo and also holds black belt rankings in Tae Kwon Do, and Ashihara Karate, the latter of which he studied under 1978 All-Japan Full-Contact Karate Champion, Kancho Joko Ninomiya. He is a certified Systema (Russian Martial Art) instructor, and is also certified by world-famous powerlifting, conditioning, and speed strength coach, Louie Simmons, to teach The Westside Method of Training.

John is also the author of STRENGH AND CONDITIONING SECRETS OF THE WORLD'S GREATEST FIGHTERS, as well as many jujitsu instructional DVD's, and is co-author with Steve Scott of THE PRINCIPLES OF SHINGITAI JUJITSU.

Today John still teaches camps and seminars on jujitsu, submission grappling, MMA, and self-defense at his Barn of Truth Dojo located on 60 pristine acres bordering the Mohican State Forest in Perrysville, Ohio. John can be reached at www.johnsaylor-sja.com.

STEVE SCOTT

and Sambo Club. He has authored several other books published by Turtle Press including TAP OUT TEXTBOOK, ARMLOCK ENCYCLOPEDIA, GRAPPLER'S BOOK OF STRANGLES AND CHOKES, VITAL LEGLOCKS, GROUNDFIGHTING PINS AND BREAKDOWNS, DRILLS FOR GRAPPLERS and CHAMPIONSHIP SAMBO, THROWS AND TAKEDOWNS, as well as the DVD, CHAMPIONSHIP SAMBO. He has also authored COACHING ON THE MAT, SECRETS OF THE CROSS-BODY ARMLOCK (along with Bill West), THE JUJI GATAME HANDBOOK (along with Bill West), PRINCIPLES OF SHINGITAI JUJITSU (along with John Saylor) and THE MARTIAL ARTS TERMINOLOGY HANDBOOK, as well as the DVD, SECRETS OF THE CROSS-BODY ARMLOCK. Steve is also active in training law enforcement professionals with Law Enforcement and Security Trainers, Inc. and is a member of ILEETA (International Law Enforcement Educators and Trainers Association).

Steve is also active in the Amateur Athletic Union's judo program (AAU Judo) and has been instrumental in the development of freestyle judo. For more information, go to www.AAUJudo.org.

Steve is a graduate of the University of Missouri-Kansas City and teaches jujitsu, judo and sambo full-time as well as CPR and First-aid. For over thirty years, he worked as a community center director and coached judo, jujitsu and sambo in various community centers in the Kansas City area. He has conducted over 300 clinics and seminars across the United States and can be reached by e-mailing him at stevescottjudo@yahoo.com or going to www.WelcomeMatJudoClub.com. For many years, he was active as an athlete in the sport of Scottish Highland Games and was a national master's champion in that sport. He is married to Becky Scott, the first American woman to win a World Sambo Championship. Naturally, they met at a judo tournament in 1973 and have been together ever since.

Steve's first coach, Jerry Swett, told him as a teen-ager that he had a God-given gift for teaching and this impelled Steve to become a coach, and eventually, an author. Steve's second coach, Ken Regennitter, helped him start his judo club and loaned him the mat first mat ever used at the Welcome Mat Judo, Jujitsu and Sambo Club. Steve owes much to these kind men. His life's work and most satisfying accomplishment has been his effort as a coach to be a positive influence in the lives of many people.

CPSIA information can be obtained at www.ICGtesting.com
Printed in the USA
LVOW09s1522230414

382934LV00012B/544/P